A *Jerry Baker* Health Book

Oddball
OINTMENTS

Powerful
POTIONS

& FABULOUS Folk
REMEDIES

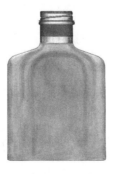

www.jerrybaker.com

Other Jerry Baker Books:

Nature's Best Miracle Medicines
Jerry Baker's Supermarket Super Remedies
Jerry Baker's The New Healing Foods
Jerry Baker's Cut Your Health Care Bills in Half!
Jerry Baker's Amazing Antidotes
Jerry Baker's Anti-Pain Plan
Jerry Baker's Homemade Health
Jerry Baker's Giant Book of Kitchen Counter Cures

Jerry Baker's Supermarket Super Gardens
Secrets from the Jerry Baker Test Gardens
Jerry Baker's All-American Lawns
Jerry Baker's Bug Off!
Jerry Baker's Terrific Garden Tonics!
Jerry Baker's Giant Book of Garden Solutions
Jerry Baker's Backyard Problem Solver
Jerry Baker's Green Grass Magic
Jerry Baker's Terrific Tomatoes, Sensational Spuds,
  and Mouth-Watering Melons
Jerry Baker's Great Green Book of Garden Secrets
Jerry Baker's Old-Time Gardening Wisdom

Jerry Baker's Backyard Birdscaping Bonanza
Jerry Baker's Backyard Bird Feeding Bonanza
Jerry Baker's Year-Round Bloomers
Jerry Baker's Flower Garden Problem Solver
Jerry Baker's Perfect Perennials!
Jerry Baker's Flower Power!

Jerry Baker's Home, Health, and Garden Problem Solver
Grandma Putt's Old-Time Vinegar, Garlic, Baking Soda,
  and 101 More Problem Solvers
Jerry Baker's Supermarket Super Products!
Jerry Baker's It Pays to be Cheap!
Jerry Baker's Eureka! 1,001 Old-Time Secrets and New Fangled Solutions

To order any of the above, or for more information on *Jerry Baker's*
amazing home, health, and garden tips, tricks, and tonics, please write to:

Jerry Baker, P.O. Box 805, New Hudson, MI 48165
Or visit Jerry Baker on the World Wide Web at
www.jerrybaker.com

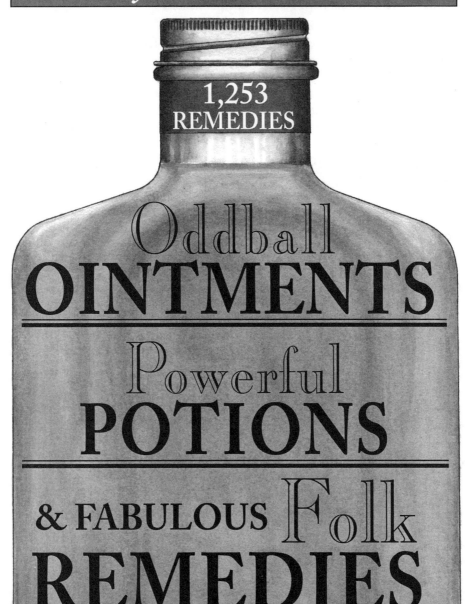

A *Jerry Baker* Health Book

1,253 REMEDIES

Oddball
OINTMENTS

Powerful
POTIONS

& FABULOUS Folk
REMEDIES

THAT'LL CURE ALMOST ANYTHING THAT AILS YA!

Published by American Master Products, Inc. / Jerry Baker
Kim Adam Gasior, Publisher

A Jerry Baker Health Book and A Blackberry Cottage Production
Editorial Consultant: Ellen Michaud, Blackberry Cottage Productions
Design: Nest Publishing Resources
Editors: Megan Othersen, Laura Wallace, Carol Keough
Writers: Jean Karen Thomas, Laura Wallace
Book Composition: Dan MacBride
Illustrator: Wayne Michaud
Copyeditor: Candace Levy
Medical Advisor and Reviewer: Elizabeth Wotton, N.D.

Printed in the United States of America

Illustrations, copyright © 2002 by Wayne Michaud

Publisher's Cataloging-in-Publication

Thomas, Jean Karen.
    Jerry Baker's oddball ointments, powerful potions & fabulous folk remedies that'll cure almost anything that ails ya /author, Jean Karen Thomas; editor, Kim Adam Gasior; illustrator, Wayne Michaud. – 1st ed.   p. cm.
    Includes index.
    ISBN: 978-0-922433-44-5
    1. Traditional medicine.   2. Self-care, Health—Popular works.   I. Baker, Jerry.
II. Gasior, Kim Adam.   III. Title.   IV. Title: Oddball ointments, powerful potions & fabulous folk remedies that'll cure almost anything that ails ya!

    RM122.5.T46 2002   615.8'8
              QBI02-200138

22 20 18 16 17 19 21 23 hardcover

Contents

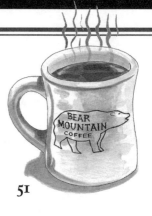

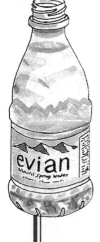

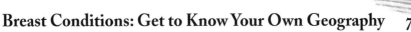

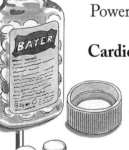

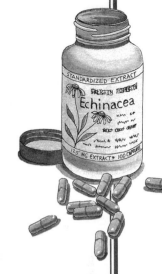

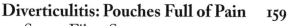

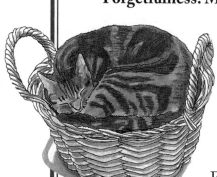

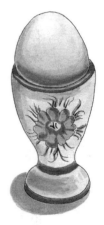

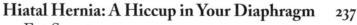

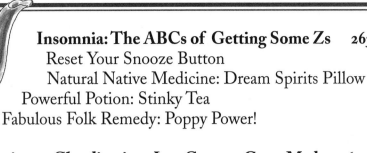

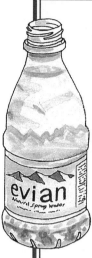

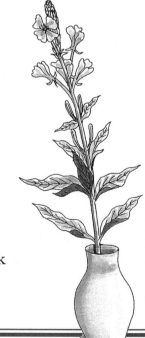

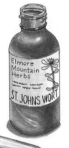

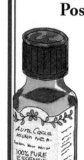

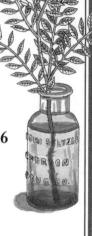

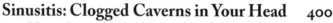

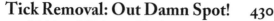

Introduction

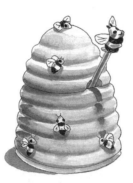

Long before Rite-Aid, CVS, or even Kinney Drugs, there was the local pharmacy in Davidson, Michigan. It might not have been much to write home about by today's standards; but back then, it seemed as grand as Walgreens does today. Just about every Saturday morning, Grandma Putt would lead me to the back of the store, through the maze of dark bottles, potent-smelling herbs, and mysterious wooden boxes, until we eventually found Mr. Ernest Hugg, the apothecary himself. I can still picture old Ernie standing behind his big oak counter—which was filled with an array of multicolored ointments and potions—busily grinding something into a powder or poultice to ease somebody's aches and pains.

A lot of folks thought Mr. Hugg was a bunch of bunk, but not Grandma Putt. When we visited, she and old Ernie would talk shop for hours, laughing, joking, trading secrets, and sharing wisdom. It was as if they had an unspoken understanding: She never bought anything, and he never asked her to. And it wasn't

because she didn't believe his tonics worked; she absolutely did!
It's just that she was a bit of an apothecary herself.

When I was growing up, it seemed that
Grandma Putt had an oddball ointment, powerful potion, or remarkable remedy for just
about anything that ailed our family—whether
it was garlic and oil for one of my
awful earaches, a hot cup of special
coffee to stop Uncle Art's asthma
attacks, or a sage-and-vinegar poultice to ease
Grandpa Putt's all-too-often bee stings. Some of these
concoctions were passed down from her Native American
ancestors. Others, she picked up from friends, neighbors,
or acquaintances—like Ernest Hugg—who knew a thing
or two about fixers and elixirs that kept the doctor away.

And did they ever! To say that I was as healthy as a
horse is like saying that I have a bit of a green thumb. I tell you, I
didn't see hide nor hair of a doctor until I was out of college, and
that was just for a routine physical. It was only after I got older
and moved away that I found myself visiting a traditional doctor
more often. It seemed that over time, the lotions, motions, and
potions that were developed in Grandma Putt's kitchen were
replaced by a variety of chemicals and prescription drugs
generated in a laboratory. And after many years of use
with only so-so results, I realized that something
had to give.

Then I met Beth Wotton, N.D. Beth is a
wonderful woman who has devoted her life to
helping and caring for others. She's a naturopathic
physician from Sausalito, California, and she just
loves to ferret out remedies that really work
for her patients. Rather than reaching for the

latest wonder drug the minute somebody sneezes, Beth combines plants, herbs, and other things with a dollop of common sense—just like Grandma Putt used to do! Imagine my surprise when I discovered that she still prescribes some of the very same things that Grandma used to use on her own family way back when.

Talking to Beth was a revelation, taking me back to much simpler time when folks relied on good old-fashioned, time-tested remedies, instead of running to the doctor at the slightest sign of a sniffle. And since I'm always on the lookout for the latest and greatest health information to share with my friends, I realized that here was an opportunity to share some of these gems—the old-time ointments, potions, and remedies—with the world. So I called my friend Jean, a New York writer who has been pawing through medical data for some 20 years now and who has written some 30-odd books about health. After discussing this project with her, I knew we were on to something—combining Beth's wide-ranging knowledge with Jean's terrific talent would result in a hard-hitting treasure trove of natural home remedies, backed by solid medical evidence. And guess what? It did!

We've worked hard over the last 2 years, gathering together the best old-time tonics and new medical marvels to help you help yourself. You want potions? We've rounded up plenty of 'em! How about ointments? We've got oodles of them, too! And what about those fabulous folk remedies that work like magic? Well, we've also uncovered a bunch of those! It's all here, in a book that's jam-packed with hundreds of tips, tricks, and tonics to keep you and your family in the pink of health. For example, you'll discover how to:

✔ Combat coughs with a triple-threat throat spray.
✔ Heal heartburn with licorice.
✔ Cure insomnia, thanks to a cup of "stinky tea"!
✔ Treat mild burns with the pizza herb.
✔ Keep bad breath at bay with a dilly of a fix.
✔ Ward off nausea with an orange.
✔ Use vinegar to relieve aches and pains.
✔ Erase age spots with horseradish and yogurt.

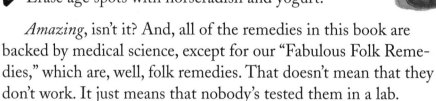

Amazing, isn't it? And, all of the remedies in this book are backed by medical science, except for our "Fabulous Folk Remedies," which are, well, folk remedies. That doesn't mean that they don't work. It just means that nobody's tested them in a lab.

The result of our efforts is one giant, easy-to-use volume that brings you the best ways to prevent, ward off, or even cure over 100 of the most common ailments and illnesses you'll ever face. While this book and our advice will never (and should never!) replace your doctor's expertise, they can help you maintain a lifetime of good health. So read on, my friends, and see if the oddball ointments, powerful potions, and fabulous folk remedies don't put the spring back in your step and the sparkle back in your eye—just like they did for Grandma Putt and me!

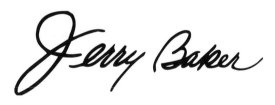

Age Spots:

Those Unflattering Freckles

I've always had freckles on my arms. But when I noticed a few larger, darker ones cropping up on the backs of my hands, I absolutely refused to admit they were "age spots."

I didn't want to look "old," and, well, age spots come with age. The only reason we develop them is because we've lived long enough to soak up a lot more sun than the neighborhood 6 year olds. Some people develop more of these freckles than others; some get them on their face, chest, or hands. The spots can pop up anywhere your skin

O·D·D·B·A·L·L OINTMENT

29¢ Spot Remover

The enzyme activity of horseradish and yogurt may help fade age spots. Mix 1 tablespoon of grated horseradish in ¼ cup of plain yogurt, and refrigerate. Dab the yogurt mixture on spots daily until desired results are achieved. Follow each application with a smear of vitamin E oil or wheat-germ oil.

Flower Face Wash

Elderflowers (*Sambucus canadensis*), known for keeping the complexion clear and free of blemishes, have their origins in folk medicine and are still used today in many commercial skin creams. Make your own elderflower water by steeping 1 ounce of fresh elderflowers in 1 pint of distilled water overnight. Strain, and use as a wash to follow your daily cleansing regimen. Refrigerated, the solution will keep for 4 to 5 days.

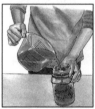

has been overexposed to the sun's destructive rays.

Medically, these spots are called solar lentigines. (There, doesn't that sound better than age spots? It has a certain . . . *panache!*) Lentigines occur because of an increase in melanocytes, the cells that contain melanin, the pigment that colors our skin. This pigment tends to darken after being repeatedly bombarded with ultraviolet rays.

SURE-FIRE FRECKLE FLATTENERS

Sick of the spots? There are many ways you can prevent lentigines from enlarging, ranging from buttermilk baths to Retin-A. You can also hide them with cosmetics—and sometimes banish them entirely. Here are a bunch of things to try:

Peel them away. There are a variety of acid-based remedies that act as exfoliants. That is, they slough off the top layer of your skin, and the lentigines with it. The spots will seem lighter on the underneath layers, and eventually, as skin layers are replaced, the lentigines will no longer be there.

Most dermatologists recommend alpha-hydroxy acids, commonly known as AHAs. These natural acids come from milk (lactic acid), sugarcane (glycolic acid), and fruit (citric acid).

The glycolic acid in sugarcane is the most common AHA. It loosens those dead cells and, at the same time, motivates new cells from lower layers of the epidermis to get busy and grow some new skin. In other words, they exfoliate—or remove—superficial pigmentation.

Over-the-counter face creams, such as Porcelana, do contain a mild acid solution, but you'll need a doctor's prescription for stronger (and more effective) alpha-hydroxy acid products. Always follow the prescription directions—applying too much can irritate your skin.

You'll know an AHA is working because you may feel some tingling at first, but that should last only a few moments. Once you've used the product for 2 or 3 weeks without irritation, it's usually okay to increase the applications to twice a day: morning and night. Dermatologists warn that you'll need to be pa-

Check Your Spots!

Most age spots are harmless marks, but always examine them carefully to be sure they're not skin cancer. If a spot enlarges, changes color or shape, bleeds, itches, or thickens, have your doctor check it out right away. Remember the easy ABCDs of melanoma from the American Cancer Society.

✔ *A* is for asymmetry: If half the mole or birthmark does not match the other, it could mean trouble.

✔ *B* is for border: Watch for irregular edges that are notched or blurred.

✔ *C* is for color: Look for spots that are not the same color all over.

✔ *D* is for diameter: If it's larger than the head of a pencil eraser or growing, see your doctor.

The Hands of Time

Most of us fuss more over our faces, but keep in mind that lentigines also appear elsewhere, especially on the backs of your hands. Your busy hands are constantly exposed to the sun and other harmful elements. So always treat them right—remember to daub on sunscreen. And wear gloves when you can, especially for outdoor tasks like gardening.

tient, however. It may take 2 months or even as long as a year before you notice improvement.

Reach for the Retin-A. There is still some controversy about the prescription vitamin acid known as Retin-A because nobody is yet sure exactly how it works. As with AHAs, when a strong dose of Retin-A is put on a lentigine, the skin will peel. After a few months of this treatment, the spot will disappear, or at least be less apparent. A 10-month study of 58 people at the University of Michigan Medical Center revealed that for most subjects, the spots were lighter after 1 month of treatment with Retin-A. After 10 months, 32 percent had at least one spot disappear, and 83 percent reported lightening of their age spots.

Some experts believe Retin-A is more effective when it's combined with other treatments. John Romano, M.D., professor of dermatology at New York Hospital Cornell Medical Center, reported that people who applied glycolic acid in the morning and Retin-A at night had the best results.

Like high-concentration AHAs, Retin-A cream is available in different strengths and only by prescription, so you'll need to visit your dermatologist. Continued use of Retin-A can make your skin more sensitive to the sun, and it may become irritated and scaly. These effects usually diminish over time, but you will still need to moisturize and use sunscreen religiously.

First, pass the test. As women who color their hair know, it's important to do a test patch first to be sure the product's chemicals won't irritate your skin. Dermatologists recommend the same precaution before you use any preparations for lentigines. Here's how: Smear a drop of the solution on a small patch of skin under your jaw. Check it the next day. If there is no sign of redness or irritation, then it should be safe to use on your face.

Apply it like a pro. First, wash your face, and pat it dry. If it's morning, apply your usual sunscreen. Then smooth the AHA over your face. Avoid your eyes—don't rub it any closer to them than the length of your eyelashes. Once your face is thoroughly dry, add your usual moisturizer and makeup. As long as there is no sign of irritation, it is probably safe to use such a preparation every day, but always check with your doctor first.

Cover and camouflage. Meanwhile, you can hide your spots with smart makeup application. Use a heavy foundation or one made especially to cover blemishes. Make sure you choose

POWERFUL POTION

BLEMISH-BANISHING TONIC

Traditional herbal blood purifiers are said to clear the skin of blemishes and spots. To try one, mix together equal parts of the dried root of burdock (*Arctium lappa*), yellow dock (*Rumex crispus*), and dandelion (*Taraxacum officinalis*). Bring 1 cup of water to a boil, and use it to steep 1 tablespoon of the dried root mixture for 20 minutes. Strain, and drink. Honey and lemon may be added to taste. **Caution:** Dandelion greens are rich in potassium and should not be taken with potassium tablets. Consult your healthcare provider if you have concerns.

the proper color, however, or you'll wind up with a mask-like look. And take advantage of store experts—ask a cosmetics pro how best to blend your makeup for the most natural look.

Bathe in buttermilk. Because AHAs come from lactic and citric acid, it isn't hard to find your own skin-smoothing acids. Next time you grocery shop, grab a quart of buttermilk. For ages, women have enjoyed lolling in milk baths and, more specifically, in buttermilk baths, because of buttermilk's high lactic-acid content. A tubful would probably mean you'd need your own cow, but many women simply bathe their face or hands in buttermilk once or twice a day.

And get some fresh lemons, too. My friend Susan cuts lemons in half and rubs the exposed fruit along the backs of her hands several times a day, and I've noticed that her age spots seem much paler. (Although I suspect she had only a mild case of lentigines.)

DON'T FRET ABOUT FRECKLES

While there are ways to minimize age spots or even rid your skin of them, remember that the best remedy of all is prevention. *Always* protect your skin from the sun to prevent any more spots from appearing.

Get serious about sunscreen—seven days a week. Most cosmetic foundations now contain sunscreen, but often in very low amounts, so be sure yours is strong enough. It's best to ask a dermatologist for the correct formula for your particular skin type. If your foundation is sunscreen-free, always apply a sunscreen to

Remember—Light Ricochets!

Reflected light that bounces off the parking lot, the deck of your boat, or snow on the slopes is actually more harmful than overhead sunlight beaming down on you, says Alex Eaton, M.D. (Dr. Eaton lives in the Sunshine State and knows sun damage!) Here are the sinister stats: Snow reflects 88 percent of light; dry sand on the beach is next; followed by concrete, black asphalt, and wooden boat decks.

your face *before* you put on makeup. Make sure to slather sunscreen on any other exposed skin, including legs, arms, and hands, too. If you have a fetching short haircut, don't forget your ears! And remember, most women forget to reapply sunscreen every time they wash their hands. It really makes a difference, so always carry a small bottle in your purse.

Make a fashion statement. Here's your chance to bat your eyelashes under a beautiful brim. A wide-brimmed hat or visor can actually eliminate half the sunlight that would otherwise reach parts of your face. So slap on a chapeau—you'll be stylish and skin savvy, too!

Boycott the blazing hours. The sun is most damaging at its highest peak. The force of ultraviolet (UV) rays is 10 times stronger at noon than it is 3 hours earlier or later. Even if you spend all day out in the sun, you'll get the biggest dose of UV radiation from 11:00 A.M. to 1:00 P.M.— when the sun is directly overhead.

Allergies:

Merely Annoying to Downright Dangerous

Every season gives us something to sneeze at. Airborne pollens pounce in the spring, grasses make us gasp in the summer, and leaf molds float merrily through the brisk fall breezes. Unfortunately, lots of other things are blowin' in the wind, too, such as increasing air pollution from industry and automobiles. Add the global warming that's confusing the seasonal clock and it's Allergies R Us!

An allergic reaction is an extreme immune response. Inhale a simple speck of dog dander, and your immune system reacts as though your body were fighting off a pack

Troublemakers

Common troublemakers for those prone to food allergies include the following:
- ✔ Milk
- ✔ Eggs (especially the whites)
- ✔ Shellfish
- ✔ Wheat
- ✔ Corn
- ✔ Nuts (especially peanuts)
- ✔ Fruits (oranges)
- ✔ Chocolate

of wolves. Racing to the rescue (when there's no real threat), your immune system cranks out quantities of a disease-fighting protein called immunoglobulin E (IgE). The IgE charges through your bloodstream like Paul Revere, signaling the release of chemicals such as histamine and alerting special cells in the lining of the throat, nose, and lungs to pump up their production of mucus. This is why your eyes and nose run.

These bothersome reactions usually occur right after the first or second time you're exposed to an allergen, but sometimes they don't happen until much later. Folks often develop allergies to their pets years after they've brought Puddly Puppy or Fuzzy Feline home from the pound. (Then, sadly enough, allergists often advise that they banish these beloved family members!) You can develop allergies at any age; and though symptoms may diminish as you get older, they never go away completely.

TRIGGERS FOR A SACKFUL OF SYMPTOMS

If you're allergic to something, you might want to blame Great-Grandpa Kerchooey for giving you his genes, since these conditions crop up more frequently in the children of allergic parents. Or go picket the local factory that's belching black

POWERFUL POTION

GINKGO TEA

Ginkgo is a celebrity herb best known for improving memory. But these pretty little leaves can help with more than just one ailment. They contain ginkgolides, a medicinal component that helps fight allergies. Try a tea made of ginkgo leaves to clear up your runny nose and itchy eyes. Steep 1 teaspoon of dried leaves in boiling water. Scoop out the leaves, cool, add some honey, and you're good to go.

Caution: Check with your doctor first if you're on any blood-thinning medication—including aspirin.

smoke—experts say that the increase in the number of people with allergies can be traced to global pollution.

And sometimes, you are what you eat. Food allergies make up a small percentage of allergic triggers. About 2 percent of adults and 5 to 8 percent of children are allergic to one or more foods. They commonly experience gastrointestinal distress, headaches, skin rashes, shortness of breath, or even asthma when exposed. In the worst cases, a food allergy can cause swelling of the skin and mucous membranes. And when that includes the mouth or throat, you're in real danger—because this can block the airway to the lungs.

Some people can tolerate small amounts of a trigger food without a problem; others need only a trace to cause a reaction, which usually comes on fast. For example, one woman I know sipped some chamomile tea. Within moments, her face began to swell and broke out in an itchy rash. (Needless to say, she's switched to Earl Grey.)

You may also be allergic to chemical substances. A few years ago, nearly everyone working in a Boston hospital got sick. After a great deal of investigation, it turned out that a new shipment of latex gloves, worn by nearly all the staff, had caused a severe allergic reaction. So take note: As more and more chemicals come into our environment, new allergies will appear.

Allergy Attack or Common Cold?

People often think they have a cold, when in fact, they are having an allergic reaction to some environmental trigger. One clue is the color of the mucus you are sneezing and coughing up. When you have a cold, which is caused by an infection, mucus is usually on the thick side and has a yellow or greenish color. With allergies, secretions are usually clear or colorless.

HOW TO DRY UP THE DRIPS

Sure, if you've got upper respiratory allergies, you could tough it out with a stoic attitude and a few doses of self-medication. After all, the medical establishment long considered these symptoms pretty trivial. But if you happen to hate having a Rudolph-the-Red-Nosed-Reindeer schnoz along with itchy, watery eyes, then you probably don't agree!

Fortunately, doctors today have a new generation of nonsedating antihistamines to offer—such as Allegra, Claritin, and Zyrtec. These drugs end runny noses and eyes, and subdue bouts of sneezing by drying membranes in the nose and sinuses. But there are drawbacks. Antihistamines can make you feel dull, sleepy, and sometimes depressed. And, basically, they only suppress the symptoms; they don't cure the allergy. That means the pattern of immune response can bounce back even stronger, so you wind up needing more and more medication.

Anti-inflammatory nasal sprays usually work, but only if you begin using them weeks before the allergy season starts. (That's fine for people with seasonal allergies, but won't do you much good if your allergies are the year-round kind.) These are designed to short-circuit allergic reactions by blocking your body's release of histamine.

FABULOUS FOLK REMEDY

Honey, Please Pass the Pollen

Bee pollen and locally made honey have long been touted as allergy preventatives. By eating bee pollen and honey *before* allergy season hits, you ingest minute amounts of the plants, grasses, and trees that may cause your allergies. By stimulating your immune system, you can build up resistance to lessen the severity of your allergies when the season is in full swing. A typical dose is 1 teaspoon of honey per day. **Caution: Never give raw honey to children under 1 year of age.**

Decongestants will clear your sinuses and shrink swollen nasal membranes, but if you take them for too long, they cause rebound congestion. That's why most folks with allergies (and with common sense) eventually turn to home remedies. Here are some of the best:

Be nice with spice. If a bowl of hot-and-sour soup or a dish of spicy chili doesn't clear your stuffy nose, probably nothing will. Spicy food is almost like a Roto-Rooter service for clearing out blocked nasal passages. The heat loosens mucus and gets it on the run, usually out your nose.

Grate horseradish for great relief. Apart from the alcohol buzz, one of the reasons a Bloody Mary feels so good is that the drink's horseradish is so stimulating. It seems to perk up the senses and clear passages from the nose right up into the sinuses. This powerful potion is best taken raw. Just grate some into a glass of tomato juice; mix it up with your favorite salsa; or, if you are very brave, eat it right off the stalk. (If you crave the celery and tinkling ice, though, make yours

IT'S AN EMERGENCY!

There's one extremely dangerous allergic reaction that's nothing to sneeze at. It's called anaphylaxis, and it can kill you. Suffering a bee sting, eating peanuts or crabs, or taking a medication that is made from mold (such as penicillin) can set off anaphylaxis in an unsuspecting person—even if he or she has never been allergic before. When this happens, the larynx swells shut, and the airway constricts. Result? Suffocation. This is a medical emergency, and the victim must be taken to the nearest emergency room. Quickly!

a Virgin Mary . . . vodka won't help your allergies.)

Sniff some eucalyptus. My daughter swears that she clears her stuffy nose with eucalyptus soap, just by using it for her daily shower. It may be that the scent permeates her nose with the hot steam or the rubbing of soap on her face helps open her nasal passages. Pick up a bar at your favorite bath shop, and give it a try.

Heat up your honker. Many people I know just place a small hot washcloth over their sinuses and stopped-up noses. Soak it in the hottest water you can stand, wring it out, and lay it across your nose and sinuses for a while. If you keep the cloth as hot as you can, it seems to work on the same principle as hot soup or spicy food: It loosens and liquefies mucus.

Natural Native Medicine

Get Steamy with Herbs

Many Native Americans use herbs to relieve nasal congestion. Here's a remedy they've inspired: Put 1 tablespoon *each* of rosemary and eucalyptus into 1 cup of boiling water, place a towel over your head to make a tent, and sniff the fumes for 5 minutes. (Be careful not to scald your face—lower it slowly over the steam.)

YOUR BEST AMMO AGAINST ALLERGIES

The best way to deal with allergies is to avoid as many triggers as possible in the first place. Here's how:

Mask your mug. Don't leave home without it . . . a face mask, that is. At least not during allergy season or in periods when air pollution is high. There was a time when seeing masked people jogging, dusting, or mowing the lawn would make us think that aliens had landed. No longer. Allergy-smart folks know that these inexpensive masks (available at any drugstore) are a great way to protect airways from allergy overload. Keep a supply of them in your car, in your office, and at home.

Seal the perimeter. During pollen season, keep the windows of your car and house closed, and stay in air-conditioned spaces whenever possible. Be especially cautious during early morning hours—pollen counts are at their highest between 5:00 A.M. and 10:00 A.M. Never hang your clothes outside to dry where they can collect pollen, and wash your hair every night to keep from contaminating your pillowcase with the stuff.

Keep it simple. Get off ebay.com, and stop filling your house with tchotchkes. Dust collectors include books, drapes, figurines, blinds, carpets, dried flowers—nearly every object in the house. Instead, develop a lean decor. Do you cringe at the thought of parting with "stuff"? Instead, try thinking: spare, spacious, low-stress, low-maintenance, uncluttered, serene. This kind of environment can be beautiful, too, so unload the unnecessary, and make it easy on yourself. And remember, when you do clean, you churn up dust in your attempt to remove it. So when you're really suffering, call in a professional housecleaning service or a non-allergic friend. (You can always

O·D·D·B·A·L·L OINTMENT

Salve Your Sinuses

When those headachy, runny-nose, sneezy allergies hit, try placing a dab of soothing salve on your temples. Choose a salve containing an essential oil, such as lavender, eucalyptus, or peppermint. The scent will soothe and relax you, while the oils open your respiratory passages and ease congestion.

barter a service in return.) And leave the house for a few hours.

Change sheets every Sunday. Dust mites are major allergens, and even the cleanest households are full of these microscopic critters. The problem is that they love to sleep in your bed, and it's full of cozy places for them to accumulate. So wash your bedding often. Have you ever seen a dust mite magnified a million times? Scary little creature! Not something I'd like to be sleeping with on a regular basis. They live in feather as well as synthetic pillows, but you can wash the synthetics frequently to drown the little mites. So unless you find a down comforter that's hypoallergenic and washable, buy synthetics for your bed.

Bag your bed stuff. Another way to minimize the amount of dust that comes from your mattress and pillows into your air space is to cover them with plastic. Most bedding stores carry zippered, allergy-proof mattress and pillow covers in a variety of sizes.

POWERFUL POTION

RAGWEED RELIEF

It's not surprising that nature provides her own springtime remedies just when allergy season hits. Spring greens and flowers often make the best potions for allergy relief. Look in your backyard for nettles (*Urtica dioica*), eyebright (*Euphrasia officinalis*), cleavers (*Galium aparine*), and elderflowers (*Sambucus canadensis*). Pick them fresh and steep ¼ cup of herbs in 1 quart of water overnight. Strain, and then drink throughout the day.

Anemia:

It's More Than Just Fatigue

Remember that old TV commercial: "Do you have iron-poor blood?" Ads for that tonic probably did more than anything else to promote the myth that any mature person who occasionally feels low on energy is low on iron. Sometimes, we all can feel as though our "get-up-and-go" had "got-up-and-gone!"

Those commercials probably sent folks who were feeling the least bit draggy rushing to the drugstore for iron supplements, which can do more harm than good. Most doctors today don't want you to take iron supplements—they can be life threatening. High levels of iron in the blood may increase your risk for heart attack as

Take Anemia Seriously

Anemia is never normal. If a doctor tells you that you are a little anemic but dismisses it as unimportant without prescribing a way to fix it, find another doctor. Any sign of anemia can indicate a problem that needs immediate attention, such as an undetected bleeding polyp.

well as cause seizures, jaundice, or gastrointestinal problems. And such ads may also have discouraged people with persistent fatigue from seeing their doctors to find out exactly what was wrong.

Although it's not as common as those old commercials would have you believe, anemia does happen—more than 400 forms have been identified. The most common, of course, is *iron-deficiency anemia,* which means that you are not getting enough iron in your diet or that your body isn't absorbing iron well. When are you most vulnerable to this form of anemia? During adolescence if you're female and after midlife for both women and men.

Pernicious anemia is the inability of your body to properly absorb vitamin B_{12}. *Megaloblastic anemia* occurs when a folic acid or vitamin B_{12} deficiency results in red blood cells that are prone to slow maturation and early destruction. And *hemolytic anemia,* which includes sickle-cell disease and *thalassemia,* is a condition in which red blood cells are destroyed faster than the bone marrow can replace them. Other forms of hemolytic anemia can be caused by chronic infection and autoimmune conditions, such as rheumatoid arthritis, and lupus, which may increase the destruction of blood cells. Sometimes, anemia means the bone marrow is functioning poorly because of infection, cancer, or exposure to toxic chemicals.

POWERFUL POTION

STRAWBERRY TEA

Strawberry leaves are berry, berry good for treating anemia. Pick a bunch of fresh leaves, and crush about 3 teaspoons of them, or use 1 teaspoon of dried leaves. Place them in 1 cup of boiling water. Let steep 5 minutes, scoop out the leaves, and enjoy the tea!

IRONWORKS

So why do you need iron, anyway? To make hemoglobin, which transports oxygen from your lungs to all the tissues of your body. This is what brings the color to your cheeks. Without iron, hemoglobin production halts, and the body gets too little oxygen. With a drop in hemoglobin, you might be easily fatigued, sleepy, or even feel occasionally dizzy. And your brain won't be functioning too well, either.

Iron plays an important role in how the liver and muscles function and is crucial to the immune system's ability to fight off infections. You can have a mild iron deficiency without being anemic, however. When this happens, you've got enough iron to fulfill your bone marrow's need to produce hemoglobin but not enough to cover your body's other needs.

Iron-deficiency anemia is almost always the result of blood loss from causes such as excessive menstrual flow or internal bleeding. Bleeding may stem from sources like an undiagnosed intestinal polyp, ulcers, or cancer. In older people, however, a poor diet is usually the culprit.

WHO'S AT RISK?

Women are six times more vulnerable than men—until the age of 65, when the gender gap narrows to about two to one. Why do men luck out? They have more blood volume than women to begin with (and they're spared the joys of menstruation, blast 'em).

POWERFUL POTION

START AT THE ROOT

Mineral-rich herbs are a good way to boost your iron levels. Use one or more of the following herbs in a tea: Yellow dock (*Rumex crispus*), alfalfa (*Medicago sativa*), and dandelion leaf (*Taraxacum officinalis*). Steep 1 heaping teaspoon in 1 cup of boiling water for 20 minutes. Drink a cup two or three times per day.

Worshiping the Great Pumpkin

If you eat pumpkin only in pie and only at Thanksgiving, think about adding it to your menu more often. Pumpkin is an excellent source of folate, the vitamin B complex component of folic acid. But don't bother nuking your Halloween pumpkins, because they won't taste very good. Look for the sweet, smaller pumpkins grown for the table. They have rich flavor and a meaty texture, and they can be prepared like squash. You can bake, mash, or grate them, or make pumpkin soup. Since 99 percent of pumpkins are grown for the jack-o'-lantern trade, you may have to search the farmers markets for fresh or stick to canned.

In the United States, 20 percent of all women of childbearing age have iron-deficiency anemia compared to 2 percent of adult men. The cause is primarily blood loss during menstruation. When women don't replace the lost iron by eating iron-rich foods, the problem gets worse. If your menstrual periods are particularly heavy or irregular, or last 7 days or more, you have a greater risk of iron-deficiency anemia.

Once they begin menstruating in their teens, some girls fail to understand that they need to make up for the iron they lose in the process. Not only menstrual blood loss but also a steady diet of junk food, irregular hours, and the emotional chaos of adolescence mean that teenage girls often neglect their iron needs. This is also the time many girls decide to go vegetarian or embark on a total fast to lose a pound and a half to fit into their size 1 jeans. Trouble is, they do this without much thought to their health.

Blood volume expands during pregnancy, so pregnant women often need extra iron. Iron deficiency in pregnancy (which should always be diagnosed with a blood test) is dangerous, because it can lead to low birth weight, premature birth, and fetal abnormalities.

One government source found that females between the ages of 12 and 50 (the time of highest risk for iron-deficiency anemia) were consuming only about half of the iron they needed.

FABULOUS FOLK REMEDY

Lemon Lifter

Ever wonder about the Southern habit of spicing up greens with vinegar? Acidic condiments, like vinegar and lemon juice, sprinkled on greens help liberate minerals, making the iron more easily absorbed by your body.

BLUE LIPS, PALE FACES, AND BELLS IN YOUR EARS

In general, if you're anemic, you'll be tired, short of breath, and have a feeling of malaise. Some people may also feel light-headed and dizzy when they stand up. Ringing in the ears is another symptom. Other symptoms are headache, insomnia, decreased appetite, poor concentration, and irregular heartbeat.

What are the outward signs of anemia? You might have bluish lips, skin that is pasty or yellowish, and brittle or spoon-shaped fingernails. The linings of your lower eyelids may be pale, and the creases in the palms of your hands, too. The color of your tongue may change, or your tongue may feel as though it were burning (this happens sometimes with anemia caused by vitamin B_{12} deficiency).

Anemic women may experience bleeding between periods or have extremely heavy periods for several months. Bleeding for more than 7 days every month may be a sign of anemia. Consult your gynecologist if you experience any of these symptoms.

GET TESTED

Because anemia can lead to serious illness and can have several causes, don't treat it by yourself until you see your doctor for a blood test. A complete blood count (CBC) will determine if the number of red blood cells and amount of hemoglobin in your blood are abnormally low. If they are, further diagnostic tests can pin down the cause so you can get treatment.

HOW MUCH IRON DO WE NEED?

Our bodies constantly use iron to build new red blood cells, but we also lose a small amount of iron each day. Things are usually in balance: Our intestinal tract is designed to protect us from

Be Wary of Ties That Bind

Spinach and rhubarb both contain oxalic acid—a substance that binds to iron and prevents your body from absorbing it. Other binders include antacids, bran, calcium, soy protein, coffee, and tannins. Obviously, you can't cut out important nutrients like spinach, calcium, and soy protein—and who wants to give up coffee or tea? But unless you have spinach every day, there's no need to worry about "binders," except if you're seriously anemic, which means your doctor should be advising you. Otherwise, just plan your meals so you don't include too many iron binders in them.

taking in too much iron—it simply stops absorbing it. But it can't protect us from having too little.

Women in their reproductive years lose more iron, an average of 1.5 milligrams per day compared to 1 milligram for men. Some researchers believe that lower iron levels caused by menstrual blood loss may explain why premenopausal women have much less heart disease than men. (Remember? Iron overload can lead to a heart attack.) Ironically, however, by protecting us from absorbing too much iron, our bodies may also leave us vulnerable to the effects of too little.

Because the body absorbs only a small percentage of dietary iron, the Recommended Dietary Allowance (RDA) calls for consuming more than we lose. Postmenopausal women and adult men need 10 milligrams a day. Women under 50 need 15 milligrams a day and a hefty 30 milligrams a day during pregnancy.

FABULOUS FOLK REMEDY

Blackstrap for Breakfast!

The syrupy substance that remains after sugarcane is processed—blackstrap molasses—is a great source of iron. In the old days, folks often slathered blackstrap on whole-grain bread for breakfast. If you enjoy the taste, you can simply swallow 2 tablespoons of blackstrap molasses. This amount contains about 10 milligrams of iron—nearly 40 percent of the daily requirement—and just 85 calories.

PUMPING UP YOUR IRON SUPPLIES

You can treat anemia from iron deficiency by eating more iron-rich foods or by increasing your iron absorption. Here's how:

Beef up your diet. Most research shows that meat sources of iron are easier to absorb than vegetable sources. Meat sources also boost the absorption of iron from other foods. Lean red meat and beef liver are good sources of iron. Organ meats like brains and kidneys are especially high in iron. And poultry, fish, and oysters are next in line.

Because meat and fish are such major sources of iron in most people's diets, vegetarians need to be especially careful to eat fruits, vegetables, and grains that offer high amounts. Here are some good choices:

✔ Green, leafy vegetables
✔ Dried fruit (more iron than in fresh)
✔ Peaches, apricots, and raisins (fresh and dried)
✔ Whole-wheat bread and wheat germ
✔ Iron-fortified cereals and pastas
✔ Legumes (dried beans and peas and canned baked beans)

Avoid anemic veggies. Remember that many nutrients are lost on the way from the farm to the table. "Fresh" veggies are usually 14 days old by the time they reach your supermarket and have lost as much as 90 percent of their nutrients. Certified, organic produce is usually best, but not at the expense of nutrients. A wilted, tired-looking head of organic lettuce is going to be iron poor no matter how organic it is. In such a case, you're better off with fresh lettuce from a nonorganic source.

Absorb more with C. Food high in vitamin C, such as citrus fruits, strawberries, and tomatoes, help your body absorb iron from food. Basically, the vitamin moves the iron through the gastrointestinal system and into your bloodstream—so it doesn't pass through to be eliminated.

Coffee, tea, or iron? If a healthy diet seems like no fun, at least make a few compromises.

BEAR MOUNTAIN COFFEE

Don't drink caffeinated coffee, tea, or cola with your meals because caffeine inhibits iron absorption, as does the tannin in black tea. And don't switch to decaf, because the acids used in that process can also inhibit iron absorption. Instead, enjoy citrus fruit juices with your meals—they'll help you absorb more iron. Other iron blockers include antacids and the phosphates found in soft drinks and ice cream.

Befriend folic acid. Folic acid is a key player in red blood cell production. You can easily add more to your diet by chowing down on mushrooms, citrus fruits, dark green vegetables, liver, eggs, milk, wheat germ, and brewer's yeast. Because folic acid is destroyed by heat and light, eat your fruits and veggies fresh, cooking them as little as possible. If you are thinking of getting pregnant, plan ahead to focus on folic acid—your need will double during pregnancy.

Raise your awareness—write it down. One of the best ways to track what you are really eating is to keep a daily record. Write down everything you eat during the day, and get a little pocket-size book that lists not only the calories but all the nutrients in most foods. This way, you can be sure you are eating enough iron-rich foods while avoiding those that inhibit absorption of iron. Soon, you'll know what to eat and won't need the diary any more.

Hop on the wagon. If you're drinking too much wine at dinner or beer at the ball game, consider what it may be doing to your iron supply. Too much alcohol can affect your iron status in several ways. It interferes with your body's ability to absorb folic acid, which you need for red blood cells. And if the problem is chronic, it usually results in poor nutrition.

Cook in cast iron. My grandmother cooked in those big cast-iron pots that lasted for generations. She had several skillets of various sizes and a big covered kettle, which I still use decades later. Grandma always believed that you get all the iron you need by cooking everything in those iron pans. As it turns out, she was right. If you cook tomatoes and other acidic foods in iron pots, you more than double the amount of iron you take in. For example, 4 ounces of tomato sauce has 0.7 milligrams of iron. But you get 5 milligrams more by cooking it in iron! Iron cookware may discolor some foods, but it won't affect the taste. Experts, however, say the iron from cast iron doesn't get absorbed into your body quite as well as iron from foods.

Vegetarians, Ferment!

Vegetarians are at risk for vitamin B_{12} deficiency. This vitamin is found only in animal sources and in a few fermented foods derived from soybeans, such as miso and tofu. Be sure to include these foods as well as dairy products and eggs in your diet. Or, if you are vegan and avoid all animal products, ask your doctor if you should take a vitamin B_{12} supplement.

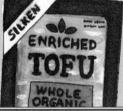

Bitter makes it better. For some reason, old folk remedies often prescribed bitter substances to stimulate digestion and thus promote better absorption of nutrients. Gentian is a bitter herb popular in Europe to treat a number of ailments, including iron-deficiency anemia. *Gentiana lutea* is the botanical name of this herb, which can be brewed into a tea or taken in the commercial form of an alcoholic extract.

Anxiety:

The Stuff Worrywarts Are Made Of

My grandmother was a chronic worrier. No matter what was going on, she was worried that something wasn't just right, somebody needed something she didn't have, or something would happen if she left the house. As a kid, whenever I spent time with her on summer vacations, she would call the hospitals and the police if I was even the slightest bit late coming home.

Grandma Dora was always pursuing remedies for a never-ending string of worries. She was also a kind and loving woman, who knew how to laugh at herself, so everybody just humored her while assuring her that everything was all right.

FABULOUS FOLK REMEDY

Treat Your Feet

Warm foot baths erase your cares and pamper your soul. Add a ½ cup of Epsom salts for relaxation and a sprig or two of fresh lavender or lemon balm to refresh your mind and calm your spirit. Those with diabetes should check with their doctor before soaking their feet in anything.

Now, when I look back, I realize she may have suffered from a generalized anxiety disorder.

Are you a worrywart, or are you truly anxious? And how would you know the difference? There is no clear dividing line between normal worry and a diagnosis of generalized anxiety disorder, according to the American Psychiatric Association. If you persistently worry every day or almost every day for 6 months or more, then you probably have anxiety disorder, and you need to get professional help.

"Anxiety is life affirming," says Linda Welsh, Ed.D, director of the Anxiety Disorders and Agoraphobia Treatment Center in Bala Cynwyd, Pennsylvania. "It gives us the energy to work through our problems." When anxiety interferes to the point at which we can't function, then we need to get help.

"All the research suggests that cognitive behavior therapy is the best treatment," says Dr. Welsh. Such therapy teaches you how to take control of your psychological and physical reactions—everything from feeling jittery and not being able to sleep, to finding it hard to draw a deep breath. Often, within 6 to 12 weeks, cognitive behavior therapy can help you outline and confront the nature and unreasonableness of fearful thinking and make it go away.

If you suspect you may have an anxiety disorder, check with your doctor to rule out other illnesses like thyroid problems. Then ask your physician to refer you to a cognitive behavioral

POWERFUL POTION

SKULLCAP SOOTHER

Along with hops, skullcap (*Scutellaria lateriflora*) is a fabulous antianxiety herb. Try combining equal parts of skullcap with lemon balm (*Melissa officinalis*) and oatstraw (*Avena sativa*) for a quick anxiety buster. Use 1 heaping teaspoon per 1 cup of boiling water. Steep for 10 minutes, and drink 1 cup twice daily.

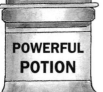

POWERFUL POTION

GRATITUDE TEA

When your worries start, reach for the chamomile tea. Studies show that it blocks anxiety-promoting brain chemicals triggered by worry. Simply measure 1 teaspoon of dried chamomile flowers (avoid the weak, store-bought kind in tea bags) into your cup. Fill the cup with just-boiled water, cover, and steep for 15 minutes. (Close your eyes, and count all the wonderful things you're grateful for while you wait.) Sip the cooled beverage and feel your worries slip away. **Caution:** If you're allergic to ragweed and other members of the daisy family, don't use chamomile.

therapist in your area. Here's what else can help get you back on an even keel:

Stop catastrophizing. Anxiety is about the future, says Dr. Welsh. Overreacting about what might be and all the "what-ifs" perpetuates the anxiety. "What if I try to speak and make a fool of myself?" "What if a bee stings me at the picnic?" Stop the fearful thinking by not projecting into the future.

Come back to the present. When you feel the what-ifs overwhelming you, try to imagine a stop sign. Say "Stop!" out loud, and stop the what-ifs in their tracks. Tell yourself that right now, you are okay, suggests Dr. Welsh.

Ground yourself. Let's say you're in your car and feeling anxious. Focus on the moment. Feel your hand on the steering wheel, be aware of your body on the seat, feel the air coming through the window. Speed up and slow down to remind yourself you are in control of the car, says Dr. Welsh. When you become more aware of what's going on all around you, you'll be less focused on the internal dialog that's a symptom of your illness.

Focus on your breathing. When you're anxious, you hyper-

How to Recognize a Panic Attack

A panic attack is a sudden surge of overwhelming terror that comes without warning and without any obvious reason. It is far more intense than everyday anxiety or stress, according to the American Psychological Association. It can happen anywhere—in the middle of dinner or during a tennis game. It feels like your body is gearing up to fight off an attacker—except that there's no real danger.

An occasional panic attack is not dangerous, but it can lead to other complications such as phobias, depression, or substance abuse. If you have had four or more panic attacks and are continually afraid of suffering another one, get professional help. Here are the symptoms of a panic attack:

✔ Paralyzing sense of terror
✔ Trembling, sweating, and shaking
✔ Difficulty breathing and a racing heartbeat
✔ Fear that you are about to die or are going crazy
✔ Hot flashes, chills, and chest pains
✔ Tingling in your fingers or toes

ventilate, and this makes your anxiety worse. When you hyperventilate, put your hand on your chest, and feel your chest moving and your heart racing. Practice breathing with your diaphragm the way singers and yoga practitioners do. Take long, slow, deep breaths. Put your hand on your stomach. If your stomach expands like a balloon, you are breathing properly. Now, breath in deeply to the count of 4, hold that breath to the count of 8, and exhale to the count of 7. Repeat the exercise four times.

Get regular exercise. Exercise will work off anxiety, and many studies have shown how exercise changes

Rethink Your Drink!

A Duke University study reveals that even low to moderate doses of caffeine can cause difficulty concentrating, nervousness, trembling, insomnia, irritability, and disorientation. Caffeine can add to the physical symptoms of anxiety and make it worse, says Linda Welsh, Ed.D. So switch to decaf, and see if you don't feel less anxious. Dr. Welsh suggests cutting back on sugar, too, because it has a similar affect on anxiety and avoiding the potent caffeine and high sugar combination of soft drinks.

your body chemistry. When you exercise, your brain releases endorphins that have a calming effect. Take a walk, a run, or a bike ride. Go dancing. Anything that gets your body moving will help. Also, getting your heart rate up because of exercise rather than because of anxiety makes you feel more in control, says Dr. Welsh.

Don't skip meals. Feeling lightheaded is a common symptom of anxiety, but it can also be caused by not eating properly, says Dr. Welsh. Be sure to eat regular, well-balanced meals to keep your blood sugar functioning normally.

Be wary of drugs. Medications such as Ativan and Xanax (benzodiazepines) can relieve anxiety symptoms rapidly, but they are addictive. And some drugs, such as Prozac, actually temporarily increase anxiety in many people, according to the American Psychiatric Association. If your doctor wants to write you a prescription, but does not suggest cognitive therapy to go with it, get a second opinion.

O·D·D·B·A·L·L OINTMENT

Lovely Lavender

A few drops of lavender oil added to your body lotion can be a source of anxiety-preventing aromatherapy all day long. For a more dramatic effect, add a drop of lavender oil to a dab of your favorite salve, and rub it into your temples or solar plexus for a reminder to relax and breathe deeply.

Arthritis:

Preventing the Pain

If something creaks when you turn your head to watch that hunky lifeguard at the pool, or part of you hops up in the morning while the rest stays in bed moaning, chances are you've joined the 43 million or so Americans who have arthritis.

They say that misery loves company, but this is ridiculous! So if you feel you've joined the creak-and-groan contingent, don't despair. There are two principal kinds of arthritis, and I'll tell you right up front that there is really no medical cure for either. But there *are* many effective ways to prevent or ease the pain.

Osteoarthritis is common

FABULOUS FOLK REMEDY

Wrap It Up!

Cabbage leaves have been used for centuries to soothe inflammations. A sturdy, outer leaf is just the right shape to place over a bent knee or an elbow. Blanch a leaf or two, and apply warm or cool to inflamed joints. Secure in place with a gauze wrap or an elastic bandage.

POWERFUL POTION

POWER-PACKED PAIN RELIEF

Use this tea during painful flare-ups. Combine equal parts of devil's claw (*Harpagophytum procumbens*), black cohosh (*Cimicifuga racemosa*), passionflower (*Passiflora incarnata*), and ginger (*Zingiber officinale*). Use 1 teaspoon per 1 cup of boiling water. Steep, covered for 20 minutes. Strain, and drink 1 cup, two or three times daily.

with age. Once you've put major miles on your joints, the cartilage within them begins to wear. Osteoarthritis announces itself with pain and stiffness, especially in weight-bearing joints such as your hips and knees. Repetitive motion is often the culprit. If you spent your youth hurling balls, you may be at risk for arthritis in your shoulders. Even relatively young skiers and runners can develop severe knee problems.

Ironically, though, being out of shape also promotes arthritis. Sitting all day is disastrous for your back, for example. (Why is lack of exercise harmful? You need strong muscles around your joints to protect the cartilage from wear.) And one thing's even harder on your joints than being a sedentary spud or fanatic jock—being overweight. Finally, if your older relatives move as though they were dragging along a ball and chain, genetics may also contribute to your risk.

Rheumatoid arthritis is fortunately much less common—yet much more painful and debilitating. This autoimmune disease can begin early in life, even in childhood. When it happens, it's as though your body had declared war on itself. The immune system becomes inflamed and eventually chews up your joints and anything around them—cartilage, tendons, blood vessels, and even bone. It can be devastating, but there's hope. Sometimes, this form of arthritis just stops, seemingly out of the blue. And in some women, rheumatoid arthritis disappears during pregnancy.

Rheumatoid arthritis usually attacks different joints from the ones osteoarthritis does, although it also begins with pain and stiffness. Eventually, the disease can deform knuckles and wrists and then move on to the shoulder, elbow, hip, ankle, and other joints.

MIRACLES MEDICINES

Because traditional medicine can't cure arthritis, most people rely on painkillers, such as aspirin and nonsteroidal anti-inflammatory drugs (NSAIDs), to reduce joint pain and stiffness. These work by blocking the production of prostaglandins, a hormone-like substance in your body that helps regulate blood pressure, fluid balance, and temperature (among other body systems), and is often implicated in inflammation and pain.

But there's a new ghost-buster on the block for osteoarthritis relief—glucosamine, which is extracted from a type of natural collagen found in chickens. This dietary supplement is said to boost the growth of cartilage, and short-term studies indicate that it also reduces pain in many arthritis sufferers. Fans say it's nontoxic, too, and produces no side effects; but keep

---

O·D·D·B·A·L·L
OINTMENT

Herbal Helper

To soothe aching joints, add a few drops of arnica oil to your favorite healing salve. Try using a warming wintergreen, lavender, or rosemary salve as a base. All three can help increase circulation to the area. For every $1/2$ teaspoon of salve, add 3 to 4 drops of arnica oil. Apply to sore joints three to four times per day. **Caution:** Arnica is for external use only. Do not use on broken skin.

The Johns Hopkins Diet for Joint Comfort

Researchers at Johns Hopkins Medical Center developed a bone-and-joint diet that, according to the *Johns Hopkins 2000* report, can help alleviate the stiff, inflamed joints common to both osteoarthritis and rheumatoid arthritis. They recommend eating two or more servings a week of cold-water fish, such as salmon, mackerel, herring, cod, and blues. The omega-3 fatty acids found in these fish enhance joint health. In a study of 41 people, the doctors observed a 25 percent improvement in swollen joints, morning stiffness, and overall discomfort in the subgroup who took the omega-3 fatty acids.

Here's a sample menu:

Breakfast: One serving of fresh fruit; one slice of bread or a bowl of cereal; one protein, such as an egg or 1 cup of yogurt.

Lunch: A fresh salad with vegetables and low-fat dressing; a protein, such as fish, chicken, turkey, tofu, or beans; one piece of bread; fresh fruit.

Dinner: One protein, such as fish, tofu, chicken, or beans; one carbohydrate, such as a baked potato, rice, bread, or pasta; 1 cup of steamed vegetables (avoiding starches like peas or corn); a salad with low-fat dressing.

Evening snack: Fruit with one graham cracker square, one low-fat cookie, or ½ cup sorbet or low-fat frozen yogurt.

in mind that no long-term studies have been done yet. Chondroitin sulfate is another popular supplement like glucosamine, but some researchers say it is not as easily absorbed through the intestines and so may not reach the cartilage. Plus, it's chemically similar to blood-thinning drugs, so ask your doctor before you take it.

Rheumatoid arthritis is a different kettle of fish. Large, even massive doses of anti-inflammatories are used to kill the pain along with drugs that whack your haywire immune system into submission. Various types of drugs used in treatment include corticosteroids to reduce inflammation and diminish the immune response, gold salts, methotrexate, and some anti-cancer and antimalaria drugs.

Unfortunately, using many of these drugs, alone or in combination, is a bit like killing fleas with a shotgun. You'll kill the fleas, but you can also damage the poor animals they're attached to. Staying on such strong drugs for pro-longed periods can be very rough on your body. But because they hit rheumatoid arthritis hard and fast, they can prevent ongoing joint dam-age and deformity.

DRUG-FREE RELIEF

Remember, macho's for movies. Sometimes, arthritis drugs are needed to make you feel more comfortable. But you may also want to give the fol-lowing alternatives a try. One or an-other may eliminate most—if not all—of your pain.

Get some good vibrations. Ex-periment with transcutaneous elec-trical nerve stimulation (TENS). A

POWERFUL POTION

CLOVER-BLOSSOM TEA

Now, clover won't cure your arthritis, but if you start the day with a cup of clover tea, it will go a long way to-ward easing some of your aches and pains. Add 1 tea-spoon of dried red clover blos-soms, crushed, and 1 teaspoon of dried alfalfa leaves, crushed, to 1 cup of boiling water. Steep for 5 minutes. Strain out the herbs, and sip. Add 1 teaspoon of honey, if you want, to sweeten it up a bit.

TENS unit is a battery-powered device, smaller than a deck of cards, that you attach to your belt or waistband. TENS delivers electrical impulses through the skin. Although it does not offer a cure, neurologist and pain specialist Emile Hiesiger, M.D., notes that TENS may relieve chronic pain. The impulses feel like mild tingling, a strong pins-and-needles sensation, or muscle contractions, depending on the intensity setting. TENS therapy also increases endorphins—your own naturally occurring narcotics—which inhibit pain impulses arising from the spinal cord to move your brain.

Natural Native Medicine

Weave Your Pain Away?

Wearing a copper bracelet has never been scientifically shown to do much of anything. Native American healers prefer a bracelet of willow root, which they claim relieves the pain of arthritis. How? The salicylic acid contained in the root may be slowly absorbed through the skin, acting as a natural aspirin.

Don't Be a Dope!

As many as 16,500 people with arthritis accidentally kill themselves with NSAIDs every year in an attempt to ease their pain. This is more than the number of people who overdose on heroin! So if your pain is not eased with your regular dosage of a NSAID, *don't take more!* Ask your doctor for a more effective pain medication, instead.

Get to the point. Many people say they find relief from arthritis pain for weeks at a time with acupuncture or acupressure, ancient Chinese therapies that are finally getting some respect from the Western medical establishment. Both healing techniques are based on *chi* (also spelled *qi*), the essential life force. Chinese medical practitioners say that *chi* circulates along energy pathways—or meridians—throughout the body. Improving your *chi* circulation en-

Soak Up the Sun

New evidence links low levels of vitamin D to the progression of osteoarthritis, says Lila Wallis, M.D, a pioneer in women's health. One study showed that people with too little vitamin D in their diets were more likely to develop osteoarthritis and three times more likely to have their existing disease get worse. Researchers now suspect that a bone-repair mechanism might not work without sufficient vitamin D.

Vitamin D is stored in body fat and manufactured naturally in your body when you're exposed to sunlight. We often rely on the vitamin D supply we build up during the summer months; but in winter, some house-bound folks may need a daily supplement. So first, try to spend more time in the sunlight. Then, if there's not enough vitamin D in your diet, add more of these foods:

✔ Milk (vitamin D fortified) ✔ Egg yolks
✔ Fish ✔ Cod liver oil

If you're considering a supplement, keep in mind that large doses of multivitamins or vitamin D can be toxic. Most multis provide 400 international units (IU) of vitamin D daily, which should be ample.

courages the harmonious balance of mind and body. This balanced flow of energy helps the healing process.

Chi is manipulated through locations on the skin called acupoints. You or an acupressure therapist can use fingers to apply deep pressure on these places. An acupuncturist heals by the same principle, but by inserting very thin needles (most say pain-

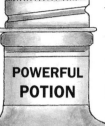

POWERFUL POTION

MEADOW MIXER FOR SUPER CIRCULATION

Combine equal parts of the following herbs: oatstraw (*Avena sativa*), horsetail (*Equisetum arvense*), yarrow (*Achillea mille-folium*), meadowsweet (*Filipen-dula ulmaria*), and peppermint (*Mentha pipertia*). Use 1 heaping teaspoon per 1 cup of boiling water. Steep, covered for 10 to 15 minutes, strain, and drink 1 cup twice daily. These herbs are rich in minerals and enhance circula-tion. Meadowsweet contains small amounts of salicylate for pain relief. This tea may be taken for 2 months or more.

lessly) into acupoints along the energy merid-ians. (Definitely not a do-it-yourself therapy!)

Because medical doctors don't understand how these therapies work, many consider acu-pressure's and acupuncture's benefits to be placebo effects. However, some Western physicians are learning these heal ing arts themselves, and study after study is proving acupunc-ture's benefits.

Your most important consid-erations? First, be sure the thera-pist is licensed. Second, verify that the acupuncturist uses only disposable needles to prevent in-fection and swipes your skin with alcohol before inserting the nee-dles. Check the professional or-ganizations such as the American Association of Oriental Medi-cine, to find a licensed therapist in your area. And talk with others who have undergone acupuncture or acupressure before you decide to give it a go.

Remember, motion's the po-tion. The bad news: Sometimes it hurts to move parts of your body when you have arthritis. The worse news: If you don't move, the pain and stiffness will increase, and you may grow weaker. The good news: When you strengthen your muscles, your joints have more support. The best news: If you walk, stretch, and adopt a moderate exercise program, your body will eventually feel better.

Swimming is the very best exercise for people with arthritis, because it puts no stress on the joints. If churning up and down the lanes is too much for you, just try gentle range-of-motion exercises in a heated pool. For example, to work your shoulder joint, immerse yourself in the warm water, and move your arm around in circles and up and down. Over time, you can extend the range to wider circles, raising your arm higher. Before you start, however, consult a physical therapist and your doctor; they'll prescribe safe and appropriate exercises for you.

Manipulate and massage. If you can't manage vigorous exercise on your own, soft-tissue massage and joint manipulation by a trained therapist can help. Massage can soothe pain, relax stiff muscles, and reduce the swelling that accompanies arthritis. And it feels so darn good! Massage and gentle stretching also help maintain your joint's range of motion. Although their techniques differ, both an osteopath and a chiropractor can carefully manipulate your spine and other arthritic joints to relieve pain and help reestablish normal use.

Turning Pain Around

Sometimes, you can help counteract the crippling effect of rheumatoid arthritis simply by turning a doorknob differently. Why? More damage is done to the outside of your wrist joint (the side with the pinkie finger), which makes it difficult to turn a doorknob to the left with your left hand, for example. So, open doors by turning the knob counterclockwise with your right hand, and vice versa with your left.

Asthma:

Waiting to Exhale

If you have asthma, you don't need me to tell you how an attack can threaten your life and scare the wits out of you! I've had asthma all my life and once had an attack so bad I was rushed to the emergency room for oxygen. They kept me there for a couple of days until everything was under control. It gave me plenty of time to think about how important it is not to let asthma get out of control.

Why the wheeze? Wheezing, chest tightness, and other asthma symptoms occur when the bronchial tubes constrict and the tiny air sacs inside the lungs—called alveoli—can't process the air coming and going through the lungs. This causes a spasm in your bronchial

---

FABULOUS FOLK REMEDY

Super Onion Soup

Onions are an old-time remedy for bronchial problems. Science has validated this use in recent years after discovering that onions are a rich source of quercetin, which is an anti-inflammatory compound. Make a pot of onion soup or eat them raw—if you dare—and feel the warmth spreading through your chest and lungs.

tubes that shuts off most of your air and leaves you gasping for breath, a sensation of drowning—you can imagine the desperate feeling.

Our airways naturally narrow a bit anyway when we're exposed to smoke, pollutants, very cold air, or substances that can harm us if we inhale them. But in people with asthma, perhaps due to a glitch in their genes, this response is exaggerated. It's also often triggered by substances or activities that are harmless to everyone else. A whiff of pollen, a little exercise, or a brisk breath of cold air can trigger an attack. And as more chemicals fill our environment, the substances we breathe are becoming more deadly, especially for people with asthma.

O·D·D·B·A·L·L OINTMENT

Take a Deep Breath

To protect your lungs during a cold or flu, use a chest rub containing menthol or eucalyptus. Better yet, make your own rub with 1 teaspoon of olive oil and 3 to 4 drops of thyme oil. The warming vapors will keep your respiratory passages open and moist even as they fight infection with their antiseptic action.

Muffle the Cold!

Asthma is often triggered by very cold air. So when the temperature is below freezing, wear a scarf or mask over your mouth to warm and moisturize the air you breathe. Breathing through your nose also warms, moisturizes, and cleans the air.

Asthma can virtually "attack" you by quickly closing down your airways, or it can do so more slowly, so you are less aware you are actually having an episode. Most people can quickly reverse an asthma attack using medication—usually a prescribed inhaler—to open the constricted airways. But sometimes an attack is more prolonged and the inhaler doesn't do much. As airways become more inflamed and often clogged with mucus, it gets harder and harder to breathe. Such episodes are a medical emergency, and you need to get to the nearest hospital emergency room—quickly. You may need an injection of adrenaline (epinephrine) and a corticosteroid drug to stop the attack. In extreme cases, you may be given oxygen to help you start breathing again.

The bottom line? Never fool around with asthma. People can and do die from this disease.

FIGURING OUT FOOD ADDITIVES

Like anyone else, people with asthma need to eat a healthful, balanced diet. This can sometimes be difficult, especially if your allergies mean you have to eliminate entire food groups. (Remember, most asthma is caused by allergies.)

Unfortunately, there is no handy list of food allergens—they vary with each individual. So if you suspect that foods may be triggering your asthma, talk to your doctor immediately. Then keep a careful record of what you eat, when you eat it, and what kind of symptoms develop afterward. After a few weeks, a pattern may emerge. Take your record to your doctor, and ask him or her to confirm your suspicions with skin or other allergy tests.

Don't Touch That Vacuum!

Vacuum cleaners can kick up 2 to 10 times the amount of allergens that normally float around your house. The extra onslaught can persist for up to 1 hour after you turn off the vac. If you have chronic asthma, look into the special vacuums that eliminate this dusty "exhaust." (They're expensive but worth it to relieve your lungs.) Or wear a dust mask when you vacuum. Better yet, swap chores with a friend.

Food additives that prevent spoilage and preserve color and texture can also trigger asthma attacks in some folks. If you are sensitive to sulfites, a sulfurous salt used as a preservative, check food labels for any ingredient ending in "-sulfite," such as potassium bisulfite. Sulfites are found in fresh shrimp, instant tea, grape juice, grapes, wine, pizza dough, dried apricots and apples, canned vegetables, corn syrup, molasses, and often in the foods in salad bars. Sulfites sometimes lead to anaphylaxis—or shock—in people who are hypersensitive to them. Other baddies include food dye and the nitrates used to cure some kinds of bacon or ham.

ASTHMA DRUGS: POWERFUL AND PROBLEMATIC

The strong drugs that doctors use to treat asthma may seem miraculous when they stop an attack in its tracks. The downside? Sometimes they pack potent side effects; and with long-term use, they may become ineffective or even addictive. In a severe attack, of course, drugs can be lifesavers— along with emergency treatment and hospitalization. Most often, though, you can avoid a trip to the ER in the first place. The

POWERFUL POTION

THE STARBUCKS SPECIAL

A few strong cups of coffee can sometimes head off an asthma attack. In one survey, 25 people said a jolt of caffeine eased their symptoms. The National Heart, Lung, and Blood Institute in Baltimore seems to back up this observation. Researchers there discovered that regular coffee drinkers with asthma suffer a third fewer symptoms than non-coffee drinkers. Nobody knows exactly why, but caffeine is a chemical that' similar to the theophylline in tea, which opens up the bronchial tubes.

BEAR MOUNTAIN COFFEE

Horehound Candy

Horehound is a main ingredient in many cough drops and hard candies. It works by helping relax the smooth muscles while clearing the lungs of mucus. Here's an old family recipe for horehound candy that you can make today.

Put 1 to 2 cups of fresh horehound leaves in a pot with 4 cups of water. Slowly bring it to a boil; then let it simmer for 15 minutes. Remove the pot from the stove, and strain out the horehound. Add 3 cups of brown sugar and 3 cups of granulated sugar, and stir with a wooden spoon until the sugar is completely dissolved.

Put the pot back on the stove, bring the syrup to a boil, then remove it from the heat. Pour your herbal batter into a greased 9- by 13-inch baking pan. As soon as the candy hardens, break it into bite-size pieces, and wrap each in waxed paper.

trick is always to use your regular medications exactly as they're prescribed. Often, they'll involve the use of an inhaler. At least 82 percent of people admitted to hospitals with severe asthma were not using their medications correctly.

Everyone reacts differently to asthma medications. In most cases, you'll need to take two types: one drug to control inflammation of the airways and a second to get you through attacks by opening the bronchial tubes. In more serious cases, oral steroids like prednisone are given. And in extreme cases, when asthma can't be controlled with any of these medications, doctors will inject adrenaline or give the person with asthma oxygen.

BREATHE-EASY RELIEF

Although asthma is a challenging condition, you can live with it. The key is to work with your doctor, follow his or her instructions, and consider the following tips:

Use your peak flow meter. This little gadget costs only a few dollars at the drugstore and, it can save your life. The peak flow meter gauges how much air you're able to push out of your lungs and may help you predict when an asthma attack is sneaking up on you. Ask your doctor what readings may signal the need to take action. Then blow into it twice a day, and compare your

Beyond Bad Breath

You've heard of acid rain? Now learn about acid breath. It was recently discovered that while *you're* having an asthma attack, your *lungs* are having an acid attack. Just as acid rain harms the world outside, pollution can also cause overly acid breath in our internal environments.

Doctors at the University of Virginia in Charlottesville reported in the American Thoracic Society's *American Journal of Respiratory and Critical Care Medicine* that during attacks, asthma sufferers' breath is a thousand times as acidic as normal. This had never been noticed before, and researchers think it may be central to the disease process of asthma and may open up a new avenue of research for better therapies.

The pH scale measures acidity on a scale of 0 to 14. Vinegar is in the 3 to 5 range. Alkaline solutions, like baking soda in water, measure above 7. The lungs of people with asthma who are sick and wheezing have a pH of about 5—as acidic as vinegar! Unfortunately, this acidity inflames lung tissue and plays a role in closing down airways.

This discovery may lead to new prevention and treatment for asthma. In fact, adjusting the pH level in your airway may some day be as easy as adjusting the pH levels in your fish tank or hot tub.

IT'S AN EMERGENCY!

If someone is having an asthma attack, call your community's emergency telephone number (usually 911). Then keep the person calm until help arrives or his medication begins to take effect. Gently massage his shoulders to help him relax and slow down his breathing. It's a bit like being a Lamaze coach for a woman in labor. Just take a soothing, not forceful, approach.

reading against your "personal best" number.

Keep moving. It used to be that if exercise triggered your asthma, you could count on becoming a couch potato. But we now know the couch is home to billions of dust mites, so you can't hang out there. Today we also know that proper exercise helps people with asthma. You need muscle tone, a stronger heart, and increased stamina to fight any disease, and asthma is no exception.

Walk away the wheeze. The best aerobic exercise for most people is walking. But we're not talking about a casual stroll. You need to walk fast enough so your heart and lungs work hard, and you work up a sweat. Obviously, if you have asthma, hard breathing can be stressful; but a consistent, steady walking program will increase your stamina. If you pick up the pace gradually over time, you'll eventually be able to handle some real huffing and puffing. Most doctors advise you to use your bronchodilator inhaler before you do any strenuous exercise.

Be ready for a rescue. Most people with asthma never leave home without their little rescue inhaler—just in case they need it. Use it before exercising or before you go out into the cold air if that aggravates your asthma. And you'll feel more confident knowing that if you do feel breathless, you can help yourself before it escalates into a real problem.

Bone up on breathing. If you, like many people with asthma, tend to breathe rapidly and shallowly from the upper chest, you may want to consider learning some new techniques. There is now plenty of evidence that proper breathing can dramatically improve your condition, according to Richard Firshein, D.O.,

Natural Native Medicine

Soothe Your Lungs

Native Americans have long been brewing a variety of herbal teas to treat asthma and other lung conditions. They use agrimony leaves, simmered into a tea, strained, and then drunk every few hours with a drop of honey. And they trust a tea made from mullein (*Verbascum thapsus*) for soothing the mucous membranes, especially during nighttime asthma episodes.

Got Milk?

If so, think about getting rid of it—and every other dairy product in your house. Milk proteins increase mucus secretion in the respiratory passages. Milk may also have allergic components, and that's why some doctors advise people with asthma to avoid it. Other doctors say the only way to know for sure is to keep a food diary. Not only milk, but yogurt, cheese, and ice cream may trigger symptoms. Check your airflow: If your peak flow is lower after downing your favorite dairy product, then perhaps you should give it up. I have never found a suitable alternative to milk products, but I've heard some people actually like Tofutti better than ice cream!

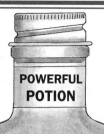

THYME OUT TONIC

Tone up your lungs with restorative herbs and vitamin C–rich rose hips. Combine equal parts of thyme (*Thymus vulgaris*), ginkgo (*Ginkgo biloba*), aniseed (*Pimpinella anisum*), rose hips (*Rosa canina*), and ginger (*Zingiber officinale*). Use 1 heaping teaspoon per 1 cup of boiling water, and steep covered for 15 minutes. Drink 2 to 3 cups per day.

who has asthma and has devoted his medical practice to treating it. Ask your doctor or respiratory therapist how to practice a healthier way to breathe.

Consider yoga. Take up yoga, which according to Dr. Firshein, is a perfect form of exercise for those with asthma. Along with strengthening and stretching your body, you will be learning deeper and more efficient breathing techniques. Find a local class and, chances are, you'll learn that someone else with asthma is in it, too.

Breathe through it. Naturally enough, when you can't breathe, you get scared. Who wouldn't? But this makes breathing even more difficult. It's important to learn to slow your breathing until you can get help. Alert your doctor or a family member for help. Then sit down, drink some water, and take long, slow, deep breaths. This is a good relaxation technique that will help combat the vicious circle of panic and respiratory distress that builds up during an asthma attack. Once your breathing slows down, the medication your doctor has prescribed will be more effective.

Blow your horn. A friend of mine's son had chronic asthma when he was young. She believed that if she taught him to strengthen his breathing, it would relieve his asthma. So she sent him for clarinet lessons. Not only did all that tootling help his asthma, but he's now a talented professional musician!

Take time for tea. The Brits are right! Tea is a great way to relax in the afternoon, but it also has many other benefits. (Even without the watercress sandwiches and Wedgwood cups.) Regular black tea is a source of theophylline, a bronchial muscle relaxant used to treat asthma. Earl Grey and all those other tea lords can do the trick. Practitioners of Chinese medicine often recommend cinnamon twig tea, mixed with white peony root, ginger, Chinese licorice, and dates. Mix equal parts of each herb with a half part of ginger. Add 1 heaping teaspoon to a cup of cold water. Bring to a boil, and simmer, covered, for 15 minutes. Strain, and drink.

Before trying any of these unusual teas, however, ask your doctor if they are suitable for you (people with high blood pressure and/or kidney disease should avoid licorice, for instance). And never take them with—or in place of—

There's Something in the Air . . .

Be aware that some seemingly beneficial aromas may be harmful to a person with asthma. The chemical "perfumes" in room deodorizers or carpet cleaners, for example, can set off an attack.

Six Foods That Help You Breathe

These foods either thin mucus, reduce airway inflammation, or dilate the airways:

- ✔ Chicken soup
- ✔ Fish high in omega-3 fatty acids (salmon, mackerel, sardines)
- ✔ Chili peppers
- ✔ Garlic
- ✔ Onions
- ✔ Mustard

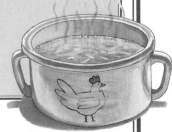

Children at Risk

Asthma has increased a staggering *72 percent* among children over the age of 5 since the early 1990s, according to the National Institutes of Health. It is now the leading cause of childhood death, especially in cities. Because all states have not yet come up with accurate tracking methods, there is no firm conclusion on the reason, but most experts agree that the increase in urban air pollution and the rise in mouse and roach infestations in poor neighborhoods are behind it.

medication prescribed by your doctor!

Treat your lungs to a sauna. Inhaling steam can unclog tight airways. Fill a teapot with water, bring it to a boil, and remove it from the stove. Hold a towel over your head and the pot, and breathe deeply. Be very careful not to scald your face. Or turn on a hot shower, and sit in the steamy bathroom for 10 to 15 minutes. Gary N. Gross, M.D., a researcher at the University of Texas, reports that steam thins the sticky mucus that clogs the airways of people with asthma. Some people like to add eucalyptus or other herbs to the hot water— just be sure you're not allergic to them.

Where there's smoke, there's . . . asthma. Naturally, sitting in a room full of cigarette smokers can precipitate an asthma attack, but so can sitting in front of a fireplace. I can't last more than 5 minutes in a room where wood is being burned. This may not affect every person with asthma, but it's important to become aware of good and bad fumes *before* you rent a vacation home with a wood-burning stove.

Athlete's Foot:

Don't Shrink-Wrap Your Toes

If your feet can't breathe, they're vulnerable to a fungus that loves dark, airless, and moist places, sort of like a creature from a Stephen King novel. The fungus cracks the skin between your toes and produces scales and bleeding. If it spreads to the soles of your feet, it will make them thick and scaly. If your feet itch, peel, and give off an unpleasant odor, this may be the cause.

The fungus is usually called "athlete's foot" because athletes, who spend so much time in sweaty socks and closed shoes, get the condition most often.

FABULOUS FOLK REMEDY

Pickle Your Toes

Good old-fashioned vinegar is an effective antifungal remedy. For best results, use white distilled vinegar. If your skin is broken or sensitive from irritation, begin with a diluted preparation of 1 tablespoon of vinegar per ¼ cup of water. Wash the affected areas twice daily.

O·D·D·B·A·L·L OINTMENT

Take a Powder

While ointments that squish between your toes may be helpful at night, for daytime walking, use herbal powders instead of ointments. Powdered marigold (*Calendula officinalis*) and oregano (*Origanum vulgare*) can be combined in equal parts and sprinkled between the toes.

Unfortunately, and unpleasantly, the fungus is related to ringworm and jock itch. (Personally, I think athletes should organize and get the name of that last condition changed) Here's how to avoid it:

Keep 'em clean. Dodge this grungy fungus by meticulously cleaning under your toenails and between your toes during your daily bath or shower.

Dry each digit. If you're prone to athlete's foot, dry each toe separately; then use a paper towel between them to absorb every drop of moisture. Or use the blow dryer on a low setting. It'll feel good!

Powder up. Once your feet are completely dry, powder them with baking soda to absorb sweat. Or you might try one of the antifungal powders available in drugstores. Dust the insides of your socks and shoes with the powder, too.

Expose yourself. Let those tootsies hang out in the fresh air and sunshine if you're not going anywhere. Just don't walk barefoot around the house. Not only will you track powder all over your rugs but you'll

Aloe There, Vera!

The desert native, aloe vera, is simply miraculous for healing skin. If you have a plant handy, break off a big leaf, mash it into an ointment or gel, and rub it on your feet. This remedy is a favorite of Native Americans.

Natural Native Medicine

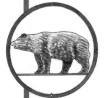

Thyme to Heal the Problem

A Native American remedy for athlete's foot is soaking your feet in hot water with a few drops of oil of thyme added to relieve the itching and burning. Then dust your feet with a mixture of myrrh and goldenseal powders in any proportion, and put on a pair of heavy cotton socks. Repeat daily for several days. **Caution:** Folks with diabetes should check with their doctor first.

plant contagious little fungus seedlings wherever you go. You don't want to be known as Johnny Fungusseed, do you?

Wick your wigglies. Socks made from the new wicking fabrics literally absorb moisture from skin and allow it to evaporate through the fiber. Wicking fabric retains 14 times less moisture than cotton. Most sporting goods stores carry these socks especially for runners. If you can't afford these fairly pricey socks, your next-best bet is cotton. Other synthetics trap moisture so your feet can't breathe. The principle applies to shoes, too. Leather, a natural material, breathes, as does cotton canvas, but most synthetic materials do not. And if you're partial to pantyhose, your feet won't thank you. They keep your feet as sweaty as if had you shrink-wrapped them.

Try tea tree oil. Tea tree oil is a cheap, safe, and effective alternative to expensive antifungal agents from pharma-

POWERFUL POTION

GARLIC WATER

If you're tired of athlete's foot, put your foot down—in a tub of garlic water! Crush several garlic cloves, and drop them into a tub of warm water with a little rubbing alcohol added. Then gently place both feet in the tub, and let them soak for about 10 minutes, once a day. **Caution: Folks with diabetes should check with their healthcare provider first.**

A Salty Solution

If you live on a seacoast, walk barefoot along the edge of the water, and let the surf wash over your feet. This highly saline environment has a cleansing affect and can hasten the cure of your soles—as well as your soul!

cies, says Andrew Weil, M.D., a holistic practitioner at the University of Arizona. Apply a light coating of tea tree oil to affected areas three or four times a day. It's important to continue these applications for 2 weeks after the infection disappears to make sure the fungus is vanquished.

Break out the bleach. Foot baths of chlorine bleach used to be a remedy for athlete's foot. In fact, the recipe was printed on the Clorox bottle in the 1950s. Doctors say there is no basis for this treatment, but some people claim it works. To try it, soak your feet in a mixture of ½ cup of bleach and 1 gallon of water twice a day. Vinegar, instead of bleach in the same recipe, may do the trick, too. Those with diabetes should not soak their feet without checking with their doctor.

Get garlic. Native American healers suggest equal portions of garlic oil mixed with olive oil as a potion for your toes. This may kill the fungus, but I'm not sure what it does for foot odor! You may not want to try this one unless you live alone.

POWERFUL POTION

TERRIFIC TOOTSIE TONIC

Severe athlete's foot must be treated from the inside out. For starters, try a tea made from equal parts of echinacea (*Echinacea purpurea*), oregano, marigold, and cleavers (*Galium arvense*). Use 1 heaping teaspoon per 1 cup of boiling water. Steep, covered, for 15 minutes, and drink up to 3 cups per day.

This concoction may also be used as an external wash. Use ½ cup per 1 quart of water. Soak your feet for 15 to 20 minutes. Then dry well!

Back Pain:

Watch Your Back!

A healthy back is easy to take for granted—until you help move your pal's sofa. Then OUCH! Suddenly, you wonder if you'll ever be able to move anything, including any part of your own body, again.

Made up of bones, muscle, and nerve, your back is somewhat like the flexible stem of a gooseneck lamp. The disks, or shock absorbers, between your vertebrae are mostly water—and they can dry out after years of sitting, walking, and bending. A disk can slip (herniate) from position and pinch a nerve root, sending pain everywhere. Vertebrae can become arthritic; ligaments can calcify. Yet, the most common cause of acute back pain isn't a disk or nerve problem: It's muscle spasm.

It's an "all-at-once acute back in-

O·D·D·B·A·L·L OINTMENT

A Tiger in the Tube

Tiger Balm is the one remedy from ancient Chinese medicine that everyone seems to know about. Rubbed into the skin, this potent salve creates heat to warm tight muscles and a tingling sensation to divert your attention from the back pain.

Take a Load Off!

I love those big lounge chairs that lean all the way back and park your feet in the air. But they just don't match the decor of my family room. Fortunately, there are some alternatives: Lie on the floor with your legs up on the couch or a chair, and place a pillow under your head. And while your at it, get some foam-rubber wedges to keep under your legs when you're in bed. Use this legs-up position to take the pressure off your back as often as possible.

jury," says Boyd Buser, D.O, a practitioner of osteopathic manipulative therapy at the University of New England College of Osteopathic Medicine in Maine. And it usually results from something as seemingly minor as dragging an object from under the bed or bending down suddenly to look under the table.

But why does a single action, such as swiftly stooping, produce such agony? "The biggest single thing that Americans *don't* do is exercise to prevent back injuries," says Dr. Buser. "You have to maintain the equipment," he adds. "It's like keeping your car running well."

Many out-of-whack backs do get better with time and a variety of remedies, such as taking painkillers, changing positions, wearing a brace, or getting a new desk chair. From health experts, here are some ideas on protecting your back and making it feel better when it hurts:

Get manipulated. Dr. Buser, a recognized expert in osteopathic manipulative therapy (OMT), says that, unlike a traditional medical doctor, the osteopath will take "a detailed structural exam of the musculoskeletal system, evaluating all of it down to the spaces between each vertebra. Medical doctors test you for motion in various regions, such as bending or turning, but they don't look at the individual vertebra—and we think that's critical," he says. Find a local osteopath who can stretch and move your soft tissues to relieve pain and reestablish normal motion. "We create conditions for the body to heal itself," Dr. Buser says. A recent study published in the *New England Journal of Medicine* found OMT as effective as other treatments for low back pain and lower in cost.

Release your *chi*. The National Institutes of Health (NIH) has endorsed acupuncture for a number of problems, including back pain, and many conventional medical doctors are now learning the technique. The theory is that acupuncture releases the body's blocked flow of energy, or *chi* (also spelled *qi*), to restore balance. To treat back pain, extremely thin needles are inserted into a dozen or more specific sites—called acupoints—on your torso, head, arms, and legs. You may be surprised to know that acupuncture is painless and even relaxing! Some therapists give the treatment in a darkened room with soft music. To get the most from acupuncture, always go to a licensed therapist. And be

POWERFUL POTION

HOT HERBAL TEA TODDY

To relieve back pain, use one or more of the following herbs in equal parts: gingerroot (*Zingiber officinale*), chamomile (*Matricaria recutita*), and peppermint (*Mentha piperita*). For muscle spasm, add skullcap (*Scutellaria lateriflora*) or valerian (*Valeriana officinalis*) to the herb mixture. Use 1 teaspoon of the mixture per 1 cup of boiling water. Steep, covered, for 10 minutes. Drink 1 cup three to four times a day. **Caution:** People with ragweed allergies may be sensitive to chamomile. Valerian should not be taken with antidepressants.

O·D·D·B·A·L·L OINTMENT

Apply Arnica— Say Ahhh!

Arnica gel is an excellent first-aid ointment for muscle or joint pain. For inflamed and irritated nerves, add several drops of St. John's wort oil. Apply frequently. **Caution:** Arnica is for external use only; do not use over broken skin.

sure that U.S. Food and Drug Administration (FDA) regulations to prevent infection are followed: Acupuncturists must use only sterile, single-use disposable needles, and your skin must be swabbed with alcohol before the needles are applied.

Aten . . . hut! Keep your shoulders back, chest out, stomach in, chin up! That's good posture, as well as a good drill for a new army recruit. Good posture means you're aligning your body so you can breathe properly and move correctly.

Shake your booty! We weren't designed to sit all day, so get up and move every now and then. Stretch and walk around. Move your head to stretch your neck muscles. And if your chair has arms, use your own arms and legs to push yourself up and out of the chair.

Don't sit on your wallet. That lump of wallet in your back pocket can do damage to your buttock nerves. It's an occupational hazard for pilots, truck drivers, and commuters. Also, don't slouch when you're driving. Use pillows, cushions, and pads for support, just as you would in a chair, so you sit upright and comfortable.

Choose comfortable shoes. If your feet are uncomfortable, your back suffers. Wear shoes suitable to what you are doing. If you are walking through the countryside or for hours on cobblestone streets, choose an excellent walking shoe or even a light hiking shoe with good support and flexible soles. And if you're a woman, remember that high heels throw your center of gravity out of whack, wreaking havoc on your back.

Use some sitting savvy. Keep your feet flat on the floor if you sit at a computer or desk all day. Your forearms should be positioned with your elbows at right angles. And set up your computer's monitor at eye level. Your chair seat should be deep enough to support your hips, but the front edge should not touch the back of your knees. The chair back should have an angle of about 10 degrees, and cradle the small of your back comfortably. If it doesn't, add a wedge-shaped cushion or lumbar pad there. And here's some back-happy news: The old-fashioned, straight-backed chair is better for your back than many of those high-tech, ergonomic extravaganzas that cost hundreds—or thousands—of dollars. You can also try a kneeler chair to see if it relieves your back pain, says Emile Hiesiger, M.D., a neurologist who specializes in chronic pain.

Be shifty. If you stand a lot, as a surgeon or a supermarket clerk does, shift from hip to hip to avoid back pain. Wear flat shoes with good support, and keep correcting your posture, advises Dr. Hiesiger. Try putting a box or step bench on the floor; and from time to time rest one foot on it, then the other. The step should be about 6 inches high.

Don't You Dare Move!

After *any* injury to your back, don't move for 1 or 2 days. Put an ice pack on your back for 15 or 20 minutes—or lie on the ice pack if that's easier—then repeat every 1 to 2 hours. This is the advice of Andrew Weil, M.D., director of the Program of Integrative Medicine at the University of Arizona. Heat will actually make the pain worse in the early stages after an injury.

POWERFUL
POTION

TUB THYME

Ease your aching back by tossing a handful of dried thyme into the tub as you run a hot bath. Soak for 10 to 15 minutes, and let the aromatic oils in this herb take your aches and pains down the drain.

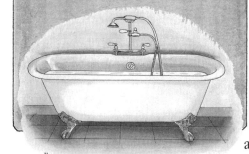

Get rhythm. In some nations, day laborers chant or sing while they do back-breaking work, such as carrying loads of freight on their heads. Hum if it helps you find a rhythm to work in, so your movements are slow and regular, not quick and jerky. Take a lesson from people who carry baskets on their heads. They walk in a balanced, undulating rhythm. Their baskets don't fall—and their backs don't wrench.

Balance the load. With the invention of backpacks, wilderness campers were able to carry amazing amounts of equipment without hurting their backs. But that's because they wore their packs correctly—both straps over the shoulders, and gear evenly balanced. Today, backpacks are popular for lugging everything from books to baby paraphernalia; but, unfortunately, many people carry them slung over one shoulder.

Some 60-pound children carry 40 pounds of books in their backpacks, and it's hip to use just one shoulder. These half-pints are growing up to gallons of back misery. When carrying heavy or awkward objects, divide them between your arms. Distribute the weight of your load, rather than toting everything in one hand or on just one side of your body, Dr. Hiesiger says.

Quit hauling. When you carry a shoulder bag, you tend to tense your shoulder to keep the bag from slipping off. This scrunched-up posture causes all kinds of muscle strain and related pain, according to Amy Klein, D.C., a New York chiropractor, who always asks to see what kind of handbag her back pain clients carry. Check out purses by designers like Liz Claiborne and Calvin Klein, who are heeding the message with new lines of short-handled carryalls. When you can't sling a bag over your shoulder, you'll be more inclined to switch the weight from hand to hand.

Always lift with your legs. Lift heavy objects by using the muscles in your legs, not in your back. Bend your knees, and lift straight up so that you feel your legs taking the brunt of the strain. Don't bend your spine, and then haul a load upright. Keep your hips and shoulders in a vertical line.

Don't be a jerk. If you sit all day in an office and then dash off for racquetball without warming up before the game, you'll jerk your muscles, tendons, and ligaments. Warm up before any physical activity, even gardening, so you gently stretch those muscles into readiness. Dragging 50 pounds of peat moss on a weekend, after days at a desk, can cause a tear or significant strain in the supporting structures of your back. But when you warm up first, your heart rate goes up gradually, increasing your muscles' blood supply, which makes your muscles more adaptable. Better yet, warming up and exercising daily will do wonders to forestall back injuries.

Avoid nighttime neck cricks. Your back is usually injured during the day, but your neck—the uppermost part of your back—is more often hurt during sleep, when you

IT'S AN EMERGENCY!

Call your doctor if back pain is causing any numbness in your groin or legs, or if you lose control of your bowels or bladder. You could have a serious spinal injury that needs immediate attention.

Soak in Some Salts

Epsom salts baths can help ease spasms and relieve pain. Add 2 cups of Epsom salts to a hot bath, and feel the relief. Afterward, place an ice pack on your back.

toss and turn. You wake up with a crick, which can signal the onset of a cervical disk herniation, says Dr. Hiesiger. If you've got a stiff neck on many mornings, discuss it with your doctor.

Pick the perfect pillow. A pillow should be soft enough to keep your neck from arching severely and large and hard enough to raise your head slightly to shoulder level. If you already have neck pain, cervical pillows may relieve it. But choose one with your doctor's advice: Many "therapeutic" pillows arch your neck and even increase the pressure on the neck's disks, facets, and joints, says Dr. Hiesiger.

Snooze on a slant. I love to read in bed. And if the book is really compelling, I force myself to stay awake to finish it. But I squirm around a lot because it's difficult to get comfortable. If I lie down flat, I'll fall asleep no matter how exciting the book. (A sure antidote to insomnia.) Few beds give us natural back protection for under-the-covers reading. When you read in bed, put pillows under the small of your back and behind your neck so your spine is not under strain, advises Dr. Hiesiger.

Face the fat facts. Excess weight causes a severe strain on your spine. As your abdomen balloons outward, you pull your spine out of alignment. In other words, a big gut pulls your back out of whack, because you've changed your center of gravity.

Encouraging patients to lose weight and exercise is "like trying to get people to stop smoking," Dr. Buser says. "When patients know you want to help them get well, they tend to take your advice. If they come back to me months later with the same problem, they feel chagrined," he notes. So let your back pain prompt you to take responsibility for the underlying conditions that caused the problem, such as being overweight or avoiding exercise.

Resist magnetic attraction. When I put some computer disks into a briefcase with a magnetic catch, my disks were erased. Whether magnets can erase back pain as easily is questionable. The therapeutic magnet industry has been raking in money from millions of people with back pain who buy magnetic shoe inserts, blankets and pads, straps—even jewelry. And while there is some evidence that magnets can help alleviate pain (without the side effects of some drugs), a double-blind study reported in the March 2000 *Journal of the American Medical Association* found no difference in pain relief between the real and fake magnets. Bottom line: Don't try magnets if you have a pacemaker or any metal hardware in your body. And certainly don't go anywhere near your computer disks!

Crunch your Abs— Not your Neck!

Naturally, you want to strengthen your stomach muscles to stabilize your spine, but if you don't do it right, you can cause further damage. If you do abdominal crunches with your hands behind your head, you can hurt your neck. Instead, try them with your hands crossed over your chest or resting at your sides.

Bad Breath:

Here's to the Freshest Mouth in Town!

Got dinosaur breath? Does your bed partner stuff his or her head under the pillow when you lean over for a good-morning smooch? In either case, you need help!

While you're sleeping, your saliva production factory is off-line, too. Busy little bacteria take over, and a few hours later, you wake up with real road-kill breath. A drop in the saliva level allows mouth bacteria to multiply and form plaque. Bad breath may also be a result of poor dental hygiene, poor diet, or a sinus or gum infection. Rarely, it can signal something as serious as kidney failure, liver disease, or diabetes. Ask your

An Apple a Day

An apple a day not only will keep the doctor away but it will keep bad breath at bay, as well. In fact, an apple is a great remedy for garlic breath. In a healthy mouth, garlic odor usually goes away after a while, but you'll speed up the process if you dilute the pungent aroma with an apple, and then brush your teeth.

doctor about persistent bad breath if you get no relief from the following reliable remedies:

Brush up on your oral hygiene. Are you brushing twice a day with a soft brush? The bedtime brushing is important, so plaque doesn't form during the night (while saliva production is off-duty). Massage your gums with the brush, too. And before you brush, floss. Flossing every day helps remove plaque—and bacteria—from between your teeth. The American Dental Association also recommends professional cleaning at least annually, and some dentists suggest twice a year.

Rake your tongue. Most bad breath comes from the wet, boggy areas in the back of your mouth, where bacteria like to breed a sulfur-smelling plaque on your tongue, according to George Preti, Ph.D., of the Monell Chemical Senses Center in Philadelphia. Before brushing, reach into your mouth as far as you can go without gagging, and scrape away the plaque, he suggests. There are plastic tongue scrapers available at most pharmacies, or you can simply use your toothbrush.

Natural Native Medicine

Chew On a Few Leaves

Some Native American traditions call for using spearmint or bergamot leaves as a quick and easy digestive aid and breath freshener. Chew a leaf or two slowly. Then make a cup of mild mint tea with 3 leaves; cool it; and use it as a gargle, rinse, or spray. Carry a sandwich bag or pouch of mint or parsley leaves, so you can chew on them periodically throughout the day.

O·D·D·B·A·L·L OINTMENT

Myrrhvalous Mouthwash

When your mouth is the source of the bad breath, consider making a mouthwash using 1 teaspoon of tincture of myrrh (*Commiphora molmol*) in ¼ cup of water.

Wash out your mouth. (But unless you deserve it, not with soap!) Use an antiseptic mouthwash that kills bacteria. Other mouthwashes just mask odor with a minty solution, but some can be quite pleasant and long-lasting. Try making your own odor-masking mouthwash with whole or powdered cloves steeped in hot water.

POWERFUL POTION

RED-PEPPER MOUTHWASH

Kill dragon breath with cayenne's fire power! Cayenne not only kills germs, but it leaves your breath feeling spicy fresh. Just dilute 5 to 10 drops *each* of cayenne tincture and myrrh tincture in a half a glass of warm water. (A tincture is a potent liquid plant extract. You can find tinctures at many health-food stores.)

Drink lots of water. Keeping yourself well hydrated is a good health practice in general, but it is especially important to help keep bad breath at bay. Drink those eight glasses a day to help keep saliva production going and reduce bacteria buildup.

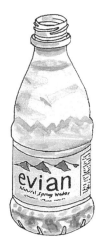

Make your own toothpaste. You can add a few drops of hydrogen peroxide to baking soda for a good, effective toothpaste, according to Native American medicine. Don't expect it to taste good while you brush; but afterward, your mouth will be wonderfully fresh.

Eat your veggies. Vegetables and fruit not only are valuable sources of vitamins and anti-oxidants, but also contain chlorophyll, a natural deodorant that sweetens your breath. So eat five to nine servings a day, for a healthy body and healthy breath, too.

And while you're at it, throw in some sour foods, such as pickles and lemons. They will jump-start the flow of saliva, helping to flush away those nasty halitosis bacteria in your mouth.

Natural Native Medicine

Spice Mix

Native Americans have a cleansing and refreshing mixture they claim clears up bad breath while brightening the teeth, and it makes a fine gargle and mouthwash. You can use this tooth powder daily, or alternate it with a commercial brand. In a small dish, measure 1 tablespoon of baking soda with $\frac{1}{2}$ teaspoon of sea salt or kosher salt, $\frac{1}{2}$ teaspoon of powdered allspice, and $\frac{1}{2}$ teaspoon of ground sage. Sprinkle this well-blended mix onto your toothbrush and brush, or stir 1 teaspoon into 1 cup of warm water and gargle.

Blisters:

How to Avoid
the Friction

Blisters are the pits. Whether they're caused by a tight shoe, a hand tool, burns, bug bites, infections or poison ivy, they're a royal pain in the you-know-what. So here's how to protect yourself from those fluid-filled sacs:

Pop it only if it's painful. You should break a blister only if it is very large or painful, or you'll risk infection. Sterilize a needle with a match, and pierce the blister gently. Let it drain, and keep it bandaged for 3 or 4 days until it heals.

Shop with fat feet. Your feet are bigger toward the end of the day. So the best time to shop for new shoes is while they're at their largest. Or shop 1 hour after working out, when your feet are still a bit swollen. That way,

Cornstarch and Petroleum Jelly

Blisters on the feet are most likely to develop if your feet are too sweaty or if the skin is too dry. If your socks are often soggy, the origin of your blister problem may be that sweaty skin. Try sprinkling a little cornstarch into your socks before you put them on, and dust some between your toes, too.

If the skin on your feet is very dry, smooth a thin film of petroleum jelly over them before you pull on your socks and sneakers.

your new shoes will be big enough and won't be burning blisters on your toes after you've been walking around all morning long.

Lace up right. When putting on running or other sports shoes, be sure to lace them up properly, so your foot is held firmly in place. Otherwise, your foot'll rub around against the inside of the shoe and create a blister.

Be sport specific. If you play basketball in shoes designed for running, they won't pivot with your feet and thus may rub and cause blisters. If you participate in a variety of activities, you need lots of different types of shoes.

Practice safe socks. Throw away all those worn-out and laundry-stiffened socks. Wear soft, cushioned socks with no ridges or seams to rub against your foot inside your shoe.

Lose the shoes. Some athletes, especially runners, like to toughen their feet by going barefoot as often as possible. Try running barefoot on the beach or in a grassy field for 10 to 15 minutes after a workout.

Reduce friction. Try this two-part friction

IT'S AN EMERGENCY!

The persistence of one or more blisters, swelling, inflammation, or bleeding can be a sign of infection, and you should see a doctor. Also, see your doctor if a blister is accompanied by fever or other symptoms of infection.

fighter: First, apply a commercial, friction-reducing gel, such as Hydropel, to your feet. Then wear silk or fine-cotton sock liners under your regular socks to further reduce friction. You can find sock liners at sports apparel stores.

Protect those working hands. Wear gloves when you work with household or construction tools. Likewise, wear gardening gloves when you're raking or pruning.

Loosen your grip. A golf club, squash racket, or tennis racket is a blister machine. So loosen your fingers, and change your grip as often as you can while playing.

Wear gloves for play, too. When you play softball or other sports requiring a bat, racquet, or club of some kind, wear gloves, like the pros always do. You can get some pretty bad blisters from sailing without gloves. Oh, how those lines burn when you're coming about in a heavy wind!

Toughen up. If you are about to embark on a home building project or other activity that will be a shock to your soft hands, get them ready. Rub denatured alcohol on your hands three times a day for several weeks before doing the manual labor, recommends Andrew Weil, M.D., director of the Program of Integrative Medicine at the University of Arizona.

POWERFUL POTION

TAN YOUR HIDE

Tannins are compounds present in many plants and trees that can strengthen the skin. To prevent blisters, soak your hands or feet in a strong, tannin-rich infusion of black tea, oak bark, or pine twigs. To make the infusion, simply soak a handful of the tea, bark, or twigs in a basin of boiled water. When the water cools, strain the infusion, and then soak your hands or feet for 10 to 15 minutes. **Caution:** People with diabetes should talk to their doctors before soaking their feet.

Blocked Ears:

Some High-Pressure Help

Next time you're speeding to the top of a skyscraper in an elevator, watch how everyone yawns or swallows at the same time to unblock their ears. At a certain height, the pressure gives your middle ear a jolt.

That's because the outside air pressure falls slightly, and it's enough to be sensed by your delicate middle ear. Inside the middle ear, the higher pressure puts stress on the ear chamber walls. Result? Ouch! To avoid the problem, try these tips:

Swallow. Swallowing opens the eustachian tubes, equalizing the air pressure in your middle ear with the pressure outside. When you feel your ears "pop," the discomfort goes away. It would be too much to expect you to keep swallowing all the way to Singapore, though, so it's a good idea to be aware of other remedies, too.

Get ready to dive. To avoid in-flight earaches, take an over-the-counter decongestant as soon as your flight is announced. Then 1 hour before the descent, use a decongestant nasal spray to help clear things up.

Keep yawning. This is a long-lasting remedy. Move your jaw gently, and yawn for as long as you can.

O·D·D·B·A·L·L OINTMENT

Put a Tiger behind Your Ear

Tiger Balm—that fabulous heating ointment—can be used to massage behind the ears. The heat increases circulation to the area, while the massage helps relieve congestion. Always massage in a downward direction to facilitate fluid flow.

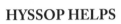

POWERFUL POTION

HYSSOP HELPS

Prefer a natural decongestant to the over-the-counter variety? Before you board your flight, locate the airport bar or restaurant. Ask for a glass of water. Then drip 1 to 4 milliliters of tincture of hyssop into it, and drink up. This natural decongestant should keep your ears cleared for both takeoff and landing.

Body Odor:

A Common-Scents Approach

Aren't you glad we're not living back when people bathed once a week—or less—and masked their body odor with heavy perfumes, powdered wigs, and lots of rarely washed clothes? I sure am. Whee-ew!

Our bodies need to sweat to regulate temperature, but perspiration's not the problem—it's nearly odorless water. The odor comes from the presence of bacteria and fungi in the sweaty areas. These busy little stinkers particularly like to get between your toes, into your armpits, and on your private parts. Our clothes can also get odorific if they're not washed often enough—from the stale perspiration they absorb.

Do keep in mind, however, that strong body odor can sometimes be a sign of a serious medical condition or skin infection. Call your primary-care doctor (or dermatologist) if an unusual odor permeates your skin, despite your best attempts to get rid of it. Here are some tips for keeping the odors at bay:

Eat sweet. Some body odor is caused by what you eat. The famous smells of garlic and onions can come right through your pores. But no need to boycott these favorites, just neutralize their potent aromas by also eating parsley and other green leafy vegetables with chlorophyll, a natural deodorant. (That's the origin of the parsley-as-garnish tradition.) If you keep it up, you'll begin to notice the difference in just a few days.

Change deodorants periodically. After years of use, your regular deodorant may no longer work as well as it used to. It may have been altered, your own body chemistry may be changing, or you may simply have developed a tolerance for the brand. Try another—change is good! You'll be using a deodorant every day for years, so why have bored armpits? If you get a rash from one deodorant, try another designed for sensitive skin. And you may want to look for a plain deodorant, because antiperspirants contain aluminum hydrochloride, which can be a skin irritant.

POWERFUL POTION

CLEAN—INSIDE AND OUT!

The skin is the largest organ of the body and an important player in the elimination of toxins. Body odor can sometimes be the result of sluggish or poor elimination. Use these gentle herbs to help clean your body on the inside. Combine equal parts of red clover (*Trifolium pratense*), yarrow (*Achillea millefolium*), cleavers (*Galium aparine*), calendula (*Calendula officinalis*), and peppermint (*Mentha piperita*). Use 1 heaping tablespoon of the herb mix in 1 quart of warm water. Steep for 15 minutes. Drink throughout the day.

Flower Powder

Powdered flowers can help absorb odors. Mix together the powdered flowers of calendula (*Calendula officinalis*) and lavender (*Lavendula officinalis*), and add to an equal part of slippery elm (*Ulmus fulva*) powder. Dust under the arms once or twice daily.

Wear clothes that breathe. Polyester and most synthetic fabrics keep odors close to your body. Cotton, silk, and some of the new wicking fabrics designed for athletes allow moisture to circulate, so it won't cling to your body or clothing. Try a sports supply or camping store for lightweight wicking underwear.

Try your fridge's best friend. Baking soda keeps your fridge odor free, so why not you? Use it as a dusting powder or body rub, or sprinkle a handful in your bath.

Go for the gold. Native Americans in the U.S. Southwest and Mexico have long used calendula flowers as skin fresheners because of their mild, pleasing fragrances and skin-soothing minerals. A cream made from these flowers absorbs well into the skin, especially during the heat of summer. Combine 1 ounce of dried, crushed calendula petals with glycerine or beeswax, distilled water, and some dried mint or bergamot. Simmer in the top of a double-boiler for about 3 hours to create a fine emulsion. Then pour it into a clean bowl, and whip it until it cools and sets. Native Americans also make a body talc by mixing crushed calendula leaves with cornstarch.

A Little Dab Will Do Ya

Splashing some rubbing alcohol under your arms may reduce the bacteria population. For a persistent odor problem, try using alcohol in place of deodorant—just not after shaving or if you have any nicks or cuts in your skin. That'll sting like crazy!

Breast Conditions:

Get to Know Your Own Geography

Your breasts are lovely wonders—they're possibly the eighth wonder of the world. If you've forgotten that, just think back to junior high. You were pressing ahead on world geography, while some poor squirming boy at a nearby desk was haunted by the notion of pressing against, well—*your* geography.

Yet your breasts are more than symbols of femininity, sex appeal, and motherhood. They are a complex and dynamic body system, vulnerable to both interior and exterior changes that you need to be aware of. The good news is that most disorders of the breast are benign. The bad news is that too many women take that for granted. Avoiding the issue means just one thing: You can miss the early signs of breast cancer. And that's a tragedy—because breast cancer is treated very successfully when it's caught early. So even if you think you're not at risk, pay special heed to the first three tips below.

More likely, however, you have a benign breast problem. Your breasts may be tender, enlarged, and painful just before your period or even during menstruation. If you're nursing your baby, your breasts may become inflamed from blocked milk ducts. But the most common, benign condition is fibrocystic breasts, or cystic mastitis, which affects 60 to 90 percent of women to some degree—and

POWERFUL POTION

EVENING PRIMROSE OIL

Evening primrose oil seems to relieve breast pain in some women, although no one's found a medical explanation as to why. It is available in health-food stores in tablet form. Follow package directions, and take the recommended dose. This oil is also one of the best-known, Native American remedies for fibrocystic breasts.

may run in families. With each menstrual cycle, estrogen and progesterone hormones stimulate the breast to develop fibrocystic changes—usually lumps. And sometimes, they're painful. Although these lumps do not lead to cancer, they can make it harder to discover a new unusual nodule among the existing lumps. Birth control pills may worsen the problem.

Examine your breasts regularly. Breast self-examination

(BSE) is a must to keep you on the alert for breast cancer. And if you have lumpy or fibrocystic breasts, knowing the particular geography of your breasts will help you sense when something is unusual. Do your BSE every month at the same time, ideally within the first 10 days of your menstrual cycle. Examine your breasts both standing and lying down. While you are standing, just look in the mirror under good lighting—checking for any breast swelling or puckering. Then lie down, and put a pillow under the shoulder on the side of the breast you are examining. Pressing your fingers against your breast, make slow, ever-widening circles all around your breast, starting from the nipple. You can also follow a petal pattern (like a daisy) around your breast, pressing from your nipple outward. If you find any unusual lump, thickening or nipple discharge, don't panic—but have it promptly checked by your doctor.

Get an annual mammogram. The number of cases of breast cancer is rising because we live longer, and there are more toxins in our environment. But with better detection, we are catching it

Try the Carrot Cure!

If your breast is inflamed (red and swollen) because of a blocked milk duct, apply a fresh carrot poultice—just grate a carrot into some cheesecloth and moisten it. Place it on the infected breast all the way up to the armpit, and cover it with a hot water bottle. Leave it on for 1 hour. A fresh poultice should be applied several times daily until the infection is resolved. If accompanied by fever and flu-like symptoms, see your doctor immediately. You may have an infection that could get worse.

O·D·D·B·A·L·L OINTMENT

Root for the Cure

Poke root (*Phyltolacca americana*) ointment encourages lymphatic drainage of the breasts. When you use it, be sure to massage up the breast and out toward your arms and chest, which is the direction of normal lymphatic flow.

in its earliest stages. The National Cancer Institute, the American Cancer Society, the American Medical Women's Association, and many other organizations recommend a baseline mammogram, or breast x-ray, at an accredited facility by age 40, and then annually after that. If you have a family history of breast cancer, start to schedule mammograms at age 35. Mammography saves many women's lives—and new digital technology will make mammograms even more accurate and easier to read.

Back it up with a clinical examination. Because mammography is not perfect—there is a 15 percent margin for error—if there's any finding, be sure it's followed up by a clinical examination. In 1992, I heaved a sigh of relief when a mammogram showed no abnormality, even though my doctor had discovered a small lump on my lower left breast, near my ribs. When I reported the mammogram results to my doctor, she examined my breasts again, and urged me to have a surgical biopsy. After some resistance, I agreed. I did indeed have breast cancer, but it was detected early enough to be cured. I will be eternally grateful for that doctor's

POWERFUL POTION

TERRIFIC TREE TEA

Chastetree berry (*Vitex agnus-castus*) helps normalize hormone levels that, when unbalanced, can contribute to breast swelling and discomfort. Drink 1 cup of chastetree berry tea twice daily. To make, use 1 teaspoon of dried berries in 1 cup of boiling water, and steep for 15 minutes.

insistence that I follow up until the lump was explained. If I had relied only on the mammogram, I might not be writing this.

Kick the coffee habit. If you have fibrocystic breasts, curb those cravings, and avoid all caffeine, including coffee, tea, colas, and (sorry!) chocolate, say naturopaths Ruth Bar-Shalom, N.D., and John Soileu, N.D. Caffeine doesn't cause the condition, but it has been found in several studies to aggravate it.

Avoid salt. When your breasts are tender and sore, any swelling can make them hurt even more. Cut down on salt to reduce fluid retention. And don't just set aside the salt shaker—read food labels, too. High sodium levels are very common in many packaged foods.

One Hot Tomato

Are you a tomato lover? Here's great news from the American Institute for Cancer Research: "A single tomato contains hundreds, possibly thousands, of phytochemicals that perform different functions to prevent cancer. Tomatoes are especially rich in the phytochemical called lycopene, which has been linked to reduced prostate cancer risk and is believed to act as a breast cancer preventive as well." Anybody want a pizza?

Twiddle your thermostat. Both heat and cold can relieve the discomfort of swollen breasts. When you're uncomfortable before or during your period, place a chilled towel or bag of ice over your breasts for a while. A warm compress held against the breast can also relieve breast tenderness. Pop a damp hand towel in the microwave for 10 seconds, or use an electric heating pad.

Sport a breast-friendly bra. A more flexible bra can relieve pain. Wear a well-fitted sports bra that is firm and comfortable, not binding and cutting.

Bronchitis:

Healing the Hack

When you have bronchitis, that bottom-of-the-well deep hacking or rasping cough that rattles your ribs feels like a tornado in your chest—and boy, does it really hurt.

Bronchitis means inflammation of the lining of the bronchial tubes, the passages that connect your windpipe and lungs. It can last 2 weeks and, without treatment, can lead to serious trouble. It can also be very contagious.

Chronic bronchitis, which many smokers develop, can lead to irreversible lung damage, leaving you vulnerable to emphysema and heart disease. Bedrest, lots of fluids, and an expectorant (not a cough suppressant) are the standard treatments.

FABULOUS FOLK REMEDY

A Bark for a Bark

The worst part of having bronchitis is not being able to sleep. Often, it seems that the coughing and hacking gets worse the moment you lie down. Wild cherry bark (*Prunus serotina*) has long been known to relax spasmodic coughs and can be used at night to sleep. Steep 1 teaspoon in 1 cup of boiling water for 10 to 15 minutes. Drink 1 to 2 cups in the evening before bed.

Make a Flaxseed Poultice

A flaxseed poultice retains heat for a long time and is ideal for soothing irritating, spastic coughs. Add $^1/_2$ cup of ground flaxseed to $^3/_4$ cup of boiling water. Continue to simmer and stir until it makes a thick paste. Spread the paste on a piece of cheese-cloth, and apply as hot as can be tolerated to the chest. Add 5 to 6 drops of an essential oil such as thyme or eucalyptus for deep penetration. Leave on for 1 to 2 hours.

Bronchitis should always be checked with your doctor, who will test your sputum to determine if the bronchitis is caused by bacteria or a virus. If it's caused by bacteria, he or she will prescribe antibiotics. If it's caused by a virus, however, some of the following strategies may help you feel better until it runs its course.

Is it productive? Coughing keeps you awake and hurts your stomach muscles. Use a cough suppressant only if the cough is not bringing up any phlegm—what doctors call an "unproductive" cough. Otherwise, it's better to loosen and cough up the excess mucus with the help of an expectorant.

Drink up. You need to drink lots of fluids to keep your lungs healthily hydrated and working at their best. So drink at least eight glasses of water a day.

Full steam ahead. Warm steam soothes the lining of the bronchial tubes and loosens secretions. Fill a bowl with very hot water, put a towel over your head, and tent the bowl. (Be careful not to scald your face.) Inhale deeply through your nose. Add a bit of eucalyptus or sage to the water to give the steam added medicinal punch. But don't use an electric vaporizer this way—they generate a concentrated stream of steam that is dangerous when used close to the face.

Avoid mucus-producing food. Milk, cheese, ice cream, and all dairy products increase mucus production or thicken the mucous membranes. This increases your congestion and makes it harder to breathe.

Hit the sushi bar. If you need to loosen up mucus, try fresh horseradish, hot mustard, or wasabi (the Japanese horseradish). All of these help break up congestion. It's impossible to eat these potent herbs without your eyes and nose running, so this is sure to help clear that clogged-up feeling in a hurry!

Blow up balloons. As we age,

FABULOUS FOLK REMEDY

Fennel Rub

Get thee to the health-food store for some essential oil of fennel. It works wonders as a chest rub to clear up congestion. Just dissolve 10 drops of fennel oil, 10 drops of thyme oil, and 10 drops of eucalyptus oil in 4 ounces of sunflower oil, and massage gently onto the chest.

POWERFUL POTION

TRIPLE-THREAT HERBAL TEA

Make a soothing marshmallow tea base by soaking 2 heaping tablespoons of marshmallow root (*Althea officinalis*) in 1 quart of *cold* water overnight. Strain, and heat 1 cup of the tea to a boil. Add $\frac{1}{2}$ teaspoon *each* of licorice root (*Glycyrrhiza glabra*) and thyme (*Thymus vulgaris*). Cover, and steep for 15 minutes. Drink 3 to 4 cups per day. **Caution:** Licorice root should not be used by people with high blood pressure or kidney disease.

our lung capacity decreases, and we are more vulnerable to respiratory ailments, such as bronchitis. A study in England examined 28 volunteers (average age 65) who had chronic bronchitis. They blew up balloons 40 times a day for 8 weeks. The result? A big decrease in their breathlessness, and they no longer got winded when walking to the mailbox. So volunteer for the next kiddie party, or sit around and blow up balloons on your own. What's a little dignity compared to the fun of breathing freely?

Chicken soup for the lungs. Inhaling the steam from a bowl of hot chicken soup will help open your nasal passages and lungs, but researchers are still looking for something else they believe is contained in this traditional remedy. According to Irwin Ziment, M.D., a pulmonary specialist at the University of California at Los Angeles, an amino acid in chicken is very similar to a drug that doctors prescribe for patients with bronchitis.

O·D·D·B·A·L·L OINTMENT

Hot Mustard

One of the oldest and most popular remedies for chest congestion is still a hot mustard plaster, which helps break up stubborn mucus in the lungs by bringing heat to the area, according to naturopath Elizabeth Burch, N.D, of iVillage's health Web site. The powder of black mustard seeds releases a potent oil when mixed with water. Mix 1 part of mustard powder with 10 parts of flour and enough tepid water to make a paste. Spread a thin layer onto a cloth. Coat your skin with some olive oil and a layer of cloth *before* you place the plaster cloth on your chest—mustard side out. Leave it on for 10 minutes or less. Remove it when your skin begins to redden to prevent blisters.

Bug Bites:

Fight Back When You Can't Bite Back!

As I write, mosquitoes are circling my head, looking for a late-night snack; a fly is keeping my cat entertained; and the *thump-thump-thump* coming from the living room tells me the fleas have attacked my dog. Fighting off these and other stinging, sucking, and biting creatures is a pain. Here's how to do it:

Make yourself repellent. Natural bug repellents are effective only if you use them frequently and there are not too many mosquitoes around. Some doctors think that the best kind are products that contain neem, lemongrass, or citronella oils. Test an area of your skin first to make sure they don't irritate you. Then spray or dab them directly onto your skin, following the package directions. Studies show that neem oil (from an Indian tree) provides significant protection from malaria-carrying mosquitoes for up to 12 hours; another study found that lemongrass and citronella oils are highly effective against most species of mosquitos.

Squish some sassafras. Sassafras, or "green twig," as the Algonquin Indians named it, is said to have insecticidal properties. Native Americans make the repellent by crushing fresh sassafras leaves with a charcoal tablet (not a brickette

IT'S AN EMERGENCY!

If you have any sign of body swelling or difficulty breathing after a sting, call your community's emergency response number (911) and have them take you to the nearest hospital emergency room. Stings can cause a life-threatening reaction in those who are allergic to the stinging insect's venom. For the future, especially if you are in an area heavily populated with bees and other stinging insects, ask your doctor for a prescription to carry emergency epinephrine that can counter the sting's effects.

Southern Mites

The fire ant is on the march throughout the South. It gives multiple stings around the original bite and, if you are sensitive, can cause anaphylaxis—a potentially fatal reaction. Want to be on the safe side? If you live in fire ant country, get desensitized with allergy shots right away.

from the barbecue!) or a small piece of charred wood from the fireplace. Then they mix it with 1 or 2 tablespoons of vegetable oil. The mixture is called sassafras squish topical insect repellent. Dab it onto your forehead and nose and around your mouth and ears; then rub it in gently. Reapply frequently.

Dress for success. Cover up your juicy body from dusk

to dawn when mosquitoes are most voracious—or stay indoors. If you're outside, wear dark or neutral-colored long pants and long sleeves—save the short-shorts for daytime. Avoid bright jewelry, too, since stinging insects are attracted to colors.

Don't smell like a rose. Or any other flower. Bees always hover around me because they like my perfume. It could be they think I smell like the pheromones of other bees or flowers. (If only men would hover that way!) So leave off the perfume when you are going to be where the bugs are. The same goes for scented hair sprays and makeup.

Foil the little buggers. Some mosquitoes don't travel far from where they hatch in water, so clean up possible breeding sites near your house. Get rid of standing water in buckets, old tires, or storm gutters, where they love to hatch. Change the water in birdbaths and wading pools often. Clean swimming pools with chlorine. And don't overwater your garden, leaving stagnant puddles around.

Learn bug first aid. Wash any bite thoroughly with soap and water as soon as possible. Apply ice to decrease swelling and the spread of venom, and elevate the bitten area. Watch for any spreading of redness, which could indicate an infection—and the need for a doctor's attention.

O·D·D·B·A·L·L OINTMENT

A Sage Poultice

You can make a great poultice using sage and vinegar. Just run a rolling pin over a handful of freshly picked sage leaves, bruising them along the way. Put the leaves in a pan, cover them with cider vinegar, and simmer on low until they soften. Remove the leaves, carefully wrap them in a washcloth, and place the pack on stings and swellings for instant relief.

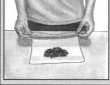

Pull a stinger out—carefully. Stinging insects, such as hornets, bees, wasps, and yellow jackets, don't transmit disease, but they do inject venom, which can cause a severe and life-threatening allergic reaction in some folks (called anaphylaxis). If you have trouble breathing after being stung, or if you've received multiple stings, dial your community's emergency number—usually 911—and breathe deeply and slowly to keep yourself calm until help arrives. If you get stung, don't squeeze your flesh to get the stinger out, or you'll force the venom farther in.

If you aren't experiencing a medical crisis, go ahead and pull or scrape off the stinger with your fingernail or a tweezer held flat

Bombs Away!

If you have pets, you may periodically also have unwanted houseguests—fleas. The bad part is you may not notice them until they have gone forth and multiplied in every carpet, cushion, and pile of laundry. By then, you need to get a professional exterminator to bug-bomb your home while you go away for a few days. Years ago, when I lived in another house, I went to the basement to do the laundry, and by the time I came back upstairs, my legs were really itchy. I looked down at my white slacks, and they were all black below the knee. It took me a few minutes to recover from my shock when I realized that I hadn't gotten dirty, I was covered with fleas!

Native Americans had the right idea by dusting their pets with ground-up sweet fern and pennyroyal. They also kept fleas from animals' bedding by stuffing it with these flea-repelling herbs.

against the skin. Some say that rubbing a bar of soap or an ice cube over the area will draw out the stinger. Even a coin or a credit card edge can come in handy. Then clean the area.

Spit and polish yourself. Southwestern Native Americans commonly chewed tobacco, and then applied the moistened juice to their skin, according to Gary Null, Ph.D. This kept bees away (and likely everybody else, too). Another "chaw" repellent is plantain, favored by the Shoshoni of the Northwestern Plains. They chewed plantain to make a paste that they then applied as a compress.

Keep your shoes on. Bees often hover just above the ground, gathering food from clover and ground flowers, so they can be hard to see. Don't go barefoot across that tempting lawn in bee season—you could step on a bee and get seriously stung.

Get smart. Knowledge is your

FABULOUS FOLK REMEDY

Put a Sock in It!

Oatmeal baths give instant relief to itching skin. Place 1 cup of oats in a sock, and hang it from the faucet while running the bath. While soaking, squeeze the sock, and let the milky water cascade over the bites. Very hot water can sometimes exacerbate the itch, so take your soak in warm water only.

Natural Native Medicine

Hold the Latte

Hazlenut coffee is delicious, as we've discovered since Starbucks and other gourmet coffee makers enlightened us. But baked hazlenuts also contain an oil that has been used by Native Americans for a variety of things, including getting rid of mosquitoes. Look for this natural repellent at your health-food store.

most powerful bug repellent. If you live in an area with harmful insects, learn all about them so you can protect yourself and treat a bite or sting properly. When you're prepared, your close encounters of the buggy kind won't live up to their painful potential.

Get shots before you fly. Be sure to make an appointment to get appropriate immunizations from your doctor before you travel to areas where disease-carrying insects are common. Then, if you do develop flu-like symptoms after a bite, get medical attention promptly.

Don't pick the flowers. At least not without checking them for bees first. Angry bees may not appreciate your cutting into their food supply.

POWERFUL POTION

ITCH RELIEF

To zap that itch, take a strong infusion of equal parts of chickweed, balm of gilead (*Populus gileadensis*), and peppermint (*Mentha piperita*). Place 1 heaping teaspoon of the herbal mixture in 1 cup of boiling water, and steep, covered, for 15 minutes. Add ¼ cup of distilled witch hazel (*Hamamelis virginiana*), chill, and place in a spray bottle. Mist onto your skin for soothing relief of itching bites.

Burnout:

How to Rekindle Your Fire

Ain't language grand? Some words really say what they mean. The term *burnout* is used to describe anything from being tired or worn out to feeling seriously dissatisfied with your life. I get burned out when deadlines mean several weeks of 12- to 14-hour days, and I get so sick of the subject that I need to do something totally different (present company excepted, of course). This is temporary burnout. Long-term burnout, however, is more serious and pervasive. If you feel burned out about your entire life, you need to seek professional help (see **Depression**). And don't be ashamed—it happens to many, many more folks than you know. Here's how to fight it and get back on the right track:

Get totally pampered. My

favorite burnout remedy is going to a day spa for a massage with hot lava rocks, reflexology, a facial, a seaweed wrap—the works! Just lying there and having somebody else do all the work feels great. All that healing touch relaxes my entire body, and the gentle music and aromas from fragrant oils soothe my soul.

Recharge your electrolytes. My friend Carol soaks in Epsom salts combined with kosher salt and a bit of potassium to replace her short-circuited electrolytes. To try her bath recipe, add 2 cups of epsom salts, 2 cups of kosher salt, and 2 tablespoons of potassium to your tub. "I sometimes add vitamin C crystals," she says.

Change the scene. Let your eyes feast on a new landscape. Are you surrounded by tall gray buildings? Take the train or bus or drive into the country for a day. Look at some fields of green. Likewise, if you're bored with a rural landscape, get to a gritty, up-tempo city. And there's nothing like being out on the ocean to give you a new perspective on the stresses in your life.

Feed your soul. My friend Larry goes to an art gallery or museum—or several—when he's burned out. He spends the afternoon looking at art because "it's good for my soul," he says.

POWERFUL POTION

RESTORE THE ROAR

Many herbs are used for their restorative actions. Using two or more of the following herbs, steep 1 heaping tablespoon in 1 quart of boiling water for 15 minutes: Lemon balm (*Melissa officinalis*), rosemary (*Rosemarinus officinalis*), vervain (*Verbena hastata*), lime blossom (*Tilia europea*), passion flower (*Passiflora incarnata*), and chamomile (*Matricaria recutita*). Cool, then sip throughout the day. **Caution:** People with ragweed allergies may be sensitive to chamomile.

Create a sanctuary. We're so busy balancing our work, home lives, and other interests that we rarely have time for ourselves. Create a restful place in your home (even a corner with a simple screen and armchair) as a private retreat. Or go somewhere that is only yours, advises psychologist Linda Welsh, Ed.D. I have a friend who sits in an empty church that she finds beautiful and peaceful. Any denomination will do. Another friend remade a room into a special place for his own interests. Me, I've always wanted a boat to hang out on, like Don Johnson on *Miami Vice*—only without the alligator.

Plug away at what you've put off. Most of us accumulate many projects that we never seem to get around to, like sorting a jumble of photos, researching the family genealogy, redecorating the bedroom, or visiting a place we are curious about. The pressure of projects left undone also adds to a feeling of burnout. One at a time, chip away at your list—and be sure to do things you enjoy as well as your chores. Being involved in

---

O·D·D·B·A·L·L OINTMENT

Lavender Oil

Lavender is lovely, and it's a wonderful restorative for the soul. Aromatherapists say it relaxes and calms. It can banish your blues and put burnout on the back burner. Try using it in an at-home spa. Fill the bathtub with warm water; then add several drops of lavender essential oil—enough so that you can smell its clean, floral fragrance. Light a candle or two, turn off the bathroom light, and slip into the water. Ahhhh!

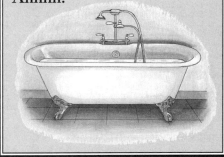

something you like will recharge your batteries. This often works for me.

Shop till you drop. Unless this will add to your worries by causing you financial ruin, go shopping for something that will make you feel special, like a new fishing rod or a silk scarf. If budget is a barrier, keep the treat inexpensive but meaningful to you.

Have a ball. Several women in Louisiana began shooting hoops after 40 years away from sports—and they're having a ball. These women were burned out from a variety of stressful circumstances, but basketball has turned their lives around. When one of the women suddenly decided to join the state-sponsored Senior Games for over-50s, the others joined her and began playing competitive basketball. They started traveling around the country, getting fabulously fit, and soaking up the cheers they missed in high school when women's sports weren't taken seriously. It has sparked a new spirit of fun for these women and added to their self-esteem.

Book a Room!

A night in a classy hotel is a great change of scenery. A woman I know loves this escape because it's the one time when someone else will clean up after her, and she can spread her makeup on the vanity without it being in someone else's space. This is a great pick-me-up, enthuses therapist Linda Welsh, Ed.D. Leave the bed unmade, indulge your inner towel-tosser, and order room service while you're at it. (Just leave a generous tip for the cleaning crew if you really mess up the place.)

FABULOUS FOLK REMEDY

Sweet Dreams

An old favorite remedy is to make an herbal pillow for restful sleep and renewed vigor. This can easily be done by stuffing a clean sock with dried herbs and placing it beneath your regular pillow. As you turn throughout the night, the herbs are crushed, and their fragrance is released. Try a mixture of lavender, hops, and lime blossoms.

Burns:

Hold the Butter

In the past, common wisdom held that if you burned your-self by touching a hot pot, you ought to smear butter over the burn. Fortunately, we're now so health conscious that many of us don't keep butter in the house!

But even if you've got a secret stash, butter's the last thing you want to apply to a burn. What you really want to do is cool down the burned skin by immediately run-ning cold water over it.

A first-degree burn injures only the outside layer of skin, such as when you touch a hot iron or laze a bit too long in the sun. No blisters will appear, but there may be mild swelling and redness. A second-degree burn goes deeper, injuring skin layers beneath the surface. It can be caused by longer

O·D·D·B·A·L·L OINTMENT

Oil Well

St. John's wort oil (*Hypericum perforatum*) can be applied to burns as long as the skin is not broken. This has the double benefit of promot-ing healing and easing pain. Apply two to three times daily.

exposure to the sun or hot liquids and will produce blisters and a red, blotchy appearance. When all the layers of the skin are destroyed, this horror is a third-degree burn. Fire, prolonged exposure to hot substances, and electrical burns are the most common causes—and safety is the best prevention.

If a burn is from a fire or chemical, if it's on your face, or if a child is the victim, get medical help immediately. But for ordinary household burns, here's what to do:

Chill out. For a first- or second-degree burn, immediately put the burned area under cold running water—or pour on any handy cold liquid such as iced tea or soda—says the American Medical Association (AMA). Apply a clean towel or handkerchief dunked in cold water if you cannot get the injured limb or body part under cold running water. By lowering the temperature of the burned skin as quickly as possible, you'll decrease potential damage to tissue.

Cover up. After cooling down the first- or second-degree burn with water, apply a *nonfluffy* sterile or clean bandage,

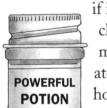

POWERFUL POTION

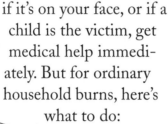

IT'S AN INSIDE JOB

Supporting the body with herbal healing agents on the inside can help speed recovery of the outside. To start your "inside job," mix equal parts of echinacea (*Echinacea purpurea*), cleavers (*Galium aparine*), prickly ash (*Xanthoxylum clava-herculis*), red clover (*Trifolium pratense*), and calendula (*Calendula officinalis*). Add 1 teaspoon to 1 cup of boiling water, and sip.

says the AMA. Cotton or a fluffy towel might leave pieces of lint on the burned area, which will only increase the risk of infection.

Keep current. Accidental burns often happen at home or work. So keep an easy-to-use, first-aid handbook in a place where you can locate it in a hurry. Because medical treatment is constantly changing, make sure your emergency

IT'S AN EMERGENCY!

For severe, or third-degree burns, head straight to the emergency room. A third-degree burn will appear charred and white. Such burns often result from contact with fire, electricity, or strong chemicals. Sometimes they don't hurt, because underlying nerves have been damaged as well as the skin. Even a lesser burn that doesn't heal in 10 days or begins to look infected, with pus or swelling, requires immediate medical attention.

FABULOUS FOLK REMEDY

Tearrific Sunburn Treatment

Good old black tea provides excellent relief from sunburn or superficial burns. Put several teabags in your bath and soak your pain away. Or place brewed tea in a spray bottle, chill, and mist on the skin as you feel the heat.

information is up to date. Toss out the handbook you inherited from the Roosevelt era and get a new one.

Anoint at your own risk. Do not apply butter or grease to a burn, and do not apply oil to an area that still feels hot. In fact, according to the AMA, you shouldn't apply any medication or home remedy without first talking with your doctor. However, many healthcare professionals do recommend applications of topical remedies to burned areas—but for minor burns only. So call your doctor *before* you put any sort of ointment on a burn.

Grow your own "burn center."
Aloe vera is called the "burn plant" because it inhibits the action of a pain-producing peptide, and it helps healing and skin growth. If you buy aloe in the form of a cream or processed gel, make sure it contains at least 70 percent aloe. Or just keep an aloe plant nearby: Simply break off a leaf, split it open, and rub the soothing juice over the burn.

Call for calendula. Calendula is noted for its healing properties—especially for skin. Ground petals combined with sunflower seed or corn oil can be rubbed on minor burns and other skin irritations, according to Native American traditional medicine.

Calendula is also used to make mild washes for healing burns. To make a wash, steep 1 heaping tablespoon of fresh calendula flowers in 1 cup of hot water until the water cools. Strain; then pour over the burn.

O·D·D·B·A·L·L OINTMENT

Soothing Cedar

Native American healers make a burn-soothing salve by mixing dried white-cedar leaves, cocoa butter, beeswax, raw honey, and a few drops of vitamin E. Cooling as it may be, white cedar is especially rich in minerals that calm irritated skin and burns.

To make the salve, chop dried white-cedar leaves, and place them in a clean glass jar. Cover the herbs with olive, almond, or sesame oil. Let the jar sit in a warm oven at 100°F for 12 hours. Then heat 1 pint of oil over very low heat, adding in 2 ounces of grated beeswax, $\frac{1}{2}$ ounce of cocoa butter, and 1 tablespoon of raw honey. Remove from the heat when melted, and combine thoroughly. Add several drops of vitamin E oil. Store in the refrigerator.

Bursitis:

Get Those Joints Jumpin' Again

Housemaid's knee, tennis elbow, and miner's elbow are all popular names for what's better known as bursitis. (My personal favorite is weaver's bottom.) And did you know that a "bunion" is really bursitis? Yup—it's an inflammation of the joint between your big toe and a foot bone.

Your bursae are tiny, fluid-filled sacs found throughout your body where a tendon passes over bone at a joint. When the bursae become inflamed, you've got bursitis. Your body has over 150 bursae, so you can imagine the painful possibilities. The most common areas for bursitis are joints that undergo heavy wear

O·D·D·B·A·L·L OINTMENT

Hot Pepper Cream

Call it chili pepper, call it cayenne, call it capsicum. Just call it—this ointment is really hot stuff! Soothe it over your sore joint, and you'll begin to feel relief. The heat from the peppers brings more blood circulation to your sore bursa, and with it, more healing oxygen. You can buy capsicum cream over-the-counter at your local drugstore or health-food store. The best creams contain 0.025 to 0.075 percent capsicum. Use it up to three times a day. But be careful—keep it away from your eyes!

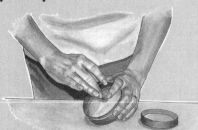

and tear, such as the shoulder, hip, and knee. Repetitive movements like rounds of tennis or days of painting can get bursitis under way, but the condition may also kick in after an accident or some unusual exertion such as moving furniture or other heavy objects. In some cases, it can accompany a systemic infection.

When bursae are damaged, calcium deposits form in them. And soon, if bursitis is in your shoulder, for example, you find you can't lift your arm over your head. But you do need a doctor's diagnosis, because sometimes other conditions, like arthritis, can be mistaken for bursitis. An x-ray will show the truth.

Once you and your doctor are sure bursitis is the problem, here are a few tips to keep you more comfortable as you heal and to prevent additional injury:

Stabilize the sore joint. Make a sling, or use a flexible bandage to keep from moving or jostling your sore joint. Most cases of bursitis will heal themselves in 7 to 10 days, according to doctors at the Mayo Clinic. Anti-inflammatory drugs, like aspirin or ibuprofen, can reduce the inflammation, and aspirin can relieve the pain. If your pain is severe, however, your doctor may use a splint to immobilize the joint completely and advise you to rest. Or your doctor may give you an injection of cortisone, a steroid, for the pain.

Use RICE. The best first aid for acute pain from an injured joint is RICE: rest, ice, compression, and elevation. Put ice on the sore joint for about 20 minutes; then remove the ice, and wrap an elastic bandage around the joint to prevent swelling. Elevate your injured limb above the level of your heart. And repeat every few hours. If you don't feel relief within 2 days, start to alternate hot compresses or a heating pad with the ice. Use 3 minutes of heat, then 1 minute of cold. Keep alternating them for 15 or 20 minutes, once or twice a day.

Minimize time on your knees. My advice is don't get on your knees for anyone. But if you are out there loving your garden or varnishing your boat deck, always wear rubber kneepads.

Widen your shoes. If you treat a bunion before it gets out of hand (or out of foot), you may be able to avoid surgery. Most bunions develop

---

FABULOUS FOLK REMEDY

Weed Out the Pain

Two common garden plants, chickweed (*Stellaria media*) and comfrey (*Symphytum officinalis*), are used traditionally to relieve swelling and pain. Pick a handful of chickweed and one to two large comfrey leaves. Blanch them both, and apply, using chickweed as the first layer and holding it in place with the comfrey leaves.

Take the Indirect Route

When you've got bursitis, you can massage *around* the sore area, but not right on it. Direct pressure may make the bursa hurt even more. But massaging the neighboring area is fine— it'll relax both your muscles and your tension.

POWERFUL POTION

BURSITIS BUSTER

Bromelain, a compound found in pineapple, and turmeric (*Curcuma longa*), are two of nature's anti-inflammatories. They are often found together in commercial preparations and should be taken between meals (approximately 200 milligrams each) for best results. **Caution:** People taking blood-thinning medications and those with sensitivities to pineapple should avoid bromelain.

after a long history of wearing tight or pointy-toed shoes, and they can actually dislocate your big toe. Wear shoes with wider, deeper toes, so your foot is not cramped. And ask your doctor if orthotic inserts in your shoes are a good idea to reduce pressure on your toe joint.

Cushion your tush. Sit on a cushion to avoid aggravating or inflaming your buttock bursa. This condition is named "weaver's bottom" because so many weavers get it from sitting on a hard surface, while swaying back and forth with the loom. Few people weave these days, but plenty of us wiggle around in uncomfortable desk chairs.

Buff up. Resistance training, or exercising with weights, will help build strong muscles. And the stronger your muscles around your joints, the better they can protect you from the kind of injuries that cause bursitis. If you've already been treated for bursitis, have your doctor prescribe an exercise program to prevent further complications.

Take more breaks. When you've got a repetitive task that can lead to bursitis, take frequent breaks. Stretching and moving around, even for just a few minutes out of every hour, can make a real difference.

Calluses:

Ease the Burdens of Your Sole

They're not cute, but they're clever. Calluses are your body's way of protecting delicate layers of skin from the effects of heavy pressure or friction. Usually found on the bottom of your feet and on your fingertips or palms, calluses are simply areas of thick, dead skin.

People who work hard with their hands usually form calluses that protect them from nicks and cuts. And as anyone who has ever tried to play a stringed instrument can tell you, learning's a painful process until you develop good calluses on your fingertips (see **Blisters** for more information).

Calluses, however, sometimes have painful nerves and bursal sacs beneath them that can cause symptoms ranging from shooting pain to aches. You need

---

O·D·D·B·A·L·L OINTMENT

Scrub 'Em with Salt

The next time you take a bath, treat your feet to a moisturizing salt rub. Moisten a handful of Epsom salts with a small amount of almond or olive oil. Then scrub your feet until the salt's dissolved and the oil has softened your skin.

your doctor's immediate attention if that happens, or if the
callus bleeds or looks infected.
Otherwise, here's what may
help:

Flavor your feet. Treat
yourself to one of the many
creams and lotions made especially for feet; they have ingredients such as peppermint and
apple-kiwi. Also, try moisturizers like vitamin E oil, cocoa butter,
or lanolin to make calluses softer and less painful.

Vaporize them. A friend rubs Vicks VapoRub on
her feet, and tells me it keeps them from getting
overly callused. She does this nearly every day before
she puts on her socks.

Soothe with a soak. Periodically soak your feet in
a pan of water with 1 teaspoon of baking soda or soap.
As the callused skin loosens, gently rub it away a bit at
a time with a pumice stone or emery board. Follow up
with lotion or cream to soften your feet. (This remedy is not appropriate for people with diabetes, who

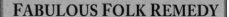

FABULOUS FOLK REMEDY

Lemon Smoother

**Lemons help soften cal-
louses. Rub a half a lemon on
your feet, elbows, and heels for
softer, smoother skin.**

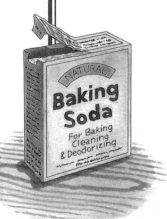

The Horse's What?

An extreme acid trip for your feet would be horse urine,
which can apparently remove calluses. But don't get any ideas
about strolling barefoot through the stable or chasing Trigger
with a bucket. Instead, try an over-the-counter cream called
Carmol 20. Made of urea, an acid derived from horse urine, it
will loosen calluses (yours, not the horse's).

may have poor circulation in their feet and thus may injure their skin.)

Go barefootin' at the beach. Those gray, gritty pumice stones we use to sand down calluses are made of volcanic rock. And while few of us have access to volcano slopes, sand on the beach acts like a pumice stone—only better! If you live near a beach, walk in the sand as often as you can. Your feet will feel fabulous.

Shop for savvy shoes. Take a good look at the shoes in your closet, especially their insides. If you find worn innersoles or seams and stitching over painful areas of your feet, out they go! Spike heels are only for glam occasions (if the torture's ever worth it). Low heels and cushioned soles that fit perfectly are best for healthy, happy feet.

Redistribute the load. Use orthotic inserts in your shoes to transfer pressure away from the callused area and absorb shock. These may help if you have calluses because of an abnormal gait, flat feet, high arches, or very bony feet. While orthotics are available in most drugstores, ask your podiatrist's advice for inserts that can be specially made for you.

POWERFUL POTION

ARNICA OIL

Native American healing traditions say you should rub your feet every morning and evening to ease the burdens they carry. Try using 4 or 5 drops of arnica oil, a homeopathic remedy that's available in many health-food stores. Simply shake the oil into the palm of your hand, and rub your feet gently for a few minutes, from the toes up to the ankle. In fact, I was so entranced with this idea that I've been doing it every day. The daily massage has softened the calluses on the heels and balls of my feet—they no longer build up to the point where my feet feel as though they were paved with tarpaper.

Cardiovascular Conditioning:

Your Pumper in Its Prime

I f there's one thing we all rely on, it's the old *lub-dub.* That's the sound of the most faithful thing in our lives. More faithful than Fido, firefighters, forsythia in spring, and fireworks in July. The heart's job one is to keep on going for us . . . and because it does, we're still here.

Think about it—your heart is a big muscle that never takes a break. It's not like arms or legs that can relax for a while. Or back muscles that get to rest every time you do. Your heart works 24/7.

So how do our hearts rebel? They do their best for as long as they can, but ultimately, if we don't take care of them, they just stop pumping. Deaths

---

FABULOUS FOLK REMEDY

Berry, Berry Good

Colorful fruits and vegetables, especially dark berries, are a rich source of bioflavonoids, which strengthen your cardiovascular system. Eat ½ to 1 cup of blueberries a day to keep your heart strong.

from heart attack have decreased since the fitness craze began and surgeons learned how to expand clogged arteries and do bypass operations. And that's great. But heart attacks and other forms of coronary heart disease (CHD) still account for 25 percent of deaths in America, making CHD our number one killer.

The good news is, you can do something about it. The Framingham Heart Study followed 5,000 men and women for 40 years, and found that the biggest risks for heart disease are factors we can control—smoking, lack of exercise, and poor nutrition. If there's heart disease in your family, you'll need to work harder to reduce your risk. But genes are just one chapter in your heart's story. If you turn around a dangerous lifestyle, you've got a much better chance of defeating heart disease.

Here's what experts suggest:

Just do it. A 5-year walking study at Harvard Medical School tracked women 45 and older who had led sedentary lives. Even those who burned only 200 to 600 calories a week cut their risk of heart attack by 30 percent if they walked every day. And if

IT'S AN EMERGENCY!

Any pain, tingling, or numbness in your jaw, chest, or left arm could indicate a heart attack. A heart attack is often confused with indigestion—and sweating, nausea, and/or shortness of breath can also be symptoms. If you have any of these symptoms, call your community's emergency response number (usually 911) immediately. Heart disease often manifests itself differently in women and men, according to Lila Wallis, M.D., a women's health expert. Angina or chest pain is often the first warning for women, whereas a heart attack itself is commonly the first sign of trouble for men. Women also have more silent heart attacks.

they stepped up the program by walking longer distances each day, they cut their risk in half. It didn't matter how slow or fast they walked, as long as they did it. You can do it, too. But check with your doctor first to see how much your heart can handle.

Pump iron. According to the American Heart Association, weight training (also called resistance training, because you're resisting the force of gravity as you work) has the potential to ward off heart trouble as well as tone your muscles and bones. It doesn't matter how old you are when you start. And even if you have a mild heart condition, more and more studies indicate that weight lifting strengthens your heart. Why? Stronger muscles mean that lifting a box of books won't put as much stress on your heart. And muscle burns more calories than body fat, so a bit of brawn keeps fighting the flab, a definite risk factor for heart disease. Some studies have also shown that resistance training can lower blood pressure and cholesterol, both risk factors for heart disease. Common sense says you should check with your doctor, however, before beginning a weight-lifting program.

POWERFUL POTION

HAWTHORN HELPER

Hawthorn is a famous heart tonic, high in bioflavonoids. Although it's European in origin, hawthorn is now common in the United States. Known to lower blood pressure, it also enhances circulation, providing the heart with extra blood, oxygen, glucose, and nutrients, improving heart function and exercise tolerance. To use, add 60 drops of hawthorn tincture to a glass of water or juice. Both capsules and tinctures are available in health-food stores.

Pump and run. The American College of Sports Medicine and the Centers for Disease Control and Prevention recommend that we get 30 minutes or more of moderate-intensity exercise on most days. It doesn't have to be all at once—10 minutes here, 20 minutes there is fine. Resistance training should account for two to three of those sessions. If you lift weights, take a day off between sessions to give your muscles time to recover and repair. Do your aerobic exercise, such as walking, jogging, or swimming, on those days.

De-stress yourself. Chronic stress increases the levels of cortisol, a hormone secreted by your adrenal gland. Along with depression and anxiety, this can have a harmful affect on your heart. Stress hormones may spike your cholesterol level, increase blood pressure, and promote heart disease. So fight stress with a heart-healthy diet, regular exercise, deep breathing when something upsets you, and relaxation techniques. For help, see **Stress**.

Take an aspirin a day. Aspirin has an anti-clotting effect that keeps your blood platelets from

Are You Full of Beans?

A study of 12,000 Americans ages 25 to 75 presented at an American Heart Association Conference showed that people who ate a variety of legumes several times a week had a 19 percent lower risk of heart disease than those who ate legumes less than once a week. Beans, peas, and peanuts all qualify as heart-healthy legumes. Researchers believe that both the protein and the fiber in legumes may be helping hearts stay healthy.

clumping together. This lowers your risk of developing a blood clot that can trigger a heart attack. Many people take half an aspirin or one baby aspirin a day to prevent heart attack. And aspirin is often given to heart-attack victims before emergency help arrives. But there are some side effects—aspirin can irritate the stomach and cause bleeding in some people, and it can even increase your risk of stroke. So talk to your doctor before you start.

Buy some Bs. You need adequate amounts of B vitamins to clear excess homocysteine, an amino acid, from your blood. Without enough Bs, the buildup of homocysteine can damage the lining of your arteries, encouraging blood clots and plaque (cholesterol) deposits to form. So take in plenty of Bs by eating beans; whole grains; and many fruits and veggies, especially orange juice and leafy greens.

Go nuts. While studies have shown that eating walnuts and almonds can lower cholesterol, a more recent report in the *Journal of the American Dietetic Association* revealed that pecans can, too. The theory is that the monounsaturated fat in nuts can protect against heart disease. But their mineral content—magnesium and copper—may be protecting the heart, as well. Just don't bake the pecans into a buttery pie, adding a million calories! About ¼ cup of nuts per day is the recommended amount.

Pick a Pomegranate

If you live in a desert area with access to pomegranate trees, pick one, squeeze, and sip the juice. An Israeli study suggests that the juice of the pomegranate prevents oxidation of the type of cholesterol that contributes to plaque formation—those artery-clogging deposits. These fruits appear now and then in supermarkets, but you can find bottled pomegranate juice in health-food stores.

Grab some garlic. Raw garlic inhibits the blood clots that can cause a heart attack. It also lowers cholesterol, reduces blood pressure, and may even make your blood vessels more flexible. Allicin, the chemical that gives garlic its potent odor, is believed to be the cause. Since garlic does have a blood-thinning effect, don't eat it on a regular basis without your doctor's okay. And be aware that garlic pills may not do the same job as garlic cloves. More research is needed before we'll know if they're just as good and (somewhat) less odiferous.

Remember the reds. Lycopene is a compound known to protect the heart, and the richest sources of it are red fruits: tomatoes, guavas, and red or pink grapefruits. Even watermelon has some lycopene. Lycopene is a carotenoid that's believed to have powerful anti-oxidant properties. A red that isn't so good for you? Red meat—which is high in saturated fats and thus a risk to your arteries.

Drink red, too. Light to moderate consumption of wine reduces your risk of developing heart disease or of dying from it. Red wine wins out over white because it contains a number of

POWERFUL POTION

A TERRIFIC TICKER TONIC

Herbs rich in compounds called bioflavonoids help boost the strength of your heart. Experiment with the following heart tonic herbs, using them alone or in combination. Especially useful are hawthorn (*Crataegus* spp.), ginkgo (*Ginkgo biloba*), and lime blossom (*Tilia europea*). Use 1 heaping teaspoon of herbs per 1 cup of hot water. Steep for 10 minutes and drink 2 cups per day. **Caution: Do not take ginkgo if you are on any blood-thinning medications without checking with your healthcare provider first.**

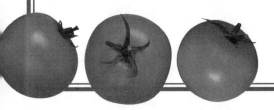

Raise Your Glass!

According to the National Institute on Alcohol Abuse, data from about 20 countries demonstrate 20 to 40 percent less coronary heart disease among drinkers than nondrinkers. Evidence suggests that people who prefer wine over other alcoholic beverages often have a healthier lifestyle: They tend to smoke less, drink less in general, and eat more nutritiously than those who prefer beer or liquor. The U.S. Department of Health and Human Services and the Department of Agriculture agree that moderate drinking is associated with lower risk of coronary heart disease in some people. The *American Journal of Cardiology* reports that the ethanol in alcoholic beverages is what lowers risk. Keep in mind that if alcoholism runs in your family, no health professional thinks you should drink.

But don't raise it too often. Sorry, six-packers, *moderate* means no more than two drinks a day for men and one for women. That's it. Alcohol is a definite risk factor for breast cancer, and it can contribute to obesity, hypertension, and abnormal heart rhythms. Drinking also increases the risks of liver disease, various cancers, accidents, homicide, and suicide. So if you have any concerns about drinking, don't use your heart as a reason to increase your intake or even to start. There are plenty of other ways to get healthier.

Get the measurements right. Pouring with abandon means you're abandoning drinking's healthy side. To stay on the safe side of alcohol, memorize this guideline from the National Council on Alcoholism and Drug Dependence. The amount of alcohol in these one-drink servings is the same: one 12-ounce bottle of beer, one 5-ounce glass of wine, and 1.5 ounces of 80-proof liquor. Remember it, and enjoy.

plant chemicals with antioxidant and anticlotting properties. The theory is that the pigment in red grape skins contains quercetin, a potent bioflavonoid. Want an alcohol-free alternative? Drink red or purple grape juice. It contains many of the same plant chemicals found in wine.

Find a cold fish. Coldwater fish are highest in omega-3 fatty acids, which researchers say play a role in preventing heart disease. Ironically, the fattiest fish with the most omega-3s—salmon, mackerel, sardines, and herring—are best for you. But all fish have some. According to the *American Journal of Cardiology,* the heart benefits of fish are so impressive that doctors should consider recommending fish-oil capsules. Aim for three or four servings of fatty fish weekly or 1 gram of fish oil a day. The Japanese, who have the lowest rate of heart disease in the world, eat fish nearly every day, along with their rice and vegetables. (And they cook with polyunsaturated fats like peanut oil.)

Go Med. The risk of heart attack among people of the Mediterranean region is half that of Americans, and they actually eat a bit more fat than we do. But it's usually unsaturated fat such as olive oil, says the American Heart Association. Your diet should contain whole-grain breads, cereals, pasta, lots of vegetables—and olive oil. This Mediterranean diet also includes nuts, seeds, and oily fish like sardines.

Avoid trans-fats. These artery-cloggers are oils—often labeled "hydrogenated" or "partially hydrogenated" on packages—that have been processed for a long shelf life. They are found in most margarines and in many fast foods and packaged snack foods. They are killers, plain and simple.

Cataracts:

Keeping the Clouds from Your Eyes

Wise old eyes. They're wonderful to look into. Yet sometimes they seem a little . . . filmy. That "film" is probably a cataract—a clouding of the eye's lens, which reduces or blurs entering light.

The biggest causes of cataracts are genes and radiation. If both your parents had cataracts, it's more likely that you will begin to develop them by middle age. Or if your work or your hobbies have meant many years in the sun (and you've not been in the habit of sporting UV-protective sunglasses)—those are risk factors, too.

Shade Those Peepers!

Sun exposure *triples* your risk of cataracts—and it's so easy to avoid! Simply wear a brimmed hat and good sunglasses every time you're out in the sun. And keep in mind that reflected light—from water, snow, or pavement—is often even more damaging than direct sunlight.

Apart from too much sun, other conditions that increase your risk include eye injury, prolonged use of certain medications, and poorly controlled diabetes. Fortunately, cataracts are painless. They progress slowly over time and are usually detected during a routine eye examination.

In the early stages, you can pretty much carry on with cataracts, as they have only a minor effect on your vision. You may find you're becoming more sensitive to light and glare and that your sight is gradually blurring. You may also discover that you need a new eyeglasses prescription more often than usual. (But do take it seriously if you are seeing double, you see halos around street lights, or your vision is actually dimming. This could be a more serious problem, such as a detaching retina, and it needs emergency treatment.)

The great news is that cataracts are almost completely curable. Modern laser surgery to remove the cloudy lens and replace it with a clear implant is now safe and effective. A skilled ocular surgeon makes an incision in the cornea and removes the opaque lens from its capsule. Then an artificial lens is inserted and fixed in place with tiny plastic loops, says Alex Eaton, M.D., an ophthalmologist who directs the retina department of

POWERFUL POTION

BILBERRY

Bilberry, a close relative of the blueberry, may help prevent cataracts or at least slow their growth. This shrubby plant is high in bioflavanoids, nutrients that enhance the action of vitamin C. Because the lens of the eye naturally contains so much vitamin C, some scientists believe a deficiency can lead to cataracts. You can find bilberry in tincture form: The usual dose is 1 to 2 milliliters two times a day. But use bilberry or supplemental vitamin C only with your doctor's consent.

the Eye Centers of Florida. But long before surgery, you can do a lot to prevent most cataracts from forming in the first place. Here are some helpful suggestions:

Eat plenty of antioxidants. Your eyes consume a lot of oxygen, because so much light comes through them. But the more oxygen we take in, the more oxidation is created. Think of a car burning gasoline. The more it burns, the more sludge gets in the engine. Oxidation creates free radicals in our bodies that muck up the works and need to be removed. Antioxidants come to the rescue by breaking down those chemicals of oxidation. Garlic is one of the best antioxidants, but eat a diet rich in fresh vegetables and fruits, and you'll also get what you need, says Dr. Eaton.

Smoke gets in your eyes. Just do it—quit smoking! Cigarette smoking increases the risk of developing age-related cataracts, and a *Journal of the American Medical Association* article suggests that quitting does reduce the risk of developing cataracts. Men who had quit smoking had a 23 percent reduced risk of cataracts and a 28 percent reduced risk for cataract extraction than men who currently smoked. If so far it's been a losing battle, ask your doctor for help. There are many new and effective ways to help you quit, and the sooner you do it, the better off you'll be.

FABULOUS FOLK REMEDY

Brighten Up, Baby!

As its name suggests, eyebright (*Euphrasia officinalis*) has a long history of traditional use in eye conditions. While it may not cure cataracts, a cool compress of eyebright tea can soothe the eyes. Drop 1 teaspoon of the herb into boiled water; then refrigerate. When cool, soak a clean cloth in the tea, wring it out, and place it over your eyes. Leave the compress in place for 15 to 20 minutes, once or twice a day.

Chronic Fatigue Syndrome:

Not Just for Workaholics

Remember the "yuppie flu"? This label landed on chronic fatigue syndrome (CFS) because the condition seemed to afflict so many people struggling to balance high-powered careers and parenthood. Unfortunately, many people with this syndrome's baffling symptoms are given short shrift by doctors unfamiliar with the disease. A 1990s study from the Centers for Disease Control and Prevention showed that CFS may be more widespread than pre-

---

FABULOUS FOLK REMEDY

Feel Your Oats

Oats (*Avena sativa*), specifically the oat "straw," are rich in minerals and can help restore a compromised nervous system. Make a cold infusion by soaking 2 tablespoons of oat straw in 1 quart of cold water overnight. Strain, and drink throughout the day.

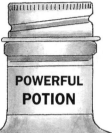

POWERFUL
POTION

GIN-ZING TEA

To add a boost to your step, bring about 5 cups of water to a simmer; then add 1 teaspoon of ground ginseng root. Cover the mixture, remove from heat, and let it steep for about 30 minutes. Then add 1 teaspoon of dried borage leaves and 1 teaspoon of dried mint leaves, and steep for another 15 to 20 minutes. Finally, add 10 to 20 drops of ginkgo biloba tincture. Strain out the herbs, and sip up to 3 cups a day. Sweeten to taste. **Caution:** Because ginseng can raise your blood pressure, do not use it if you are taking high blood pressure medication without checking with your healthcare provider first.

viously thought—even more than double previous estimates, according to a Harvard Medical College study.

CFS usually begins with cold or flu-like symptoms, but it can strike all at once. The chronic, disabling fatigue lasts at least 6 months and sometimes years. Frequent symptoms include intermittent low-grade fever, muscle and joint pain, memory loss, and insomnia. But it doesn't doom you to inactivity. Consider Michelle Akers, 34, a former member of the U.S. Women's Soccer Team. She's had CFS for years, but still manages to play championship soccer.

Doctors now know that CFS is an infection, but they don't yet know which organ it targets. CFS can be mistaken for hypoglycemia, an allergy syndrome, or chronic mononucleosis.

Other possible causes can be quite serious. Your doctor will want to rule out thyroid or adrenal diseases, lingering infections, mononucleosis, a thyroid condition, arthritis, lupus, cancer, and depression. According to diagnostic criteria from the Centers for Disease Control and Prevention, to confirm the syndrome, the chronic fatigue and at least eight other nonspecific symptoms must persist for at least 6 months.

If you're diagnosed with CFS, you'll need to take the best possible care of your health. Be vigilant about regular exercise and reducing stress—and get your body back in shape. Follow a healthy diet: You need ample starches, fruits, and vegetables for energy and lean meat and other protein foods to build and maintain muscle tissue. Here's what experts suggest:

Know your nutrition. Ralph Ofcarcik, Ph.D., nutritionist and guest education manager at the Red Mountain Health Resort in Ivins, Utah, says he regularly meets folks with CFS who come to the resort to focus on their health. "Good nutrition may be the single most important strategy for whipping CFS," says Dr. Ofcarcik. "Since the immune system is functioning at less than an optimum level, it makes good sense to focus on 'nutrient-dense,' or unprocessed, foods—typically roots, tubers, grains, beans, fish, and poultry."

Eat your veggies. Dr. Ofcarcik believes you will benefit by eating mostly natural plant foods supplemented with a reputable multivitamin and multimineral—preferably one that contains extra magnesium. "As simple as this strategy appears," says Dr. Ofcarcik, "I personally have seen dozens of CFS sufferers

Stop and Smell the Primroses

According to one study, 85 percent of a group of people with CFS reported some improvement after 15 weeks of taking a combination of evening primrose oil and fish oil supplements. Start with 1,500 milligrams, two times a day. Check with your doctor before trying other herbal remedies—some cause side effects that may increase the effects of CFS.

who unshackled their balls and chains by simply eating more vegetables."

Sleep well. Everyone needs a good's night rest, but with CFS, it's got to be a real priority. Establish a regular sleep routine, and sleep for 7 to 9 hours a night. Ask your doctor for help if you're having serious problems sleeping.

Simplify your life. This may be the time to delegate housekeeping or line up more babysitters. If you have a spouse and children, work out a plan to share the chores. If you can afford to hire help, spend money on that, and cut back on things that matter less.

Don't lug your luggage. Invest in a wheeled suitcase or duffel bag, and buy a lightweight folding cart you can toss in the backseat and use for groceries or even as a briefcase. Have groceries and other supplies delivered whenever possible, so you can conserve your strength.

Control the phone. Screen your calls with an answering machine, and answer only when you feel up to it. Constant interruptions add stress and make you feel defeated. Establish a habit of returning phone calls when you are not busy or feeling exhausted.

POWERFUL POTION

FATIGUE FIGHTER

Combining tonic, relaxant, and restorative herbs may help ease fatigue and improve immune function over time. Use equal parts of lavender (*Lavendula officinalis*), lemon balm (*Melissa officinalis*), licorice root (*Glycyrrhiza glabra*), skullcap (*Scutellaria lateriflora*), wood betony (*Betonica officinalis*), and vervain (*Verbena hastata*). Steep 1 heaping teaspoon in 1 cup of hot water for 20 minutes. Strain, and drink 2 cups a day. **Caution:** Licorice root should not be used by people with high blood pressure or kidney disease.

Colds:

Commonsense Cures for the Common Scourge

When my friend Carol gets a cold, she likes to rent some videos, buy a bottle of champagne, and retire to her couch for the duration. Her significant other prefers an old Russian remedy of raw garlic sandwiches on black bread. "I can always tell when he's feeling under the weather," Carol says "All I have to do is sniff."

The common cold is actually 1 of about 200 mild virus infections of the upper respiratory tract. Whichever virus we catch, it creates pesky symptoms, including runny or stuffed nose, sore throat, laryngitis, teary eyes, sneezing, wheezing, and heavy breathing (not that kind!). A cold also blunts our senses of smell and taste, and it can bring on a mild headache and a general

Hail Mary!

To cure a cold, make a Bloody Mary, with or without the booze. To the tomato juice, add some lemon, a celery stalk, and horseradish—and drink it quick. Tomato juice is full of vitamin C, but it's the horseradish that really does the trick. Its powerful fumes will loosen mucus congestion, making your cold more bearable.

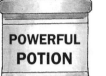

POWERFUL POTION

HERBAL THROAT SPRAY

Here's a blast of natural relief for a sore throat: First, buy yourself a new plant mister. Then brew up a triple-strength tea with 3 teaspoons *each* of dried slippery elm, echinacea, and licorice in 3 cups of water. Bring it to a full boil; then reduce the heat, and let it simmer 10 to 15 minutes. Strain out the herbs, and pour the brew into your new spray bottle. Open your mouth, stick out your tongue, and spray the back of your throat as needed during the day. Ahhhh, relief! **Caution:** Licorice shouldn't be used by folks with high blood pressure or kidney disease.

feeling of lassitude. Until it runs it's course, here's what you can do to make yourself more comfortable and the cold feel unwelcome:

Get steamed. Steam will kill cold germs on contact if water temperatures are 110°F or more. Herbs, such as eucalyptus, add a penetrating scent and disinfect. Put fresh leaves in a bowl, pour boiling water over them, and make a towel tent over your head and the bowl. Lower your face over the bowl (carefully—you can scald yourself if the steam is too hot), and breathe in. You can also add a few drops of oregano oil to the water. It's nice—a bit like diluted Vicks—but pricey.

Don't dry out. The Brits found that when you're in artificially controlled environments with really dry air, such as like offices and airplanes, your nasal membranes dry out and the passages may form tiny cracks that invite viruses. The best defense? Drink plenty of liquids, and use nasal saline spray often to hydrate these tender membranes.

Snooze with booze. Try a hot toddy as a cold rescue. Before hundreds of cold remedies became available at the local drugstore, certain home remedies were probably a lot more fun to take. And if you took enough, you absolutely got rid of

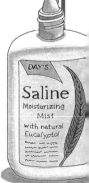

DAY'S

Saline
Moisturizing
Mist
with natural
Eucalyptol

your cold, because pretty soon you couldn't feel it anymore. There are many variations on the hot toddy, which apparently originated in Scotland. Start with juice, honey, or tea, and add the liquor of your choice. A Jewish musician says his grandmother's remedy for a cold was warm milk and honey with a little booze.

Suck up some C. I love to drink gallons of orange and other citrus juices when I have a cold (which is hardly ever anymore). Perhaps it's the vitamin C in the citrus that feels so cleansing. Or maybe just the idea of C—even if it's a placebo effect—works for me. While no one has yet proven that vitamin C can cure a cold, some say it acts like interferon, a natural body chemical that stops virus growth. It's most effective if you take it at the first sign of a sniffle. Most health professionals agree that vitamin C does have a slight antihistamine affect, so drinking more citrus juice or taking a supplement may help reduce nasal symptoms.

Take echinacea. Echinacea, or purple coneflower, has a strong reputation as an herbal cold fighter; it's available at most drugstores. Take it according to package directions at the very

---

O·D·D·B·A·L·L OINTMENT

Rub on the Oil

Using poultices when you have a cold is a good way to make yourself rest. Make your own chest rub by adding 3 to 4 drops of an essential oil (try eucalyptus, lavender, or thyme) to 1 tablespoon of olive oil. Apply liberally to your chest, cover with a clean cloth, and settle into a comfy chair with a cozy afghan and a nice good book.

first sign of a cold. This immune stimulant battles cold germs after they enter your body. In fact, studies show that it will decrease the length of your cold and cut the severity of your symptoms in half. **One caveat:** Echinacea should be avoided by people with autoimmune conditions, such as lupus or rheumatoid arthritis.

Try chicken soup for the nose. Why did the chicken cross the road? To get into the soup pot? Nobody knows exactly what chicken soup does—but it helps colds. Most doctors believe that the steam from the hot soup promotes drainage and thus makes you feel better. Some believe that neutrophils, the immune cells activated by the cold virus, are slowed down by something in chicken soup. Many people know this remedy as Jewish penicillin—it has been in use since the twelfth century.

Add some spice to your life. Spicy foods, like hot peppers and chili con carne, contain capsaicin, a substance that can help reduce nasal and sinus congestion. Try garlic, turmeric, and other pungent spices for a similar effect. Some cold sufferers add these strong spices to chicken soup to promote drainage. Cold or no cold, any hot soup or hot spice will help get your eyes and nose running.

Peel Me an Onion

Whenever you peel an onion, you cry a river. That's because the chemicals released by an onion are attracted to water. The trick for weepless peeling is to turn on the tap, and hold the onion close to the water as you peel. On the other hand, if you want to let onion fumes help fight your cold, peel a big onion, and hover over it. The fumes will have their way with your mucous membranes and help clear your congestion.

Root it out with ginger-root. The oil in ginger is similar to the capsaicin in peppers. It is slightly irritating and thins out mucus. You can clear your head with ginger in several ways. Cut the root into pieces, brew a tea, and then inhale the vapors as you sip; grate it up, and toss it into a salad dressing; or chop it into a super supper stir-fry.

Take tea and see. A hot cup of regular tea with honey usually feels great when you have a cold. You can also try other types, like red pepper tea, which are meant to loosen up the mucus. Lemon and honey, added to weak tea or even plain hot water, also ease head pain and help break up congestion.

Sink it with zinc. After the Cleveland Clinic evaluated zinc as a cold remedy, sales of zinc lozenges soared. The study found that people who began taking the lozenges within 24 hours of when their symptoms began were free of cold symptoms after about 4½ days. But the poor placebo group stayed sick for 7½ days. According to doctors at the Mayo Clinic, there is evidence that zinc may prevent colds; but scientists aren't sure why.

FABULOUS FOLK REMEDY

The Vigor of Vinegar

Appalachian healers make the following remedy from common, household ingredients: Mix a dash of cayenne pepper and a pinch of salt into 1 ounce of apple cider vinegar, and drink it three or four times a day. Another remedy some folks use for colds is 1 tablespoon *each* of honey and lemon juice. Sip it three times a day.

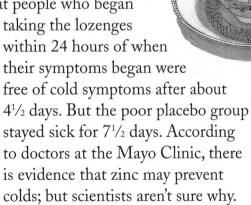

Respect your Elders!

An Israeli study found that elderberry extract attacks cold and flu viruses. You can find a variety of elderberry products in your local health-food store.

They suspect it may keep the cold virus from reproducing, or it may increase the body's own immune response. As with any immune stimulant, overuse can cause problems, so take only as directed. Good food sources of zinc include wheat germ, dried peas and beans, oysters and other seafood, meat, poultry, tofu, and dairy products.

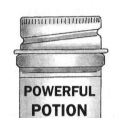

POWERFUL POTION

IMMUNE SYSTEM STIMULANT

Immune-stimulating and astringent herbs can help ease the discomforts of a cold. Combine equal parts of yarrow (*Achillea millefolium*), lemon balm (*Melissa officinalis*), licorice root (*Glycyrrhiza glabra*), gingerroot (*Zingiber officinale*), eyebright (*Euphrasia officinalis*), and rose hips (*Rosa canina*). Use 1 heaping teaspoon of the herb mix per 1 cup of boiling water. Drink 2 to 3 cups per day. **Caution:** Licorice root should not be used by folks with high blood pressure or kidney disease.

Keep your nose (and hands) clean. Hardy cold viruses can live for hours on doorknobs, faucet handles, books, money—all the things we touch every day. Frequent hand washing is the single best way to avoid catching a cold or spreading your own. Unfortunately, the habit is in decline. The American Society of Microbiology (ASM) and the Centers for Disease Control and Prevention (CDC) watched 8,000 people in restrooms in several cities. Only 67 percent stopped at the sink. In a related survey, only 40 percent of women reported washing hands after sneezing or coughing, and men were even worse—just 22 percent. (They were also asked if they washed their hands after changing a diaper or petting an animal—and believe me, you don't want to know.)

Dispose of the germs. Bacteria and viruses live on cloth towels and sponges for hours, so try to use paper towels, tissues, napkins and other disposable items when someone in the house has a cold.

Disinfect dirty surfaces. Frequently wash places that are constantly touched in the home, such as stair railings, telephones, countertops, and doorknobs. And children's toys are common culprits, too. Wash them in warm, soapy water to kill the bacteria and viruses they collect.

Laugh it off. It is now widely known among doctors that positive emotions strengthen the immune system by increasing gamma-interferon, an immune-system hormone that activates other infection-fighting compounds. So next time you have a cold, make your video rental a snicker fest, and laugh off the symptoms.

Lay off the dairy. When you've got a cold, stick to juices, water, and hot beverages. Avoid milk and milk products, because moo juice promotes mucus formation. If you do dairy during a cold, not only will you get a milk moustache but you'll also get more congested.

FABULOUS FOLK REMEDY

Keep Vampires Away!

Garlic (*Allium sativum*) has long been used for its potent healing effects, and it doubles as a cold preventative because it keeps other people at a distance! Surprisingly, garlic tea doesn't taste as bad as it sounds. Chop 2 medium cloves, and simmer in 1 cup of water for 10 to 15 minutes. Add 2 to 3 slices of fresh gingerroot to improve the taste and increase the warming action of the garlic. Honey and lemon are optional. Drink 2 to 4 cups per day. **Caution:** People taking blood thinning medications should steer clear of garlic unless given the green light by their physicians.

Constipation:

Relieving the Inner Gridlock

A hundred years ago, people blamed constipation for everything from crime to bad skin to baldness and—if you can believe it!—suicide. The theory? Backed-up "rot" was seeping into their blood, poisoning body and mind. Some startling remedies appeared, too, including abdominal vibrating machines and gut massage. This obsession with digestion was directly responsible for the birth of the Kellogg's company in the 1920s—their fiber-rich cereal was aimed at eliminating elimination problems. And get this, even as late as 1986, the National Institutes of Health had to issue pamphlets

---

FABULOUS FOLK REMEDY

Lemon Aid

Lemon juice is a powerful cleanser and helps jump-start the digestive system. Just thinking about it makes my mouth water—and the mouth is where good digestion begins! Simply add a squeeze of lemon juice to $\frac{1}{2}$ cup of warm water, and sip before every meal.

explaining that we do not absorb poisons from blocked fecal matter.

Our food is digested and passed through more than 20 feet of intestines to the colon, where the remaining water is absorbed through the intestinal wall; the solids stay behind. Constipation means that the feces are too hard to pass through your digestive system, causing traffic jams. Normally, it takes 24 to 48 hours for our food to become waste. Elimination can take a day or a week, depending on your age, diet, activity level, medications, emotions, and personality. (Ever heard someone described as "anal retentive"?)

The most common causes of this intestinal gridlock are bad diet, lack of exercise, emotional tension, chronic use of laxatives, and certain medications. Pregnancy, advancing age, and sometimes diabetes or an underactive thyroid can also contribute to the problem. When constipation alternates with diarrhea, it could be irritable bowel syndrome (see **Irritable Bowel Syndrome**). If constipation bothers you, check with your doctor;

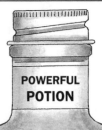

POWERFUL POTION

DANDELION JUICE

To make a dandy drink that'll relieve constipation, purée some dandelion leaves in a blender with water, and pour the juice into a glass. Drink up to three glasses of this tonic. Just be sure your leaves come from a lawn that has not been blasted with chemicals. **Caution:** Dandelion is rich in potassium and should not be taken with potassium tablets. Check with your healthcare provider.

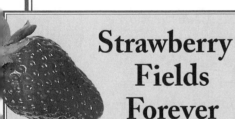

Strawberry Fields Forever

Here's an old Native American remedy that's a pleasure to try. Many believe that eating fresh strawberries will clear up constipation. It makes sense, too, since fruit is a soluble fiber, which does ease the passage of waste through the colon.

then see if these tips might help:

Jog it loose. Get into the habit of regular exercise. It's good for lots of things that ail you, including constipation.

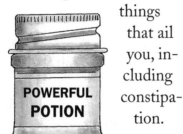

POWERFUL POTION

ROOT IT OUT

Make an anticonstipation decoction by simmering 1 teaspoon *each* of burdock root (*Arctium lappa*) and dandelion root (*Taraxacum officinale*) in 2 cups of boiling water for 20 minutes. Remove from the heat and add 1 teaspoon of peppermint (*Mentha piperita*). Cover and steep for another 10 minutes. Strain and sip ½ cup first thing in the morning and before each meal. If constipation is due to stress, add 1 heaping teaspoon of catnip or lemon balm to the mixture. **Caution:** Dandelion is rich in potassium and should not be taken with potassium tablets. Check with your healthcare provider.

IT'S AN EMERGENCY!

If feelings of discomfort or bloating persist after a bowel movement, or if constipation persists after you've tried to treat it, call your doctor. Persistent abdominal pain or fever, a change in the color or consistency of stool, or blood in the stool could be signs of obstruction or disease.

Exercise helps food travel through your intestines more quickly and reduces stress and anxiety, which cause you to tighten up in more ways than one.

Sip. A lot of constipation is caused simply because we don't drink enough water. Make sure you drink 8 to 10 glasses a day.

Ditch commercial laxatives. Regular consumption of laxatives is self-defeating, yet Americans spend $847 million a year on these products. Some laxatives work by irritating the bowel. Over time, they cause your bowel to wait for artificial stimulation to do its business, rather than respond to natural body signals. Some over-the-counter and

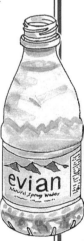

herbal remedies contain the same irritant—senna. Compounds containing mineral oils are a poor choice, too, as they interfere with the absorption of fat. Citrate of milk of magnesia and milk of magnesia draw large volumes of fluid into the intestines—and this effect is too drastic.

Have a triple cocktail. Prunes, bran, and applesauce are frequently mixed together in hospitals to get things going. To make your own cocktail, mix 4 to 6 chopped prunes with 1 tablespoon of bran and ½ cup of applesauce. Try it just before bed.

Toot on some muscial fruit. Beans will move anything. They're loaded with fiber and will jump-start a stalled gut. Try ½ cup a day to keep chronic constipation at bay.

Soften with psyllium. Many doctors recommend powdered psyllium, a type of seed that is available in drugstores and health-food stores. Take 1 to 2 tablespoons of powder stirred into a glass of water or juice. Follow this with another full glass of water. You can take psyllium once a day, but drink lots more water throughout the day, or the psyllium will form a new obstruction, adding to your problem.

O·D·D·B·A·L·L OINTMENT

Belly Button Massage

A gentle belly massage can help wake up your intestines and send them the message that it's time to move! Using your favorite massage oil, start at your belly button, and begin to massage in little circles in a clockwise pattern. Gradually, let the circles get bigger, until you are massaging along the edges of your entire abdomen. **Caution:** If you experience pain of any kind that does not respond to a change in hand pressure, consult your healthcare practitioner immediately.

Cough:

Amen to Ahems

Ever wonder why so many people start coughing as soon as the play is about to begin? Can't they cough before they enter? Do they all have colds? Is the air in the theater particularly dusty? Or do they just crave attention? Okay, now that's off my chest (so to speak) . . .

A cough is your body's reflex action to clear excess mucus or foreign matter from the linings of your air passages. The air a cough propels carries out dust; food particles; pollutants; and anything that is irritating your larynx, trachea, or bronchial tubes. A cough can also indicate boredom or a means of getting attention. (This must be what happens to some people in the theater, but I'd

POWERFUL POTION

CATNIP TEA

Catnip makes your kitty go crazy, but this herb can also make your cough just go! Fix up some catnip tea by steeping 1 or 2 table-spoons of dried catnip leaves in 1 cup of boil-ing water for 10 to 15 minutes. You can drink up to 3 cups a day.

never say so.) Any cough that lasts more than 1 week or produces blood should be checked by a doctor. But for those minor ones that pop up during colds or when you're watching a play, here's what to do:

Check out your cough clues. Before you treat yourself, see if you can figure out whether your cough is from an infection, an allergy, or something in your environment. A dry, unproductive cough, for example, could be simply due to an overheated home. A hacking cough could be bronchitis. Or if you cough up lots of phlegm, you could have an infection or allergic response. The phlegm's color also offers a clue: Yellow or darker mucus may indicate an infection, while a colorless fluid may be a sign of an allergy. Once you've done some basic detective work, you're ready to choose the appropriate relief.

Pick the right remedy. Depending on its cause, you'll want to either suppress the cough or encourage it to clear mucus from your lungs. Coughs caused by chest colds are helped by expectorants, which loosen mucus. But breathing in some steam with a towel over both your head and a bowl of very hot water will do the same

FABULOUS FOLK REMEDY

Healin' Honey

Honey, mixed with onion juice, was widely used during the Great Depression, when few folks could afford drugstore remedies. And to this day, people tell me about it. Honey or sugar is used to draw the juice from an onion, forming an effective cough syrup. The onion, it is said, stimulates saliva flow, which clears the throat and perhaps reduces inflammation. Here's what you do: Slice 1 onion into rings, and place them in a deep bowl. Cover them with honey, and let stand for 10 to 12 hours. Strain out the onion, and take 1 tablespoon of the syrup four or five times a day. Or chop 1 onion finely, and mix with $\frac{1}{2}$ cup of granulated sugar. Let stand overnight. Take 1 tablespoon of the resulting syrup every 4 to 5 hours. **Caution:** Never give raw honey to a child under 1 year of age.

thing. The vapor acts as an expectorant, too, so you can cough up the loosened mucus. Dry coughs, often from too much dry heat or dust, may keep you awake at night, so an over-the-counter cough suppressant, such as dextromethorphan, may be helpful. But bear in mind that over-the-counter cough suppressants frequently contain alcohol, so never take them with sleeping pills. It can be a deadly combination. One tip: The pediatric versions of cough syrups frequently have no alcohol added.

Warm your wine. A friend from Belgium told me her mother's remedy for cough was hot red wine with lemon, cinnamon, and sugar added. She said it puts you right to sleep, so you don't know if you're coughing (and probably don't care, either). Alcohol is a component of many cough medicines, but use it cautiously—too much will weaken the immune response, which you need to fight infection.

Lie up, not down. When your chest is congested, and you're coughing up a lot of mucus, pile on several pillows, or sleep on a foam wedge. Sleeping with your head raised 6 or 8 inches will prevent the mucus from pooling in your bronchial passages, thus promoting more peaceful sleep.

Hydrate a hack. Any time, but especially when you've got a cough, is the right time to drink lots of fluids. Enjoy a cup of hot tea or a tall glass of lemonade with honey—these are also good at loosening the mucus.

Take a Bite Outta Your Bark!

How often do you use those little packets of hot mustard that accompany Chinese takeout? Well, don't throw away the extras—they can come in handy when you have a cough. Work this super-hot mustard into salad dressing or perhaps a chicken salad to liquefy mucus and stop your barking.

Crow's Feet:

How to Make 'Em Fly Away

Personally, I can't get too worked up about a few lines. Those crinkles at the corners of our eyes are the natural result of years of smiling or squinting. (Especially if you've been squinting at cigarette smoke.) To quit squinting, smoking, or hanging out in places where smoking is permitted is one solution, of course. But if you really want a line-free face, you could quit smiling and laughing, too. And I wouldn't recommend that.

Really phobic about crow's feet? You could try a fairly radical treatment—Botox injections. Normally used to treat neurologic disorders, Botox temporarily paralyzes the muscles you squint with, according to Randall Bjork, M.D. This allows the wrin-

---

FABULOUS FOLK REMEDY

A Honey Dew Mask

Honey has been used since ancient Egyptian times as a beauty aid. Applied as a mask, it moisturizes skin and leaves your face soft and dewy. Just smooth it over your face, and leave it there for 20 minutes or so. Then rinse with warm water.

kles to gradually fade or disappear. A dermatologist or cosmetic surgeon can do it for a mere—mere!—$400 to $900.

Of course, there are a few risks, such as permanent eyelid droop. And the injections are not recommended if you are pregnant, allergic to a whole bunch of things, or have a neuromuscular disorder. So if Botox seems too brutal, here are some suggestions that can help prevent those pesky lines to begin with:

Take sunscreen seriously. Certain skin types are more vulnerable to the sun, and over time, radiation damage really adds up. Sunlight damages the cell layers that generate the connective tissue that gives your skin strength and elasticity. But you can prevent further damage—and even reverse some existing damage—by using sunscreen religiously. Always (and that means year-round) wear sun-

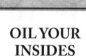

OIL YOUR INSIDES

Essential fatty acids are essential to skin health. Fatty acid deficiency can leave skin looking dried out and wrinkled. Make sure you eat one serving of omega-3 oils every day (salmon, almonds, and sesame seeds are good sources), or take it in capsule form. You can find flaxseed oil, black currant oil, borage oil, and evening primrose oil at your natural foods store. Take 1,000 milligrams once or twice daily.

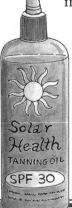

screen. If you use makeup, choose products with added sunscreen. Apply a product with a sun protection factor (SPF) of at least 15, and give it about 20 minutes to start working before you go outdoors.

Keep your beauty brimming. When you go out in the sun, plop on a wide-brimmed hat. Not only will it give you a touch of glamour but it will shade your eyes and the vulnerable skin around them from overhead sun. (Consider it a supplement to, not a substitute for, sunscreen. Remember that reflected glare bouncing off the sand, the sea, or even the parking lot pavement still reaches your face.)

Sport some shades. You'll look cool—and the skin around your eyes will stay relaxed—when you shade your eyes with sunglasses. (Along with radiation damage, it's those constant muscle contractions that form wrinkles.) Get in the habit of wearing shades every time you go out. And be sure to choose sunglasses that block UV light. Wraparound styles and those with wide side pieces offer extra protection to the crow's-feet area.

Skip the smokes. In addition to disease, death, and other forms of disaster, cigarette smoke is a major culprit in prematurely wrinkled skin. In addition to damaging skin cells, smoking also causes you to spend hours every day squinting. That's why smokers usually have much deeper crow's feet than other folks do. (Not to mention more wrinkles of all sorts.) So if you smoke, see your doctor for help in quitting. Smoke gets in your eyes—and that's nothing to crow about!

O·D·D·B·A·L·L OINTMENT

Feed Your Face

You'd be hard pressed to find a more emollient fruit than avocado. Its high fat content makes it an ideal base for a mask. Mash ½ of an avocado; then add ½ teaspoon of vitamin E oil and 1 tablespoon of plain yogurt. Mix well and apply, paying close attention to the fine lines around your eyes and mouth. Leave on for 20 minutes; then rinse with warm water.

Dandruff:

Shake Those Flakes for Good

Ever feel as though you lived inside one of those little snow globes? All around you, people might be strolling through spring, summer, or fall—but for you in your new dark suit, it's winter all the way. Maybe you should just wear your galoshes on your shoulders?

Many people shed a dandruff flake or two now and then, especially in winter, when the scalp tends to dry. More serious dandruff, however, results when tiny oil glands at the base of the hair roots run amok. The scalp's skin normally replaces itself once a month; but if you have dandruff, somehow this shedding process gets accelerated. Hair becomes greasy, and those tell-tale crusty, yellowish flakes sprinkle your shoulders. Chances are, they're not your favorite fashion accessories.

POWERFUL POTION

DANDRUFF-B-GONE

The B vitamins, particularly biotin, are essential to a healthy scalp. So make sure your multivitamin contains biotin, or find a B-complex vitamin that contains 300 micrograms of biotin.

Another type of dandruff occurs when the scalp's sebaceous glands become plugged. Hair loses its gloss, and the dandruff flakes are dry and grayish. Because more men than women have dandruff, doctors suspect that the male hormone testosterone may have something to do with it.

Other factors that can give you a case of the flakes include family history, food allergies, excessive sweating, alkaline soaps, and yeast infections. And although no one knows exactly what causes dandruff, stress does provoke it, according to Alvin L. Adler, M.D., a dermatologist and instructor at the New York Hospital-Weill Cornell Medical Center and Beth Israel Medical Center, also in New York. See a doctor if you are losing hair, your scalp seems inflamed, or you have itching, scaly skin on other parts of your body, which may indicate a more serious problem like psoriasis. Otherwise, there's a lot you can do to control dandruff. Here are some options:

O·D·D·B·A·L·L OINTMENT

Steam Clean

Steaming the scalp with nutritive herbs gives a deep, cleansing treatment for dandruff. Mix together equal parts of fresh or dried leaves of rosemary (*Rosemarinus officinalis*), nettles (*Urtica dioica*), and peppermint (*Mentha piperita*). Use 2 tablespoons of dried herb ($^1/_2$ cup fresh) in 2 cups of hot water, and steep, covered, for 10 minutes. If using fresh nettles, be sure to wear gloves while preparing the infusion to avoid getting stung. Strain the infusion, cool slightly, and apply carefully to the scalp. Cover your hair with a shower cap, and wrap your head in a hot, wet towel. Leave on for 30 minutes; then rinse with an herbal rinse.

Find the right shampoo. A good, dandruff-fighting shampoo reduces scaling of the scalp and allows medication to penetrate, reports Dr. Adler. Look for shampoos that list tar or salicylic acid among the ingredients, he advises. Although there are many over-the-counter dandruff shampoos, the U.S. Food and Drug Administration (FDA) has approved only five active ingredients as safe and effective against dandruff: coal tar, pyrithione zinc, salicylic acid, selenium sulfide, and sulfur. The FDA also recognizes a combination of salicylic acid and sulfur as effective.

Use it daily. Wash your hair every day. This breaks up larger flakes of dandruff, making them less noticeable. It also prevents the buildup of hair spray, gels, and other hair preparations—some of which can look a lot like flakes as they wear off the hair. Massage the shampoo into your scalp, and let it sit for 3 to 5 minutes—longer if your dandruff is severe. Rinse thoroughly to get all the shampoo out.

Squeeze a lemon. After shampooing, rinse your hair with lemon juice or—if you can stand the smell—vinegar. Dilute each with enough water (say, 2 ounces of lemon juice or vinegar to 1 quart of water) so you don't feel a burning sensation on your scalp. This hair treatment is popular with many folks, because it leaves your hair shiny and squeaky clean. Rinsing or dabbing these weak acids right onto your scalp helps remove dandruff flakes, too.

Natural Native Medicine

Hops to It

It flavors beer—that's how most of us know about hops. Yet the wild hops plant is found all over the world, and Native Americans use it as a cure for dandruff (among other things), according to Gary Null, Ph.D., host of the *Natural Living* radio show. You don't need to comb the fields and woods for hops, however—just rinse your hair with beer or add a good squirt of the suds to your regular shampoo.

Get to the roots. Native American healers use roots of the yucca plant, pounded and whipped with water, to treat dandruff. Yucca roots contain soapy substances called saponins. For a simpler approach, try a ready-made yucca root shampoo, which is available in some health-food stores.

Hang up your hair dryer. Whenever you can, let your hair dry naturally, rather than blowing it dry. When you must have extra volume for a special occasion, be sure to use a lower setting. That hot wind really dries out the scalp, making you more vulnerable to dandruff.

Flake out. Using a natural-bristle brush, brush your hair from the scalp outward with steady, firm strokes. This carries excess oil away from your scalp, where it can cause dandruff, to the hair strands, where it gives your hair a healthy shine.

Style with sense. When you're perfecting your hairdo, use only nonoily gels or mousses. Greasy hair fixatives can make a dandruff problem worse, according to Dr. Adler.

Thyme Out for Dandruff

If you'd like to try an herbal approach to dandruff control, dab some thyme oil diluted with olive oil (4 drops of thyme oil per teaspoon of olive oil) on your scalp 1 hour before washing your hair. Then, after shampooing, it's thyme for an antidandruff rinse. To make the rinse, boil a handful of dry thyme leaves in 1 quart of water, strain, and cool.

FABULOUS FOLK REMEDY

Blonds Have More . . . *Marigolds*?

Herbal rinses add sheen to the hair shaft while relieving scalp irritations. Traditional herbs include rosemary and sage for dark hair, chamomile and marigold for blonds, and cloves for auburn or red hair. Make a strong tea using 4 tablespoons of herb to 1 quart of boiling water. Steep for 15 minutes, and add ¼ cup of apple cider vinegar to restore the scalp's proper pH. Use as a final rinse after shampooing your hair.

Depression:

Chasing the Blues Away

Sometimes, in the ocean of life, the surf is calm and regular. Other times, it's so savage, it takes your breath away. Life is an ever-changing series of cycles and events that can take us up or down. After all, if we didn't feel down now and then, we wouldn't be human. But it isn't normal or healthy to be depressed for a long period of time. Grief and sadness over particular events in your life, such as a divorce, losing a loved one, changing jobs, or facing an empty nest, are just part of the human equation. Depression, on the other hand, may feel like a long-term state of mind.

Depression affects your physical health, too, and has always been linked to heart disease. Johns Hopkins researchers found that depressed people

---

FABULOUS FOLK REMEDY

Hold the Thistle

Blessed thistle (*Cnictus benedictus*) is an old-time remedy for melancholy, typically extracted in wine or alcohol. Make an infusion using 1 teaspoon of dried thistle per 1 cup of boiling water. Steep for 10 minutes, and drink 1 to 2 cups per day.

were four times more likely to have a heart attack than those who said they were not depressed. And a study of middle-aged women found that those who had depressive symptoms (sleeping problems, lack of energy, frequent boredom, and crying) and who also felt unsupported by their friends and families had low levels of high-density lipoproteins (HDL), the "good" cholesterol—another risk factor for heart disease. So it's important to learn how to deal with the blues. You should always see your physician if the doldrums last more than a few days, or head for the emergency room if you have any thoughts whatsoever of suicide. Otherwise, here's some help:

Make sure it's not physical. See your doctor for a complete examination to rule out a medical reason for your depression, such as anemia, a thyroid abnormality, hormone imbalance, diabetes, or another condition that could be affecting your mood. Once you're in the clear, follow a preventive lifestyle to stay healthy.

Go see a pro. Depression is a biological disease, not a sign of weakness—and you should never hesitate to get help. If you're clinically depressed, your doctor may prescribe an antidepressant

POWERFUL POTION

HERBAL CHEER TEA

Native American healers have a basic herbal cheer mix made of St. John's wort flowers, passionflower, and devil's club bark. To try it, combine equal amounts of *each* herb in a glass jar, mix well, seal, and make a tea when you're feeling low. Put 1 tablespoon in a mug, add boiling water, cover, steep for 10 minutes, and strain. Drink 2 cups a day. Before using this tea, be sure to read the cautions concerning St. John's wort (in the potion box on page 146).

and refer you to a professional for one of many "talk therapy" options, ranging from in-depth psychoanalysis to group therapy, behavioral therapy, and a variety of newer techniques. Both short- and long-term treatments are available. One tip: Studies show that psychoanalysis alone is not that effective for depression. The use of antidepressants combined with cognitive therapy or interpersonal therapy is.

Eat mood food. Try a turkey sandwich to ease the blues. Tryptophan, an amino acid abundant in turkey, converts to serotonin in the brain. Serotonin is a natural brain chemical that works as a neurotransmitter and hormone to enhance your mood. You also can get tryptophan from other meats, fish, and dairy products as well as from choline, part of the B-complex vitamins.

Go fish. Research at Harvard Medical School reveals that fish oil may help mood disorders. In particular, it's the omega-3 fatty acids found in blue fish and other oily cold-water fish, such as salmon, mackerel, herring, and sardines. There is no positive proof, but all evidence points in

O·D·D·B·A·L·L OINTMENT

Take a Deep Breath

Scent has a powerful effect on our mood as the olfactory nerve connects our nose to the limbic system—the part of the brain that rules our emotions. Find a scent that appeals to you, and experiment with ways to incorporate it into your life—via a body lotion, perfume, atomizer, candle, or bath oil. Essential oils are better than synthetic preparations. Some oils to consider are chamomile, clary sage, jasmine, lavender, lemon balm, rose, and ylang ylang.

that direction, the researchers say. A study at the Laboratory of Membrane Biochemistry and Biophysics, a branch of the National Institute on Alcohol Abuse, shows that the less fish a nation consumes, the more clinical depression its citizens experience. So enjoy fish several times a week to keep depression at bay.

Fake it until you make it. Remember the famous restaurant scene in the movie *When Harry Met Sally,* when Meg Ryan noisily shows Billy Crystal how she can fake an orgasm? "I'll have what she's having," said a nearby patron (whose part was played by Crystal's mom!) You can fake yourself out to lift your mood, too. Put on your favorite music, dress in your best clothes, stand up straight, and go about your day as if it were the best day of your life. But if your depression is severe, be realistic, and get help. Putting a happy face on a serious problem is denial— and that's unhealthy.

Talk about it. Depression is far more common in women than in men (or maybe, women just own up to it more often). In our culture, women are encouraged to talk about their feelings. Thankfully, more men are

POWERFUL POTION

FLOWER POWER

Flowers do more than make our world a more beautiful place: Their fragrance, color, and chemical makeup can also lift our mood. Passionflower (*Passiflora incarnata*), lavender (*Lavendula officinalis*), vervain (*Verbena hastata*), borage (*Borago officinalis*), rosemary (*Rosemarinus officinalis*), and skullcap (*Scutellaria lateriflora*), with their beautiful purple and blue flowers, can be just the thing for chasing the blues away. To beat the blues, try making a tea with just one of the herbs or use two to three in combination. Steep 1 teaspoon of the dried herb (or 1 teaspoon of mixed herbs) in 1 cup of boiling water for 10 minutes. Drink 2 to 3 cups per day.

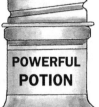

POWERFUL POTION

ST. JOHN'S WORT

Today, many people take St. John's wort for mild depression. Unlike some psychotropic drugs, this herb is not addictive, but you must take it consistently for 3 to 6 weeks to feel its full effect. Check with your doctor about whether this herb is safe and appropriate for you—especially if you are already taking antidepressant medication. Once you get the okay, take the recommended dose: 300 milligrams, two to three times a day.

learning to do this, too. So don't deny your pain—that just keeps you in an emotional prison. Seek advice from a trusted friend who can help you run a reality check on your complaints. Or see a counselor for a more objective view. What happens when you bottle it up? For men, unexpressed emotional problems are likely to show up as substance abuse or violence. And remember, you're hardly alone: A National Depressive and Manic Depressive Association panel estimated that 24 percent of women and 15 percent of men suffer from clinical depression at some time in their lives.

Get some space. Although taking a vacation is not a cure-all for depression, a few days off and a change of scene may help. Sometimes, you can think things through more easily when you're away from your usual surroundings. You can take stock of the situation that has you down and plan more useful strategies. From a distance, you may find you see things more clearly.

Exercise those endorphins. Vigorous exercise not only boosts your physical well-being but rearranges your brain chemistry and lifts your mood faster than a drug. In fact, you can consider exercise a free antidepressant! So don't sit there in the doldrums. Get out and run, do a few laps in a pool, or just walk briskly for a block or two. As your body releases its own feel-good hormones, called endorphins, you may think more rationally and come up with more effective ways to deal with what's bringing you down.

Researchers at Duke University studied 55 people with depression who did short, but strenuous workouts for as little as 8 minutes. No matter how depressed they'd been beforehand, participants felt more vigorous and energetic after their workouts. And no marathons are required—a regular brisk walk will do!

IT'S AN EMERGENCY!

It is important to distinguish between a passing feeling of the blues or sadness and the symptoms of a major or clinical depression. Untreated depression can lead to suicide, which is the third leading cause of death for teenagers and the fifth leading cause of death in adults aged 25 to 64. If you have any thought of suicide, are depressed for more than 2 weeks, can't concentrate, feel guilty, can't sleep or sleep too much, or have a noticeable change in weight, get professional help right away. If you have recurrent thoughts of suicide, head straight for the emergency room at your local hospital.

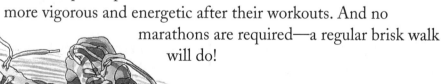

Diabetes:

Managing a Complex Condition

Folks who don't have diabetes may think the biggest deal is the daily fingerstick or, worse yet, having to give yourself a shot. But ask anyone with diabetes, and chances are they'll tell you the biggest hassle is having to be more disciplined about their diets—all the time—than most celery-stick supermodels.

The biggest problem people with diabetes face is the challenge of keeping the condition under control, says Karen Nichols, D.O., who practices in the Chicago area. "It's always there. There are no days off. You always have to behave," she says. Looking down a long road of constant

---

FABULOUS FOLK REMEDY

A Berry Good Tincture

Bearberry (*Arctostaphylos uva-ursi*) has been traditionally combined with bilberry (*Vaccinium myrtillus*) in a tea to treat diabetes. Add 2 parts bilberry tincture to 1 part bearberry tincture. Take 10 to 20 drops of the mixture in a glass of water between meals.

attention to diet, exercise, and blood-sugar levels creates stress for many people with diabetes. "It's a challenge," Dr. Nichols adds.

Diabetes is serious, but in most cases, it's controllable. It develops when the pancreas either doesn't produce enough insulin, or the insulin that's available is ineffective, or both. If insulin levels are inadequate, glucose and fatty acids accumulate in the bloodstream and trigger early symptoms of excessive thirst, excessive hunger, increased urination, and weight loss. Insulin resistance may have subtler symptoms and a slower onset, but both types have devastating systemic effects when not treated properly.

Many people can manage their diabetes with diet and exercise. Others may need oral medications or injected insulin to regulate their blood sugar. Uncontrolled diabetes damages eyes, kidneys, nerves, gums, and blood vessels—and sets the stage for heart disease and stroke.

A PREVENTABLE EPIDEMIC

There are two types of diabetes. Type 1, or "juvenile-onset" diabetes, generally begins in childhood or in young adulthood and is considered an autoimmune disorder. Type 2, or "adult-onset" diabetes, accounts for 95 percent of cases and is becoming an epidemic in the United States, says the American Diabetes Association (ADA). There was a 33 percent increase in type 2 diabetes from 1990 to 1998—and for

IT'S AN EMERGENCY!

If your blood sugar levels soar too high or dip too low, it can be an emergency. If you begin to feel sluggish or as though you'd been drugged, get emergency medical help immediately.

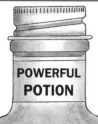

POWERFUL POTION

EVENING PRIMROSE OIL

Evening primrose oil can be used to treat a wide range of ailments, including diabetes. It seems to balance hormones, boost the immune system, keep cells strong, and reduce inflammation. The best way to take evening primrose oil is in capsule form—1,000 to 2,000 milligrams a day—after checking with your healthcare provider.

the first time in history, so-called adult onset diabetes showed up in young people. What's more, experts estimate that there are about 5 million people with the disease who haven't yet been diagnosed.

The biggest risk factors? Being overweight and a lack of exercise. Unfortunately, however, we're just getting fatter. Currently, 16 million Americans have diabetes: 1 in 10 people over age 50 and 1 in 5 people over age 65. And now, younger people, particularly obese teenagers, must also deal with this problem. And for kids, diabetes is a serious risk because they must live through many years of potential complications.

If you're one of those trying to handle this devastating disease, here's how you can work with your doctor to stabilize blood-sugar levels and help keep type 2 diabetes under control:

About-face! More than half of Americans are overweight—and every excess pound raises the risk of diabetes by 4 percent! Fight back by deciding once and for all to lose those extra pounds, and make exercise an everyday event. A healthy weight and two 15-minute walks a day can make the difference between being able to do what you want in old age and living as an invalid.

Maintain a positive attitude. Hate testing your blood? Dr. Nichols believes the best approach is to take it one day at a time and to create your own positive reinforcement along the way. When your diabetes is out of control, she says, you need to check your blood-sugar level as often as four times a *day*. However, when you stay on top of the disease, you often can limit the finger-sticking routine to just three times a *week*. So keep at it, and give yourself a pat on the back when your discipline pays off.

Personalize your plate. Dr. Nichols urges her patients to see a registered dietician to work out a diet that includes their personal preferences. That way, you'll be more inclined to stick to the plan and not let your eating get out of control. You also need to learn your own individual responses to what you eat, Dr. Nichols says.

Go natural. There is a movement now among desert Native Americans to return to their original diet of plants such as beans, squash, cactus, and mesquite. These low-fat, low-sugar, high-complex-carbohydrate foods are more healthful than today's highly processed, packaged foods. Studies have shown that people on such a diet in Arizona and Australia have more stable blood-sugar levels and lower cholesterol than most of us who eat a "normal" diet. (High insulin levels mean your body isn't using sugar effectively or that you're bombarding your system with too much sugar.)

The lesson here, however, is not to start munching on cactus—it's

POWERFUL POTION

BILBERRY BREW

Bilberry (*Vaccinium myrtillus*), goat's rue (*Galega officinalis*), fenugreek (*Trigonella foenum-graecum*), and devil's club (*Oplopanax horridum*) can be used to treat diabetes. Mix together equal parts of the herbs, and use as a tea. Steep 1 heaping teaspoon of the mix in 1 cup of boiling water for 15 minutes. Drink between meals. **Caution:** When using any therapies that may alter blood sugar, you must monitor your blood-sugar levels morebfrequently than normal. Check with your physician if you are taking any blood sugar–altering medications.

that a natural whole-foods diet heavy on grains is far more likely to help blood sugar than one of fast food and refined sugar.

Don't march to the starch. A Harvard study in the *Journal of the American Medical Association* noted that people who eat lots of starches to avoid fats may unwittingly set themselves up for diabetes. Study participants drank a lot of soft drinks and crowded their plates with potatoes, white bread, and white rice—all of which have almost no fiber. The result? They had 2.5 times the rate of diabetes found in people who ate less of these foods and more fiber, specifically from whole-grain

A Little Something for Your Nerves

A new screening device—a nylon fiber on a handled tool—can help identify undetected nerve damage in the foot caused by diabetes. A doctor pushes the filament against different parts of the bottom of the foot and notes when you feel the pressure. Regular screening with this device can help prevent *50 to 90 percent* of amputations caused by diabetes, according to the U.S. Health Resources and Services Administration.

cereals. The carbohydrates in refined foods, such as white bread and white rice, are quickly absorbed, causing a big surge in blood sugar. This, in turn, triggers the islets of Langerhans, found in the pancreas, to secrete high levels of insulin. Ounce for ounce, these starchy foods increase glucose levels more than if you simply ate pure sugar. So don't let a fat phobia overload your diet in favor of carbs. Ask a registered dietician to explain the proportions—and portions—that will help keep your blood sugar balanced.

Measure your meals. Buy an inexpensive scale (such as a postage scale), so you can measure ounces of cheese and fish, advises the ADA. Keep measuring cups and a set of measuring spoons handy. Use them regularly, and you'll develop a visual memory of appropriate portion sizes. Then, when you eat out, you'll know how much to have. Soon, it'll be second nature to recognize that your favorite eatery just served you pasta for three!

Butt out. Nicotine raises blood-sugar levels on its own, so it's definitely time to quit smoking. If it's been a while since you tried, see your doctor. Today, there are all sorts of new stop-smoking aids available, and one of them can work for you.

Just do it. Vigorous exercise helps improve your sensitivity to insulin. If you exercise regularly, you can even lower your need for injections. Exercise withdraws glucose from the blood for energy, which lowers your blood-glucose levels. It also delays or even halts cardiovascular disease, the leading killer of people with diabetes. The ongoing Nurses Health Study at the Harvard

Ginseng Breakthrough

A Canadian study published in the *Archives of Internal Medicine* shows that taking 3 grams of American ginseng with meals can lower blood sugar by 20 percent! This is a breakthrough study because it was the first to test an herbal product using accepted scientific criteria. The theory is that ginseng may slow digestion, decreasing the rate of carbohydrate absorption into the bloodstream. Researchers also believe American ginseng may modulate insulin secretion, but they don't yet know whether Asian ginseng will give the same result. If you have diabetes or high blood pressure, talk with your doctor before using ginseng.

School of Public Health shows that moderate activity, such as walking, protects you as well as tougher workouts as long as you burn around the same number of calories. (so if you want to walk instead of run, just exercise longer.) If you already have diabetes, walking will help control your blood sugar and manage your weight.

Stay hydrated while you huff and puff. Drink lots of water to prevent dehydration, and replenish the fluids and nutrients you lose during exercise. Drink a glass of water before exercise, and take a break every 20 or 30 minutes for more. This common workout wisdom is especially important for people with diabetes. A high-glucose sports drink can help prevent your blood sugar from dropping too low, according to the ADA, and you can use it like water when you are working out.

Be a sugar scout. Always be prepared. Diabetic coma and hypoglycemia, two life-threatening complications of diabetes, can usually be avoided with regular urine testing. When levels change, you can adjust your insulin, diet, and exercise accordingly. To be safe, a person with diabetes should always carry a few lumps of sugar or a candy bar. This is especially important when you are exercising or more physically active than usual, which may sometimes cause a change in your balance of sugar and insulin. Also, be sure to wear a medical alert bracelet, carry a diabetic identification card—or both.

Diarrhea:

Slowing Down the Urge

Ugghhh. An attack of "the runs" when you're away from home. We've all been there—and we'd prefer not to go back, thank you very much. When you're in the grip of the diarrhea demon, you need a clean, quiet bathroom so you can suffer in peace. A little moaning and groaning always helps, too.

The frequent, watery bowel movements of diarrhea usually result from a bout of food poisoning, dysentery, certain foods, caffeine, or alcohol. Emotional stress also can bring it on. Some women experience a mild diarrhea at the beginning of their menstrual

Natural Native Medicine

Blackberry Bliss

Blackberry is the most common diarrhea remedy used by Native Americans, says Gary Null, Ph.D., author of *Secrets of the Sacred White Buffalo*. Squeeze some juice from the berries—fresh or frozen—or make a tea from the leaves. Sip 2 to 4 cups a day.

Stop Chewing Gum!

Many gums are made with the artificial sweetener Sorbitol, which can cause diarrhea. If you want to chew gum, read labels to find a Sorbitol-free brand or give in to a few calories, and chew a stick made with real sugar.

cycle and at the onset of labor (at least *that* doesn't happen every month). Sometimes, diarrhea can be caused by over-the-counter indigestion remedies made with magnesium.

There are nonprescription remedies that contain loperamide hydrochloride, like Imodium, which may stop the diarrhea if taken according to instructions. However, this is only a stop-gap measure. If your diarrhea continues, you need medical attention. But, here's some help to get you on the road to recovery:

Do the dungeon diet. Well, try crackers and water (we're talking modern dungeons here). According to the Centers for Disease Control and Prevention, if your diarrhea is severe, you should take in only fluids and salty crackers until it's under control.

Pick the right liquids. You'll need to give up milk and other dairy products until you're feeling better. When you have diarrhea, your intestines are temporarily impaired in their ability to digest milk and other

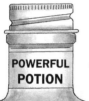

POWERFUL
POTION

CLOG UP THE WORKS

When nothing else has seemed to work, let carob and applesauce come to the rescue. Mix 1 teaspoon of carob powder in $1/4$ cup of applesauce, and eat slowly. Two or three doses may be needed throughout the day.

How to Avoid the Globe-Trotter's Trots

Traveler's diarrhea is usually caused by *Escherichia coli,* a bacterial toxin that damages the fluid-absorbing function of the colon. It is often found in unsafe water systems, especially in developing nations. So be a savvy traveler: Don't drink any water or anything made from the water, such as lemonade or ice cubes. Drink only bottled water and beverages. If cans and bottles have been chilled in buckets of ice cubes, wipe them clean to prevent contamination from unsafe ice water. Other tips to travel by:

Peel your own. Don't eat any fruit or raw vegetables (such as in salads) that you cannot peel yourself. A mango or banana is okay. Any produce that has been washed in local water may be contaminated with *E. coli.*

Drop some acidophilus. Take acidophilus tablets with meals. This will give you a supply of good bacteria to combat the bad ones you may pick up.

Give bacteria the brush-off. Brush your teeth, gargle, and rinse—all with bottled water. And remember not to wet your toothbrush under the tap before you brush, either.

Be sus-fish-ious. Be cautious about seafood. Fish available in markets and restaurants is not necessarily safe to eat. Regulations differ from one part of the world—or the country—to another. Very often fish, especially shellfish, is contaminated by pollution in the lake, bay, or ocean in which it was caught. Ask where the fish came from before you indulge.

Boil the water. If you run across a situation in which there's no bottled water available, simply boil water in a clean container to disinfect it. It must come to a full boil and stay there for at least 10 minutes.

Rice Water Relief

Rice water soothes an irritated intestinal tract, while providing hydration. Boil ½ cup of brown rice in 1 quart of water for 15 to 20 minutes, stirring constantly. Strain, and add honey if desired. Drink throughout the day.

dairy products. Likewise, you'll want to avoid citrus and vegetable juices, alcohol, and caffeine, which also make things worse.

Be a BRAT. This acronym helps you remember a diet of bland and binding foods: banana, rice, apples, and toast. These are the most widely recommended foods to eat while you recover from diarrhea, doctors say. Another option is eating chicken-and-rice soup to replenish the sodium and potassium you've lost.

Stick to it. It may be dull, but it will help you get better. Keep on eating the BRAT diet until you're completely well. Many, if not most, other foods can aggravate diarrhea or cause it to start all over again.

Check with your doctor. If you have chronic diarrhea; if diarrhea persists with fever, chills, and cramps; or if there is blood in your stool, see your doctor. Children, the elderly, and people with chronic diseases who are on medications should check with their doctor whenever diarrhea starts.

POWERFUL POTION

PEPPERMINT TEA

Peppermint is a natural menthol and antispasmodic. Try a cup of calming peppermint tea to relax the muscles of your digestive tract and relieve the spasms that trigger diarrhea. Just stir 1 teaspoon of mint leaves (fresh or dry) into 1 cup of boiling water, and let it simmer for 10 minutes. Strain out the leaves, and enjoy. Drink as many as 3 cups a day after meals.

Diverticulitis:

Pouches Full of Pain

Painful, irritated pouches in the colon, caused by constipation—bleecchh! But before we get to the grimmer details, let's entertain ourselves with a little Latin. Ready? Here's a brief diverticulitis dictionary: One pouch is called a *diverticulum*. More than one are *diverticula*. If you have them, your condition is called *diverticulosis*. When an infection flares, the acute condition is called *diverticulitis*.

Don't worry—there's no quiz. But you might want to keep these distinctions in mind the next time intestinal pain sends you scuttling to your doctor.

A diet of highly processed, low-fiber foods can catch up with us in many ways, including constipation.

FABULOUS FOLK REMEDY

Super Spasm Solution

Chamomile tea (*Matricaria recutita*) has been used as a digestive herb throughout history. Its gentle astringent action and antispasmodic effects relax and heal the gut. Use 1 teaspoon per 1 cup of hot water. Steep 3 to 5 minutes, and drink 2 to 3 cups per day. **Caution:** People with ragweed allergies may be sensitive to chamomile.

And constipation, in turn, has consequences, with the infection called diverticulitis among the nastiest.

The main cause of excess pressure on the colon, constipation can create small pouches in the colon wall. Half of us over age 60 have them, and nearly everybody over age 80 does, says the American Digestive Diseases Clearinghouse (ADDC). Sometimes, these pockets bulge outward through weak spots in the colon, like an inner tube poking through thin places in a tire. And when the pouches become infected or inflamed, as they do in 10 to 25 percent of folks with diverticulosis, they make their presence known—painfully.

A diverticulitis attack can develop without warning. Suddenly, severe abdominal pain strikes along with tenderness in the left side of the lower abdomen. Fever, nausea, chills, and other symptoms may also occur. Unless the infection is treated with antibiotics, an abscess may form and lead to further complications, including peritonitis and emergency surgery, says the ADDC. Once your doctor has diagnosed and treated diverticulitis, here's how to prevent a recurrence:

Let it heal. If you have been treated for diverticulitis, your doc-

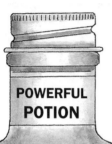

POWERFUL POTION

SLIPPERY SOOTHER

This slippery concoction soothes and eases inflamed intestinal tissues and softens stools. Grind equal parts of marshmallow root (*Althea officinalis*), flaxseed (*Linum usitatissimum*), and slippery elm (*Ulmus fulva*) (this is often found in powder form) in a coffee grinder. Stir 1 rounded teaspoon into an 8-ounce glass of water, and drink immediately. Repeat one to two times daily, following each dose with another full glass of plain water. For an added benefit, mix in unfiltered apple juice for the bowel-soothing pectin content.

Secret Fiber Source

It shouldn't be a secret. But unless you read nutrition labels in the cereal aisle, it's a big one. That's because although most cereals—including whole-grain cereals—have only a few grams of fiber per serving, there are a few that have 13 or 14 grams of fiber per serving. Which ones? You'll have to read the labels to find out!

tor will probably suggest you remain quiet for a few days. In addition to taking antibiotics, you'll need to restrict your diet to low-fiber foods, avoiding whole-grain products and all fruits and vegetables. This respite allows your colon to rest and heal. Once you're better, you can gradually restore your healthy, high-fiber diet.

Eat more fiber. Soluble fiber, found in apples and other fruit, keeps your stool soft for an easier passage through the colon. Insoluble fiber, found in whole grains and vegetables, adds bulk, decreasing the pressure on the colon walls. So bulk up your diet with these good-for-you foods. (As a bonus, you may find that your hips will lose some bulk, too.)

Drink it. The American Dietetic Association recommends 20 to 35 grams of fiber each day. In addition to high-fiber foods, your doctor may also recommend a daily fiber supplement, such as Citrucel or Metamucil. Drink one of these products mixed with 8 ounces of water or juice, and you can add 4 to 6 grams of fiber to your diet.

IT'S AN EMERGENCY!

Call your doctor if you have severe abdominal pain, constipation, or fever or if you notice blood in your bowel movements. When diverticulitis is severe, it can rupture the colon and cause peritonitis, a life-threatening infection of the abdominal cavity that requires emergency surgery.

Add fiber gradually. When you add fiber to your diet, do it gradually to avoid uncomfortable bloating and gas. A high-fiber diet helps form bulkier stool, which requires less muscle contraction and pressure to move through your bowel. "Think of a tube of toothpaste; you don't have to squeeze as hard to get the toothpaste out when the tube is full compared to when it's nearly empty," says the ADDC.

Fill up on fluids. A high-fiber diet requires lots of liquids, according to the Mayo Clinic. Fiber acts as a sponge in your large intestine. So if you don't drink enough, you could become constipated. Aim to drink at least eight glasses of water every day.

Don't be scared of seeds. Until recently, many doctors suggested avoiding foods with small seeds (such as tomatoes and strawberries) and stringy foods (like celery) because they thought particles might lodge in the diverticula and cause inflammation. This is now a controversial point and no evidence supports it, according to the ADDC. So enjoy these seedy, fiber-rich foods—they're good for you!

Heed the call. When you feel the urge to move your bowels, head right for the throne. According to the Mayo Clinic, putting off a bowel movement can lead to impacted stool. When that happens, you'll need more force to move things along, which increases the pressure on your colon.

Dry Eyes:

Cry Like a Crocodile

Eyes are the windows to our souls, limpid pools, and all that, right? Well, sometimes they're far from it. Instead, try hot, gritty, red, swollen—and dry. Tears are our eyes' only natural moisturizer, our best defense against dry-eye syndrome. The bad news is that as we age, tear production decreases. (Although I find this hard to believe because I'm sure I now cry more than ever.)

Long-term contact lens wear is the most common cause of dry-eye syndrome. And some medications may dry your eyes, including decongestants, antihistamines, high blood pressure medications, and tran-

Pull Down the Shades!

If you have a fan blowing near you, wear sunglasses or regular glasses, even indoors. Breezes can evaporate moisture on the surface of your eye. Any glasses will help, but wraparound shades offer the best protection.

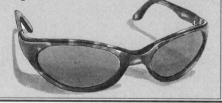

quilizers. Or living in a dry, dusty, or windy climate can result in that desert-eyes feeling. Dry eyes are also more common in women than men, which may be due to hormonal fluctuations, according to doctors at the Mayo Clinic. Sometimes, dry-eye syndrome also can be a symptom of a systemic disease, such as rheumatoid arthritis or lupus. If home remedies bring no relief, and your eyes are still uncomfortably dry, see your doctor. Here's what may help:

Drip some drops. There is no cure for dry-eye syndrome, but it's best to treat it with soothing remedies. Use "artificial tears" eye drops regularly to restore the film of moisture over your eyes. But ask your doctor which products are best and how often you should use them. Some eye drops can blur vision, so choose those made with saline (salt) or synthetic cellulose. Some contain vasoconstrictors that help with bloodshot eyes, but these products can dry your eyes further and increase redness and soreness when used for more than 3 days, according to the Mayo Clinic.

Try a warm compress. Heat opens clogged oil glands in the eyelids, so placing a warm compress over your eyes may induce some moisture. Just run some hot—but not too hot—water over a small towel, wring it out, and lay it over your closed eyes.

Rinse your face and eyes. When you are in a dry, dusty climate, rinse your face and eyes often with cool, clean water. This

will ease irritation and add some moisture to offset the arid atmosphere.

Goggle up. Use goggles when you swim—especially in chlorinated pools. Chlorine can irritate your eyes and dry them out. Ever noticed how red people's eyes look when they've been in the pool too long?

Put some moisture into your air. Use a humidifier if you live in a dry climate or work in a place that is very dry. Adding moisture to the air will help combat the effects of the dryness. Be sure to keep the humidifier clean so you don't add allergens, such as mold spores, to the air, which act as another irritant to your eye environment.

POWERFUL
POTION

BERRY THE
PUFFINESS

Bilberry (*Vaccinium myrtillus*) has a long history of use in eye complaints. High in bioflavonoids, bilberry helps strengthen tissues and reduce swelling there. Make a tea using 1 teaspoon per 1 cup of hot water. Steep for 10 to 15 minutes, and drink 2 to 3 cups per day.

Don't get parched. Drink lots of water to keep your body well hydrated, especially if you live in a dry place where your body moisture evaporates quickly. This will help keep your own natural tear supply flowing freely.

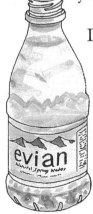

Cool it with the blow dryer. Avoid blow-drying your already dry eyes when you style your hair. Direct the air flow away from the eye area, and avoid any and all blasts of heat.

Dry Hair:

No More Bad Hair Days

I used to condition my hair periodically with mayonnaise. I smooshed the gloppy stuff into each strand, piled my hair up on my head, covered it with a shower cap, and let it sit for half an hour or so. Then, a shampoo and rinse—and voilà!—healthy hair.

Now, there are so many hair care products that I get dizzy just shopping for them. Unfortunately, each comes in about 16 variations, and every time I look at the drugstore shelves that hold these products, I feel I need a graduate degree in chemistry!

Why do we need conditioners? Well, hair dries out when it is overprocessed with coloring, perms, or relaxers, or if it—like mine—is heated with the blower dryer, sprayed, and moussed. Fortunately, hair can easily be returned to health—even if you don't have a degree in chemistry. Here's what to do:

Let natural oils out. Before you color your hair, avoid shampooing for 3 or 4 days to build up the natural oils on your scalp. They will protect your hair from becoming too dry from the processing. Also, because the wrong dye can harm your hair, investigate before you color, even if you only ask your friends or doctor, or check the Web site of the hair-color company. A patch test for allergy is also critical if you have not used a particular product before.

Don't let your hair get thirsty. Add lots of moisture to your hair if it is over-processed. The more, the better. This will make your hair stronger and more resilient. Do a deep conditioning several times a week.

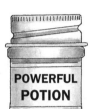

POWERFUL POTION

BLACK BEAUTY

A 500-milligram capsule of black currant oil, twice a day, is the remedy for dry hair recommended by Andrew Weil, M.D., a recognized expert in alternative medicine. It takes 6 to 8 weeks, according to Dr. Weil, to see the difference. Once your hair is in better condition, you can cut the dosage in half.

FABULOUS FOLK REMEDY

Marshmallow Rinse

Marshmallow (the herb, not the candy) makes a great natural moisturizer for dry hair. Instead of using a store-bought conditioner, try this rinse: Put 2 teaspoons of dried marshmallow root into 1 cup of boiling water. Simmer about 15 minutes. Strain out the herb, and let the liquid cool in the refrigerator before using it to rinse your hair. You can easily keep a week's supply in the refrigerator without it losing any of its *amazing* moisturizing abilities.

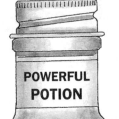

POWERFUL
POTION

HEALTHY HAIR HERBS

Like fingernails, hair health is a reflection of internal health. So make it a practice to drink nutritive teas, rich in minerals, to optimize your skin and hair health. Use one or all of the following herbs daily: nettles (*Urtica dioica*), oatstraw (*Avena sativa*), horsetail (*Equisetum arvense*), and red clover (*Trifolium pratense*). Steep 1 heaping teaspoon in 1 cup of hot water, and drink 1 to 2 cups daily. **Caution:** Be sure to wear gloves when handling fresh nettles so you don't get stung.

Keep shampoo and conditioner separate. The products that claim they clean and condition in one application really can't do a great job of either. It's better to use a gentle shampoo designed for dry hair and to follow with a conditioner intended for the same thing. But give yourself an hour or so to find them on the store shelves!

Forget hairdryers. They dry out your air. Instead, let your hair hang free and dry naturally.

Don't let the sunshine in. Constant sun exposure weakens and dries your hair, so wear one of those big-brimmed hats like the old movie stars used to parade in. Also, use shampoo, conditioners, and other hair products that contain sunscreen protection.

Go herbal. Eggs are rich in protein and make an excellent conditioning pack for hair. Beat an egg until it's light yellow, and then apply it to your hair. Leave it in for 10 to 15 minutes, and then rinse your hair thoroughly, using cool to tepid water.

Dry Skin:

Soften Up Your Birthday Suit

nlike the woman on TV who's so pal-sy with that alligator, most of us hate dry skin. It itches, it looks dull, and it's just no fun to live in. Right now, as I write, it's so humid that I don't need any moisturizer. In fact, makeup rolls right off my face (the TV model doesn't seem to have that problem). But with winter will come my city apartment's dry central heat, and then my skin will be a thirsty sponge. Dry skin, medically known as xeroderma, can result from cold weather, frequent bathing, sun exposure, or chemicals that leach the natural oils from our skin. What you need to do is replenish moisture—inside and out.

If your skin is dry, itchy, and flaking, it could be an allergy or in-

Vermont Country Milk

O·D·D·B·A·L·L OINTMENT

Roses and Herbs

Put a handful of rose petals into a 1-pint glass jar. Then add a sprinkling *each* of dried calendula (leaves or flowers), chamomile, comfrey, and lavender. Then fill the jar nearly to the top with vegetable oil. Twist the lid on tight. Stash the jar in a warm place, maybe near your stove. Every morning, give the jar a vigorous up-and-at-'em shake. Do this for a couple of weeks, then open the jar, and strain out the herbs, using a fine-mesh sieve. Finally, add a few drops of lavender essential oil. You now have your very own massage oil to rub into your dry skin each day.

fection, or a systemic condition that needs your doctor's attention. Some dry skin, known as ichthyosis, is an inherited condition and linked to a poorly functioning thyroid or lymphoma. This condition is beyond basic dryness, though—it means the skin is rough, scaling, wrinkled, and itching.

Here's how to get the moisture back and get comfy in your birthday suit:

Watch the soaps. Some soaps irritate the skin. I absolutely cannot use that famous "99 percent pure" one, because it totally dries out my skin. On the other hand, moisturizing soaps give me a rash, as do some deodorant varieties. If you have similar reactions, you might try my recent discovery—French milled soaps. They are big and heavy and extremely expensive—until you realize they last about six times longer than the others. These mild, high-fat soaps have a subtle, fresh aroma and leave your skin feeling wonderfully clean but not parched. And the lovely scent lasts all day.

Moisturize slowly. We are often so rushed that we barely have time to apply moisturizer after a shower when our bodies are damp. Give yourself a few more minutes for a mini-massage, and rub a moisturizer all over your body. Take your time. The massage will stimulate blood flow to your skin, which helps the moisturizer be more effective.

Bathe with bath oil. Add a fragrant bath oil to your bath water, soak, pat yourself dry, and finally moisturize. Be careful not to slip in the tub. Experiment with bath oils to find ones that feel best to you. In places where your skin is extremely dry,

Be Delicious—Inside and Out!

You can visit most any spa today to be massaged and moisturized with a variety of household foods. Apricots, with their ample vitamin A, are blended into a cream to moisturize and revitalize dull skin. They soften it, too. Coconut oil locks in moisture. Another popular moisturizer is jojoba, a natural oil made from beans found in southern Arizona. Jojoba is similar in structure to natural body oils. Avocado oil is also used to moisturize skin. Even lipid-rich Shiitake mushrooms can moisturize your skin, although I can't get too turned on by the notion of rubbing a fungi over my body. (A commercial mushroom moisturizer is Serum Vegetal de Shiitake.)

With a bit of imagination, you can even make your own body moisturizers. Just whir some of these ingredients in a blender with added honey, olive oil, or even milk until it reaches the consistency you like. Store in the refrigerator. If it's a chilly day, just warm the moisturizer by letting it sit in a sinkful of warm water as you bathe. If it's a hot day, take it directly from the refrigerator, and smooth it all over.

such as your feet, rub on some additional moisturizer. Then wear socks to bed so you won't get your sheets greasy.

Just the fats, Ma'am. Dry skin, especially in the winter, can be the result of too little fats—the right kind of fats. Our skin is the place where water and oil meet, and both are essential to good skin health. Make sure your diet includes one or more servings a day of omega-3 fats found in cold-water fish (salmon, mackerel, sardines), nuts (almonds, walnuts, pecans), and seeds (sesame, flax, sunflower).

Don't let your bubbles burst. While a long soak may feel so relaxing and soothing that you never want to leave the tub—especially if you have some music or a good book with you—don't overstay your welcome. A bubble bath and even some bath oils can dry out your skin if you stay too long.

Keep your internal rain barrel full. You need lots of water to keep all parts of your body working well, including your skin. It's really quite simple: The more water you drink, the more water is available to pump up and out to your epidermis. So don't be stingy with the water—drink at least 8 to 10 glasses a day—and carry a water bottle with you when you're exercising or out in the heat.

> ## O·D·D·B·A·L·L OINTMENT
>
> # Slather on the Oatmeal
>
> Treat yourself to a whole-body mask. Make a big pot of oatmeal, cool slightly to a tolerably warm temperature, and slather it on from head to toe. Leave on 20 minutes, or until dry, and rinse. Better yet, soak it off in a warm tub. For ease of removal, lightly oil your skin before applying the oatmeal body mask.

Dry Vagina:

Dealing with the Discomfort

Of all things to dry out! Yet a dry vagina often results from diminishing levels of estrogen at menopause. It doesn't mean all your love juice is gone forever—just that you need to help it along. Without estrogen, the vagina gradually returns to its prepuberty state, becoming shorter and narrower with less elastic walls and fewer secretions, according to Lila E. Nachtigall, M.D., a professor of obstetrics and gynecology at New York University (NYU) School of Medicine and Director of the Woman's Wellness Center at NYU. Here's how you can keep things moist:

Use it or lose it. If you can,

O·D·D·B·A·L·L OINTMENT

Sweeten Up!

Good, old-fashioned honey can be used to gently moisturize vaginal tissues. While you may need to use it daily at first, over time, you should be able to decrease the frequency of use. For ease of application and extra benefit, add several drops of vitamin E oil to it.

Heat Up; Then Chill Out!

Calendula flowers (*Calendula officinalis*) have a gentle healing effect on the skin and mucous membranes. Use a strong infusion of calendula (steep 1 cup of fresh flowers in 1 quart of water for 15 minutes, strain, and add to the bath) in alternating hot and cold sitz baths to increase circulation to the pelvic organs, soothe irritations, and tone tissues. Prepare a warm sitz bath, and immerse yourself up to your belly button. After soaking for 5 to 10 minutes, get out of the tub, and apply a cold wet towel like a diaper. Leave the towel on for 3 to 5 minutes. This may be repeated two to three times in a session. The greater the contrast between the hot and cold, the greater the tonifying effects.

stay active sexually as you age. It helps keep your vagina more elastic, flexible, and lubricated. According to those famous sexologists Masters and Johnson, intercourse at least once or twice a week over a period of years will keep a woman of any age wonderfully slick. The stimulation encourages the production of mucus secretions, helps maintain muscle tone, and preserves the shape and size of the vagina. (By the way, even if you've been celibate for a while, your vagina will quickly adjust to renewed sexual activity, so "lose it" isn't quite as dire as it sounds.)

Go easy on antihistamines. Antihistamines and decongestants that are designed to dry nasal membranes also tend to have the same effect down below, according to Dr. Nachtigall. Other drugs, including cardiovascular medications, antidepressants, atropine drugs, and diuretics can also have a drying effect on vaginal membranes. Talk to your doctor if you think a medication may be the cause of your vaginal dryness.

Learn about lubricants. Lubricants, such as K-Y jelly, Astroglide and Lubrin are available at your drugstore. (There are also vaginal suppositories such as Lubrin and Lubafax.) To be safe, a vaginal lubricant must be water soluble and oil free. The only exception is vitamin E oil, which doesn't dry or cake and may possibly have a beneficial effect on the vaginal lining. But stay away from almond oil, coconut oil, and other flavored oils. Their high sugar content encourages fungal infections, according to Dr. Nachtigall.

Never use a lubricant that is not designed for vaginal lubrication, because it can compound your problems, advises Dr. Nachtigall. Most cosmetic creams, for example, contain perfumes and alcohol that can irritate tender tissues. Petroleum jelly and baby oil can cake and dry, causing irritation or damage. They also provide a habitat for bacteria and block the release of your own secretions. Worse yet, petroleum products can destroy latex condoms and damage diaphragms.

Try moisture gels. Even more effective than lubricants are nonhormonal moisturizing gels, such as Replens and others sold over-the-counter. They hydrate the cells of the vaginal lining and allow them to build

O·D·D·B·A·L·L OINTMENT

Yogurt Works

If you need a lubricant now and can't dash off to the pharmacy, you may find help in the fridge. Yogurt is an excellent vaginal lubricant and nonallergenic for most people, according to Lila Wallis, M.D., a recognized pioneer in women's health. This remedy is meant to be used only in a pinch (or clinch) when you have no commercial gel or lubricant on hand. Keep in mind that, although yogurt can do the job, it's not necessarily sterile.

up a continually moist protective layer. In most cases, these products significantly increase moisture, acidity, and elasticity after a few months of use, according to Dr. Nachtigall. Each application lasts up to 3 days. To use, insert the moisturizer into the vagina with the disposable applicator about three times a week, preferably in the morning.

Ask about estrogen. Vaginal estrogen cream, which is absorbed by vaginal tissues, reverses the degenerative changes, encourages lubrication, and relieves dryness in a few days. How much cream to use and how often depends on your individual requirements. Some women need more than others because they may absorb it less efficiently. A vaginal ring is worn like a diaphragm and delivers a small dose of estrogen through the mucous membranes. Unlike a diaphragm, however, it needs to be changed only every 3 months. Keep in mind, though, that estrogen cream is still estrogen. So if you feel you are at particular risk for breast cancer, ask your doctor to help you decide if the cream is safe for you.

POWERFUL
POTION

**FROM THE
INSIDE OUT**

Black cohosh (*Cimicifuga racemosa*), red clover (*Trifolium pratense*), partridgeberry (*Mitchella repens*), and chastetree berry (*Vitex agnus-castus*) have been used to reduce perimenopausal symptoms in general. Mix equal parts of the herbs together; then place 1 heaping teaspoon in 1 cup of boiling water, cover, and steep for 15 minutes. Drink 2 cups daily. This is a tonifying tea; and for best results, it should be taken for several months.

Earache:

Muffle That Pain

Everybody seems to have a favorite remedy for the common earache. My friend Sue told me her Italian mother would roll a newspaper into a cone, light the wide end, and put the pointed end into the ear. She apparently never burned down the house or set anyone's hair on fire.

This remedy is not as far-out as it sounds. Native American healers have been using "coning" for centuries to treat earaches. They place herbs and beeswax on a piece of muslin, roll it into a tapered cone, insert it in the ear, and light it. The warm, dry smoke is supposed to draw out wax and excess fluids, while the vaporized beeswax and herbal essences in the smoke fight infections in the ear, the sinuses, and the lymph system. Some

Natural Native Medicine

Licorice for Your Ears?

Licorice leaves are a traditional Native American remedy for earache. The plant is plentiful in the Northwest, and its dried leaves are found in many health-food stores. Soak a big handful of leaves in hot water, shake off any excess water, and place them over your ears and nearby areas.

healers add yerba buena to the mix.

Not interested in the firey approach? Can't say that I blame you. Most physicians will treat an ear

infection with antibiotics—even if it appears to have a viral cause—since they don't want to risk letting an infection damage your hearing. Here's what you can do until you get to the doctor:

Fix your nose first. Over-the-counter antihistamines, decongestants, or nose drops may help decrease nasal secretions, shrink the mucous membranes and open the eustachian tube, doctors suggest. Be sure to follow package directions, and don't use them beyond the recommended period. **Caution:** If you have high blood pressure, check with your doctor or pharmacist before taking any antihistamines.

Warm up your ears. Warmth is probably the most common

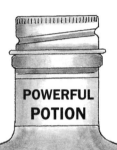

POWERFUL POTION

MULLEIN DROPS

To ease the pain of ear infections, crush a couple of mullein leaves in a sieve, and collect the juice. With a dropper, put 2 drops of mullein juice right in the painful ear, and seal it up with a cotton ball. This method also works with bottled mullein flower oil (made by steeping flowers in olive oil), which you can keep in the refrigerator. The only thing you do differently is warm the dropper by rubbing it in your hands first, so your ear isn't shocked by the cold! Mullein oil helps kill the bacteria that caused the ear infection.

remedy for earache. Doctors note that a warm heating pad or warm water bottle can reduce discomfort. You can also try placing a cotton ball saturated with warm oil into—but not far into—the affected ear. Some people use a blow dryer to blow warm air into the ear. (A better version might be a warm person who could whisper sweet nothings into your ear! That warm breath might help your pain, not to mention what it will do to your libido!)

Gargle and pop. According to Andrew Weil, M.D., director of the Program of Integrative Medicine at the University of Arizona, gargling promotes healing of an ear infection by bringing more blood to the eustachian tube. Gargle several times a day with 1 teaspoon of salt in a glass of water that's as hot as you can tolerate.

Muffle your ears. To keep your earache from feeling worse, keep your ears covered on cold days. Most body heat is lost through your head, so you need to keep your head warm and that includes your ears, too. Wear hats with ear flaps, a scarf that covers your ears, or good old-fashioned earmuffs.

O·D·D·B·A·L·L OINTMENT

Garlic Ear-Oil

Chop 2 garlic cloves, place them in a clean jar, and cover them thoroughly with olive oil. Seal the jar, and place it in a cool, dark place for 3 to 4 days, turning it once or twice a day. Strain, and store the oil in the refrigerator. Warm the jar under hot running water for several minutes before placing 2 to 3 drops of oil into the affected ear. Repeat two to three times daily. Keep the oil in the refrigerator between treatments, and discard after 1 month.

Erectile Dysfunction:

New Treatments, New Hope

When Bob Dole lost the nomination for president in 1996, he began a new career as the poster boy for Viagra—and he probably made lots more money than he would have as president. Viagra, a medication to restore male potency, was the biggest hit and most widely sold drug since aspirin.

The National Institutes of Health estimate that 10 to 20 million American men between the ages of 40 and 70 suffer erectile dysfunction (ED), but fewer than 10 percent of these men do anything about it. Before Viagra, most believed ED was the near-inevitable result of aging and diminishing testosterone levels, which start to fall around age 40. Many men are familiar, too, with an enlarged prostate, which often causes sex problems and even compete impotence after age 65. Sadly, few realized ED could be medically treated.

Erectile dysfunction can also occur after back or prostate surgery or after radiation treatment for prostate cancer. But more commonly, it results from other health problems such as diabetes, high blood pressure, and spinal cord injuries. Smoking, alcohol abuse, and some medications for conditions such as high blood pressure, excess stomach acid, depression, insomnia, and anxiety can contribute to the problem.

In addition to Viagra, there are many nondrug treatments available, such as penile implants, injections, and vacuum devices. These tips may also help:

Order pasta to go. Why are Italian men reputed to be such great lovers well into their 70s and 80s? Is it just their dark good looks, or do they know something other men don't? According to James F. Balch, M.D., studies of Italian men show they eat pizza and many other foods with lycopene-rich tomato sauce. A Harvard University study reported in the *Journal of the National Cancer Institute* that increased lycopene levels help maintain prostate health, which, in turn, promotes performance. To get more lycopene, you should eat five servings of cooked tomato products a week, according to Dr. Balch.

POWERFUL POTION

MANLY TONIC

This tea was specially created for guys. Drinking 1 or 2 cups a day may help keep prostate problems at bay! Mix 1 teaspoon *each* of saw palmetto berries, hawthorn berries, fennel seeds, marshmallow root, and licorice root together. Then put them in a pan with 6 cups of water. Bring to a boil, and let simmer 25 minutes. Allow the tea to cool, strain out the herbs and then bottom's up! **Caution:** Licorice root should not be used by people with high blood pressure or kidney disease.

Shuck those oysters, guys. Are oysters really an aphrodisiac or simply a sexual placebo? Men who slurp them off the half-shell in the hope of extra sexual vigor may find themselves succeeding because they believe it will work. But it's interesting to note that oysters are rich in zinc, which the prostate needs to manufacture seminal fluid, according to urologist Marcus Loo, M.D. You can also load up on zinc by eating other shellfish, poultry, wheat germ, vegetables, grains, and yogurt.

See a sex therapist. If you are troubled by frequent ED, ask your family physician to recommend an expert in the condition, then schedule a few visits. It could make all the difference.

Talk with your partner. When a man's penis doesn't cooperate, it can be an embarrassing experience. This is, after all, your chief barometer of manhood. But don't try to resolve the prob-

The Stamp Test

How do you know whether your problem is physical or emotional? Take the postage stamp test to find out. Before you go to sleep, wrap a strip of gummed postage stamps around your penis. (The self-stick kind may not work.) If you wake up in the morning with the strip intact, it means your penis did not become erect during the night (it normally enlarges during sleep). This implies a physical problem. If the strip of stamps broke apart, however, your penis was probably enlarged during sleep, and your ED is more likely due to a nonorganic cause.

lem all by yourself. Be sure to involve your partner in the process as well. She's got as much at stake as you do. If she doesn't understand what's going on, she's going to be less than enthusiastic about sex—and the last thing you need is an inhibited partner.

Bust a gut. Erectile dysfunction increases in direct proportion to your waistline. A study recently presented at the annual meeting of the American Urological Association revealed that 34 percent of men aged 51 to 88 had ED. After adjusting for age, smoking, and hypertension, the researchers found that men with larger waistlines were more likely to suffer from ED than their slimmer buds. In fact, men with waists of 42 inches are twice as likely to have ED than men with 32-inch waists.

Motion is the potion. Inactive men are also more likely to have ED than those who exercise at least 30 minutes a day. "Even though ED affects an estimated 30 million American men, little research has been done about how modifiable lifestyle factors may contribute to the condition," says Eric Rimm, Sc.D., of the Harvard University School of Public Health in Boston. He said the study, reported at the American Urological Association annual meeting,

FABULOUS FOLK REMEDY

The Ginseng Option

Ginseng (*Panax ginseng*) has had a reputation of being an aphrodisiac throughout the history of folk medicine. I'm not sure that's justified—and research has only begun to scratch the surface of this potent herb. If you'd like to try it as a tonic, drink 1 cup of tea daily using 1 heaping teaspoon per 1 cup of hot water and steeping for 15 to 20 minutes. If you try ginseng, be sure to check with your doctor first, especially if you have high blood pressure. Also, be aware that ginseng makes some men jittery.

"indicates that ED may be correlated with lifestyle factors, re-inforcing once again how important adequate exercise and a healthy diet are to overall good health." The bottom line? Make exercise a priority, and you're more likely to make love.

Get happy. If you're depressed, you're twice as likely to have ED, according to a study of 1,200 men between the ages of 40 and 60 that was reported in the journal *Psychosomatic Medicine*. The study used data from the Massachusetts Male Aging Study conducted by New England Research Institutes between 1986 and 1989 with grants from the National Institute on Aging and the National Institute for Diabetes and Digestive and Kidney Disorders. If you are down in more ways than one, see your doctor about getting some help for depression.

Keep circulating. High-fat foods clog the arteries to your heart as well as the arteries to your penis—and the latter are a lot smaller and thus clog up quicker. Smoking impedes blood flow, including blood flow to the penis. Good health and good sex belong together, so cut out the fats and the butts to keep your blood circulating to all the right places.

POWERFUL POTION

GET GINKGO

Ginkgo (*Ginkgo biloba*) is used to increase circulation and may be helpful in some cases of erectile dysfunction. Combine it with two or three male tonics such as saw palmetto (*Serenoa repens*), horsetail (*Equisetum arvense*), and true unicorn root (*Aletrium farinosa*). Make a tea using 1 heaping teaspoon per 1 cup of boiling water. Steep for 10 minutes, and drink 1 to 2 cups daily. Tonic herbs are slow acting, and you may need to take the tea for several weeks before seeing improvement. **Caution:** Do not take ginkgo if you are on blood-thinning medications without checking with your health-care provider first.

Eye Bags:

Temporary Stowage Available

Hey, on Jim Lehrer of PBS fame, they're kinda cute. But most of us would rather leave those saggy-looking pouches under the eyes to the basset hounds.

Eye bags have two causes. They can be a temporary result of fluid retention, or they may actually be fat deposits that have accumulated over the years. Unfortunately, there is no diet or exercise that can diminish the latter kind. For a permanent solution to fatty eye bags, cosmetic surgery is probably your best bet. To flatten the temporary pouches that result from fluid buildup, see **Fluid Retention**. Meanwhile, these short-term solutions can be useful:

Minimize them with makeup. The skin on your baggy lower lids is usually darker than the rest of your eye area. If this is the case, use a concealer there that is one tone lighter than your regu-

---

FABULOUS FOLK REMEDY

Bag the Bags!

Black tea with its astringent nature makes an excellent remedy for baggy eyes. Simply wet two black tea bags, and place one over each eye while you rest for 20 minutes or so.

lar foundation. Or, if you don't wear foundation, match the concealer to your skin color. Use a small brush to apply the concealer before blending it lightly with your finger. Once you add foundation or powder over it, the concealer will set for a longer lasting look.

Scope out the shelves. There are a number of de-puffing products available in most drugstores to help reduce eye bags. Most require chilling or freezing before you apply. If you keep them in the fridge, they have an effect similar to chilled cucumbers—an age-old remedy for puffy eyes. Most of these products are a bit pricey, however, so you may actually want to stick with cucumber. (If you do, simply lie down with your eyes closed. Place a 1-inch thick slice of chilled cucumber over each eye, and relax for 15 or 20 minutes.)

POWERFUL POTION

FABULOUS FENNEL

A cold compress made with fennel tea can reduce the swelling around puffy eyes. Just pour 1 cup of boiling water over 2 teaspoons of fennel seeds. Cover, and allow the brew to steep for 10 minutes before storing it in the refrigerator overnight. In the morning, strain out the seeds, and your eye-pleasing medicine is ready!

To use, dip a paper towel into the fennel tea. Find a quiet place to lie down, shut your eyes, and put the moistened paper towel over them. In 10 minutes or so, your eyes will sparkle and look refreshed. This recipe makes enough for five daily treatments.

O·D·D·B·A·L·L OINTMENT

Potato Patties Prevail

Make a potato patty compress by grating raw potato and wrapping in clean cheesecloth or gauze. Place over your eyes for 20 minutes while resting. A simpler method is to thinly slice a raw potato, and apply the potato directly to the skin. Follow with your favorite eye skin cream, taking care not to stretch the delicate skin around your eyes.

Flatulence:

Turning Off the Gas

Ever seen that TV commercial where the man and woman get in their car after dining out, and their overstuffed bodies inflate like air bags? Of course, this is a pitch for an over-the-counter gas remedy, which they take so they can go right out and gorge on dessert.

But flatulence isn't an unnatural thing. Almost every food, except possibly rice and lean chicken, can cause it. It's just part of the process of food and air going through the digestive system. When babies and household pets pass gas, everybody laughs. Try that as an adult? You'll be blushing, but never mind—nobody will see it, since they've all left the room.

FABULOUS FOLK REMEDY

Cast Off the Pain

When gas pains persist, ease the discomfort with an old-fashioned castor oil pack. Saturate a clean cloth with castor oil, and place against your skin, taking care to cover your abdomen completely. Cover with plastic wrap (castor oil stains clothing!), and then place a hot-water bottle on top—wrapped in cloth so it won't burn your hands. Leave it in place for 1 hour or so.

Here's how to deflate the embarrassment before it starts:

Eat like Ms. Manners. When you gobble a meal on the go, you're bolting air along with the food. And the more air you swallow, the gassier you'll get. Slow down, chew thoroughly, and take a break at mealtime. On average, you normally pass gas 13 times a day. Eating too fast just ups the ante.

Don't suck up bubbles. Pick a bubble-free beverage—carbonated drinks are full of extra air. And when your beverage arrives with a straw, open one end of the wrapper, crumple it short, place it over one end of the straw, and blow it at your meal mate. Then set the straw aside. Drinking through a straw pulls lots more air into your digestive system.

Take an after-dinner stroll. Go for a walk after meals. Regular exercise promotes bowel function and helps your body digest food. Flopping your butt down on the couch after dinner encourages food to ferment, creating gas.

Don't boycott the broccoli. Some flatulent folks fear veggies cause gassiness. Cabbage, broccoli and Brussels sprouts do rank high—but they don't cause much more gas than most other vegetables do. And you need veggies—

POWERFUL POTION

BEE BALM TEA

Have tea with the birds. According to Native American healers, 4 ounces of hummingbird digestive tea before a meal aids digestion and relieves gas. Hummingbird tea is made from bee balm—a favorite flower of hummingbirds. To make a tea, crush 1 tablespoon of dried bee balm leaves with 1 teaspoon of powdered marshmallow root. Put the mixture in a tea ball, and steep in hot water for 5 to 10 minutes. Add 1 teaspoon of honey or maple syrup to ½ cup of tea in a small glass, and drink it before each meal.

their healthful nutrients prevent disease. So don't avoid them, just add more vegetables to your diet in gradual doses. Given a chance, your body will get used to them, and they won't worsen flatulence.

Savor seasoned veggies. Add anise, fennel, or ginger to "gassy" vegetables like Brussels sprouts, broccoli, and cabbage. Along with enhancing flavor, these herbs offset the gassy effects of these healthy foods.

Reach over-the-counter. Beano is made from a plant enzyme that breaks down the sugars in the food. Put a few drops of liquid Beano on your first bite of food, or take a Beano tablet before eating. You'll enjoy your meal without that bloated feeling. Activated charcoal products will also absorb gas but could also absorb any medications you take. So check with your doctor before using this alternative.

Get some culture. Live cultures, that is. Yogurt with live cultures (called acidophilous) breaks down milk sugars and keeps a bal-

---

IT'S AN EMERGENCY!

If you have persistent flatulence accompanied by abdominal pain for more than 3 days, it could be a more serious problem, such as appendicitis, gallstones, ulcer, or a malabsorption problem. Call your doctor immediately.

O·D·D·B·A·L·L OINTMENT

Rub It Out

Relieve gas pains with a simple belly rub containing antispasmodic herbs. Add 4 to 6 drops *each* of lobelia tincture (*Lobelia inflata*) and catnip tincture (*Nepeta cateria*) to 2 tablespoons of olive oil. Then gently massage it into your abdomen in a clockwise pattern.

ance of healthy bacteria in the digestive channels. So read yogurt labels to be sure it contains acidophilous, and eat it often for better digestive health.

Avoid the big offenders. Deep-fried foods and other highly fatty dishes are relatively difficult to digest and thus cause gas. Choose a healthy, low-fat diet of fruits, vegetables, and whole grains instead, with some fish or lean meat if you like. Also avoid sorbitol, a common sugar substitute. Since you're eating healthier anyway, those few calories saved aren't worth the bloat.

Snack on after-dinner seeds. Chew ½ teaspoon of fennel seeds at the end of a meal when you feel gassy, advise Native American healers. They also like to chew dill, caraway, coriander, or aniseeds to ease digestion. For a refreshing after-dinner (and antigas) drink, steep about 1 teaspoon of aniseeds in 1 cup of hot water for 10 minutes, and enjoy.

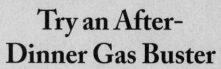

POWERFUL POTION

TUMMY-TAMER TEA

Poor digestion, especially poor fat digestion, can leave you feeling gassy and bloated after meals. Carminative herbs contain oils that help release spasms and relieve gas pains. Mix equal parts of caraway seeds (*Carum carvi*), fennel seeds (*Foeniculum vulgare*), and anise seeds (*Pimpinella anisum*). Then slightly crush 1 teaspoon of the seed mixture and add to 1 cup of boiling water. Remove from the heat, and steep, covered, for 20 minutes. Strain, and drink after meals.

Try an After-Dinner Gas Buster

A gas-busting, after-dinner drink is cinnamon tea. Steep a stick of cinnamon in boiling water for about 10 minutes, and let cool. Pitch the cinnamon, and sip the tea.

Flu:

It's Nothing to Sneeze At

Flu has become a catchall word for any malady from a bad cold to a stomachache that hits us in the fall or winter. But influenza is caused by a very specific group of viruses classified as type A, B, or C.

These viral strains have been known since the 1930s and 1940s. The worst is type A, which killed 20 million people in a global epidemic in 1918. Type A is also to blame for the 1957 Asian and the 1968 Hong Kong flu epidemics. Type B is also serious, but does not cause such widespread epidemics. Type C is the mildest form, and that is what most of us have experienced at one time or another.

FABULOUS FOLK REMEDY

Chamomile Calmer

Chamomile (*Matricaria recutita*) is one of our most versatile herbs and has been used historically in the treatment of various disorders. It is an antimicrobial, eases pain, calms the stomach, and induces relaxation. Use 1 teaspoon per 1 cup of water, and steep, covered, for 10 minutes. Drink 1 cup three times per day. **Caution: People with ragweed allergies may be sensitive to chamomile.**

The flu can hit you quite suddenly with fatigue, muscle pain, headache, fever, runny nose, and sore throat. A dry, hacking cough can follow congestion as the other symptoms progress. You may feel weak and tired for weeks after the flu has left the building. Here's how you can both sidestep and handle the flu:

Avoid crowds. The flu is highly contagious. If you happen to be in the same room with a person who sneezes or coughs, the airborne bug can literally bomb you with flu. At the height of flu season, boycott crowded places such as subways, theaters, and parties as much as you can. Airplanes aren't the best idea, either.

POWERFUL POTION

EUCALYPTUS OIL

To prevent passing the flu bug by hand-to-hand contact, clean those high-touch household surfaces, such as phones, countertops, and toilet handles. You can disinfect them with a few drops of eucalyptus oil mixed into a pint spray bottle. It will also unstuff your poor red nose as you work.

IT'S AN EMERGENCY!

If you have chest pain, wheezing, difficulty breathing, or are coughing up green or yellow sputum, these can be signs of pneumonia. This means the virus has infected your lungs or compromised your immune system. People over 65 are at serious risk for pneumonia, especially if they have other chronic conditions—such as diabetes, cancer, or heart or lung disease—and if they are in a hospital or nursing home. See your doctor promptly if any of these symptoms arise.

Hands off. Flu is also contagious through indirect transmission. This means that the virus can live for hours on telephones, faucets, or anything infected people who have not washed their hands have touched in passing. Once the bug enters a particular community—such as a school or nursing home—it spreads like a wildfire. So wash your hands frequently throughout the day during the flu season to reduce your chances of contamination. And make sure you wash them every time you return home.

Don't skip the shot. If you're very young, very old, have contact with the chronically ill, or just plain don't want the flu, you need to get a flu shot. It's best to get it in the fall to give the vaccine time to take effect. In North America, influenza season is from December to March and peaks in February. (It has been known to start before Thanksgiving.) In the tropics, flu thrives year-round. One caveat: Most doctors agree that those who are allergic to eggs should not get the shot. If you're in doubt, talk to your doctor before you do.

Be sweet to yourself. When preventive measures fail, and you're felled by the flu, make yourself as comfortable as you can. Influenza just has to run its course—usually 3 to 7 days. If you treat the symptoms, you'll at least feel better while your natural antibodies destroy the virus. Take acetaminophen or over-the-counter pain medications to fight the fever and ease the aches and pains while you rest and drink lots of fluids. (But avoid aspirin and never give it to a child who has the flu. It can bring on a condition called Reye syndrome, which can be fatal.)

O·D·D·B·A·L·L OINTMENT

Get Well with Garlic

Garlic (*Allium sativum*) has immune-stimulating and antiviral activities. If you don't mind the odor, you may want to try a garlic foot rub. Coat the soles of your feet with olive oil. (Better yet, have someone else do this for you, and enjoy a soothing foot massage!) Slice a clove of garlic in half, and rub the cut end on your well-oiled feet. Put on a pair of clean socks, and go to bed. **Caution:** The oils in garlic can cause burns, so it is imperative that you oil your feet well before applying the garlic to them.

Fluid Retention:

Pop That Water Balloon!

Some days—particularly hot, humid ones—we retain so much fluid that our bodies feel more like water balloons than flesh and bone. The problem is usually too much salt in the diet, food allergies, medications, or our body's own obnoxious way of getting ready to menstruate. In some cases, it can be heart or kidney disease.

How do you know which is which? You don't. But if you press your fingers into your flesh, and an indent remains

The Chinese Melon Cure

The Chinese use watermelons, cucumbers, and other melons to reduce fluid retention. These foods contain cucurbocitrin, which is said to increase the natural leakiness of tiny blood vessels, or capillaries, in the kidneys. This means that more water escapes into the kidneys for elimination.

O·D·D·B·A·L·L OINTMENT

Wrap It Up!

Make a strong infusion of yarrow (*Achillea millefolium*) and peppermint (*Mentha piperita*) by steeping 1 table-spoons of *each* in 1 pint of water. Strain and chill. Meanwhile, prepare several lengths of gauze, muslin, or cheesecloth. When the infusion is thoroughly chilled, saturate the cloths, wrap them around your lower legs, and relax—with your legs elevated—for 20 minutes or so. This will leave your legs refreshed and help discourage fluid retention there.

for a few moments, you're retaining fluid. If the fluid seems to hang around for a couple of days or return often, check with your doctor to make sure it's not caused by heart or kidney problems. Otherwise, when you're feeling a little plumped up, here's what may help deflate the problem:

Don't dehydrate. Rather than cutting back, you actually need to drink more water. The amount of fluid you drink has nothing to do with the fluid that bloats your body. Plenty of water every day actually helps drain excess fluids trapped in your body's tissues.

Skip the salt. Don't add extra salt to the foods you cook—too much makes your body hold on to water. You get a lot of salt in most prepared foods, so read labels for low-sodium alternatives, and take that shaker off your table.

Make like Peggy Lee. One of the torch singer's most famous songs is called "Black Coffee." If you don't drink coffee often and have trouble with fluid retention now and then, try a cup—black. Parsley and asparagus are also natural diuretics, so add these to your plate when you feel as though your decks are awash.

Balance your electrolytes. Potassium and magnesium counterbalance sodium and help reduce fluid in your body. To get

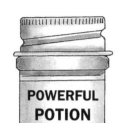

plenty of potassium, enjoy grapes, orange juice, vegetable juices, and—of course—bananas. Most of us get enough magnesium in the food we eat; but if you suspect you don't, add some wheat germ, whole grains, and nuts to your diet.

Put up your feet. If your ankles swell, that means fluid is pooling in your legs. But sitting down with your legs raised will allow the fluid to be moved more easily by your circulatory system. If ankle swelling is a chronic problem, check with your doctor—and keep a footstool handy.

POWERFUL POTION

BLOAT-BUSTING TONIC

To enhance lymphatic flow, combine equal parts of the following herbs: hawthorn (*Crataegus* spp.), horsechestnut (*Aesculus hippocastanum*), ginkgo (*Ginkgo biloba*), cleavers (*Galium aparine*), and dandelion leaf (*Taraxacum officinalis*). Steep 2 tablespoons of the mixture in 1 quart of water for 15 minutes, and drink, cool, throughout the day. **Caution:** Dandelion is rich in potassium and should not be taken with potassium tablets. And people on blood-thinning medications should consult their physicians before using ginkgo.

FABULOUS FOLK REMEDY

Pull the Plug

An old-fashioned remedy for fluid retention is the plant called pellitory of the wall (*Parietaria officinalis*). Steep 1 heaping tablespoon in 1 pint of water for 10 to 15 minutes. Drink $1/4$ cup once or twice daily.

Food Cravings:

Must-Haves No More

These days, if I don't have Ben and Jerry's Cherry Garcia frozen yogurt in my freezer, I panic.

But my cravings tend to change periodically. For about 7 years, I couldn't face the day without a bagel with my coffee every morning. Then one morning, I woke up and never wanted to see another bagel again.

Does this mean that someday I'm going to dump Ben and Jerry as well? It's hard to imagine, but the truth is food cravings can change, says Doreen Virtue, Ph.D. In most cases, they're triggered by hunger,

---

FABULOUS FOLK REMEDY

Craving Calming Tea

Food cravings that have their origins in emotional upheaval may respond to an herbal tea containing wood betony (*Betonica officinalis*). It is both a nervine and a digestive tonic that can be used long term, with no adverse effects. Make a tea using 1 teaspoon per 1 cup of hot water. Strain. Drink 1 cup twice daily.

hormonal changes, nutritional deficiencies, or some buried emotional issues that have never been addressed. And they may be connected to stress, fear, feeling blue, or unmet needs for fun. Or maybe they're tied to love, too much work (that one struck home!), or lack of appreciation.

If you have extremely bizarre cravings for nonfood objects like laundry starch or paint chips, particularly during pregnancy, they can be caused by magpie disease, or pica, which is named for the magpie bird—which eats anything. So if your cravings seem odd, check with your doctor. Otherwise, here are some commonsense ways to handle them:

Give in. Whether the craving is caused by repressing your feelings or by a nutrient deficiency, denying the craving will only make it worse, notes Dr. Virtue. That's why it's better to give in to it, unless it's something that can hurt you. So have a piece of chocolate or a scoop of ice cream when you feel the need.

Pass the pickles. The old joke about pregnant women waking up in the middle of the night craving pickles, or sometimes pizza, is not as far-fetched as it sounds. When you are pregnant, your digestion slows, perhaps creating a craving for vinegar or spicy foods. So if you're pregnant and craving a pickle or another very sour food, enjoy. On the other hand,

O·D·D·B·A·L·L OINTMENT

Temper Your Tastebuds

Food cravings are often a reaction to stress. So when you're feeling tense, temper your taste buds and relax your mind with aromatherapy. Rub a drop or two of essential oil of peppermint (*Mentha piperita*), chamomile (*Matricaria recutita*), or lavender (*Lavendula officinalis*) into your temples. Because essential oils can irritate sensitive skin, however, you may want to apply a thin layer of vegetable oil or lotion before putting on the essential oil.

if you find yourself craving ice, check with your doctor, because this seemingly innocent craving may indicate an iron deficiency.

Chow down on chocolate. The *Journal of the American Dietetic Association* reports that some people may crave chocolate to compensate for a magnesium deficiency. When you're stressed, your body uses more magnesium than it would normally, depleting your supply and leaving you feeling low. So, go ahead, have a little chocolate—it may regulate your mood and your magnesium. (How wonderful! Those dark chocolate chunks in Cherry Garcia really are good for me!)

But detour around too many sweets. If you anticipate your craving ahead of time, you may be able to get around it. For example, if you always crave sweets as your menstrual period approaches, be sure to eat high-starch foods or fruits. (They're part of your healthy daily diet anyway, right?) These foods raise your blood-sugar levels, so you won't crave the empty calories of sweets so intensely.

POWERFUL POTION

FEEL BETTER WITH BITTERS

Herbs that tone the digestive system can help normalize your eating patterns. Try a bitters formula taken warm before meals. Mix equal parts of dandelion root (*Taraxacum officinale*), centaury (*Centaurium erythraea*), chamomile (*Matricaria recutita*), and fennel (*Foeniculum vulgare*). Steep 2 teaspoons in 1 cup of hot water for 20 minutes; then strain. Drink ¼ to ⅓ cup before meals. **Caution:** Dandelion is rich in potassium and should not be taken with potassium tablets. Also, people with ragweed allergies should steer clear of chamomile.

Forgetfulness:

Mind over . . . *What?*

Excuse me, I'm having a senior moment. It's the latest witty line and may seem like a hip way to face the dilemma of forgetfulness. But I know personally that it's also a bit of black humor. Most of us fear losing our minds more than anything else that could conceivably happen with age. Okay, we could walk with a cane or two, give up marathon running, or even sport a hearing aid—but lose our brain power? Yikes!

The good news is, we can be forgetful for many reasons other than approaching dementia. Forgetfulness at midlife is more often a result of being busy, stressed, or short on

---

FABULOUS FOLK REMEDY

Remember Ginseng

Ginseng (*Panax ginseng*) is a whole-system tonic that helps you withstand stress, increase endurance, and improve mental performance. Steep 1 teaspoon of the herb in 1 cup of hot water for 15 minutes. Drink 1 to 2 cups daily. Take for no longer than 6 weeks at a time. If you have high blood pressure, check with your doctor first.

sleep. Estrogen loss in menopause may have some small effect, as can too much caffeine or a drop in blood-sugar levels. Clinical depression is a frequent cause of forgetfulness. And then there are some things that we may just not want to remember.

Memory is about attention. Just as we clean out our filing cabinets, we do the same with our mind's "memory files." Some things just become less important over time. Here's how to keep those memory files from disappearing too soon:

Fuel your memory banks. Memory loss is most often attributed to low blood sugar and fatigue. Be sure to eat nutritious, well-balanced meals—especially a good breakfast of protein and complex carbohydrates like whole-grained cereals and breads. You may find that your spells of forgetfulness come less often.

Eat Italiano style. An Italian study of diet and cognitive decline reported in *Neurology* found that cognitive impairment was less common among elderly people who ate a

Forget Hormones!

If you're a woman going through menopause, don't take hormone-replacement therapy (HRT) because you think it will keep your mind sharp. Studies have shown that it makes little difference, despite the long-held belief that menopause makes muddy thinkers. (It may just be interrupted sleep from all those hot flashes that makes us too tired to think straight!) The Harvard Nurses Health Study tested more than 2,000 nurses ages 70 to 74 and found no difference in memory function among those who did or did not use HRT. Other studies have supported these findings.

Mediterranean diet, which includes lots of olive oil—a monounsaturated fat. As their "healthy fat" intake increased, their risk of memory problems declined.

So when you cook, swap the saturated, brain-fogging fats like butter and marbled meats for healthy monounsaturated fats—like olive and canola oils. Use them not only on pasta, but also in salad dressings and hearty soups.

Find some folate. If you don't get enough folate (folic acid), your brain could atrophy, according to a recent study. Folate, as well as vitamins B_6 and B_{12}, may keep your gray matter going by keeping homocysteine levels in check. Elevated homocysteine, a by-product of methionine metabolism, is associated with Alzheimer disease. So pad your diet with folate-rich orange juice, broccoli and other cruciferous veggies, avocados, and legumes. Vitamin B_6 is found in meat, poultry,

POWERFUL POTION

GINKGO TEA

This lovely tea may not turn you into a wizard, but it will certainly give your brain a healthy workout. Combine 2 parts of ginkgo (*Ginkgo biloba*) with 1 part *each* of rosemary (*Rosemarinus officinalis*), yarrow (*Achillea millefolium*), and hawthorn (*Crataegus* spp.). Use 1 heaping teaspoon of the mixture per 1 cup of hot water, and steep, covered, for 15 minutes. Drink 1 to 2 cups per day. **Caution:** People on blood-thinning medication or aspirin should consult their doctors before using ginkgo.

whole grains, and green leafy vegetables; and vitamin B_{12} is mostly found in meat.

Balance your blood sugar. Dutch researchers recently found that the risk of dementia quadruples if you have a blood-sugar problem. In the Rotterdam Study, these researchers spent 5 years studying 6,370 people who were at least 55 years old. They were stunned to find that the risk of dementia is highest in those on insulin therapy. Both high and low sugar levels appear to make the problem worse. If you have diabetes, that means that tight control of blood sugar is even more important than you might have thought. If your blood sugar tends to spike highs or lows, talk to your doctor about new ways to monitor and control it.

Try food for thought. Remember hearing about brain food—eat a brain to get a brain? (Yuck!) Well, folklore aside, our brains need lecithin, which is found in beans, egg yolks, and cabbage, to produce chemicals that act as messengers for our thoughts and memories. We also need minerals like magnesium, potassium, and

Life's a Bowl of What?

Eating ½ cup of blueberries a day may clear the sludge from your memory banks and improve your balance and coordination, reports a Tufts University study. Blueberries are reported to have the highest antioxidant level of any fruit or vegetable. The berry's blue color comes from a pigment called anthocyanin, an antioxidant. So keep bags of frozen blueberries on hand, and add them to your oatmeal, smoothies, and salads for a brain-boosting treat.

boron, which are important for mental alertness. Millet, dark leafy greens (such as collards, kale, and broccoli), and figs are full of these minerals.

Take vitamin E. Reporting in the journal *Neurology*, doctors at New York City's Weill Cornell Women's Health Center concluded that supplements of vitamin E and C had a significant protective effect against vascular dementia (loss of cognitive function due to atherosclerosis). The study subjects performed better on tests, too. And in a 1997 study, vitamin E slowed the mental decline of patients with Alzheimer disease. Just one caveat: Vitamin E supplements may not be advisable if you are also taking aspirin, garlic, or other blood thinners.

Curb the stress. Stress makes your adrenal glands pump out a hormone that can lead to difficulty retrieving long-term memories. A study reported in *Nature Neuroscience* showed that chronic stress floods the body with cortisol. The cortisol overload is associated with memory problems, fuzzy thinking, and difficulty in concentrating and making decisions. Do all you can to control the stress in your life—and consider some counseling if you just can't seem to relax. Check out **Stress** for more helpful ways to create a little bit of breathing space in your life.

Bust a move. If you're serious about getting your exercise, you're more likely to be mentally sharp, too. Physical activity boosts the production of brain chemicals. A study of sedentary individuals who began taking brisk walks showed that they improved in both mental agility and concentration. So add a brisk daily walk to your routine. Well supplied with oxygen, your brain will remember better—and the rest of you will feel better, too.

Use it or lose it. Studies of healthy people, according to the Weill Cornell Women's Health Center, suggest that ongoing mental stimulation—such as work, continuing education, extensive reading, mentally challenging games, and crossword puzzles—can keep your mind sharp. Scores of laboratory studies link mental activity and the production of protective neurotrophins. Even Alzheimer disease is less common among the well educated (although many smart people do suffer it). The explanation? Mentally active folks may have an increased brain reserve, more neurons, and a more complex cell-to-cell communication system to draw on if some brain cells sustain damage. So take out the chessboard (or learn if you've never played), write in a journal, or design that gadget you've always wished you had.

Chose brains over brawn. Consider taking another look at that shy guy who always has his nose buried in a book. The same Women's Health Center study revealed that living with an intellectually stimulating spouse enhances you mentally, too. (Let the boy toys and material girls have each other, so you can make a wiser, more adult choice.)

Keep on the sunny side. If you're happy with your relationships, you're

IT'S AN EMERGENCY!

If your forgetfulness is constant and causing serious problems, see your doctor to rule out a systemic problem, such as low blood pressure or chronic fatigue syndrome.

less likely to develop dementia, according to a study reported in *The Lancet*. Researchers questioned 1,200 people who were at least 75 years old about three aspects of their social lives: whether they lived alone, had friends, and had satisfying relationships with their children. Over the following 3 years, those older adults with the poorest social networks were 60 percent more likely to develop dementia than those who had only one unsatisfactory area or who had a rich, extensive social network. So keep your

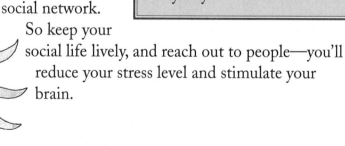

social life lively, and reach out to people—you'll reduce your stress level and stimulate your brain.

Be a Fat Head!

Brain cells are 60 percent fat, which is needed to transmit the impulses that carry thought. In a healthy brain, the omega-3 fatty acids predominate. In fact, low levels of omega-3s have been linked to depression and to the risk of Alzheimer disease. How do you get these healthy fatty acids? They're plentiful in oily fish, walnuts, and flaxseed. To benefit your whole body, add a handful of nuts, a serving of fish, or 2 tablespoons of freshly ground flaxseed to your diet every day.

Gallstones:

Lighten the Load

Like many overweight, middle-aged women, my friend Pam is prone to gallstones. She nearly scared us to death when she was rushed to the hospital with severe chest and stomach pains after eating a swordfish dinner. Her family thought she'd had a heart attack. But what Pam had was a gallbladder that was already gangrenous because her doctor had refused to take seriously her previous complaints of pain.

Here's the inside story on gallstones: After a meal, your gallbladder releases a greenish brown fluid called bile that helps you digest and absorb fats. Gallstones form when the bile hardens into crystals

IT'S AN EMERGENCY!

A gallbladder attack can often be mistaken for a heart attack. Gallstone pain begins in the lower right abdomen, and shoots upward to the shoulder and around the back to the right shoulder blade. If you have any unusual abdominal pain that won't go away, fever, sweating, chills, yellowish skin, yellowing of the whites of your eyes, or clay-colored stool, see your doctor immediately.

Lovely Lavender

When gallstones cause gall-bladder spasms, place a few drops of lavender essential oil in a hot tub of water. Soak your whole body until the water cools or the spasms pass.

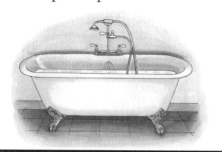

that can range in size from a grain of sand to a golf ball. Since bile is made of cholesterol and other substances, gallstones are actually hardened cholesterol.

Oddly, though, cholesterol-lowering drugs can increase your risk of gallstones, because they increase the amount of cholesterol secreted in the bile. Other risks include diabetes, dieting, and high levels of serum triglycerides. Excess estrogen from pregnancy, hormone-replacement therapy, or birth-control pills also may increase the amount of cholesterol in the bile. And for some people, there's a genetic risk. Here's how to prevent gallstones before they start:

Roll the stones away. Since women have twice the risk of gallstones than men do, it pays to get moving. Increase your exercise routine to 2 to 3 hours a week—studies

POWERFUL POTION

SPASM STOPPERS

To tone, relieve inflammation, and release spasms in the liver and biliary tract, try dandelion root (*Taraxacum officinale*), milk thistle (*Silybum marianum*), artichoke (*Cynara scolymus*), greater celandine (*Chelidonium majus*), butterbur (*Petasites hybridus*), or even peppermint (*Mentha piperita*). Put 1 teaspoon of any one of these dried herbs into 1 cup of hot water. Steep for 15 minutes, strain, and drink 1 cup, warm, between meals. **Caution:** Dandelion is rich in potassium and should not be taken with potassium tablets.

FABULOUS FOLK REMEDY

Dandelion Salad

Old-timers used to pick young dandelion leaves in early spring to cure what ailed 'em. The powerful compounds in the leaves act like a mild laxative and digestion stimulator. And it's a long-held belief that these same compounds can bust up those painful little stones. If you're prone to stones, it probably wouldn't hurt to toss a few dandelion leaves with some salad oil once in a while and serve 'em up at dinner.

show you'll be much less likely to develop gallstones than your sedentary sisters. Need more motivation? Think about 20-20 (not the TV show). Walk briskly for *20 minutes* a day, 5 to 7 days a week, and you'll reduce your chances of developing gallstones by *20 percent,* according to recent studies. The more active you are, the less your gallstone risk.

Suck up the C. One study examined data from 13,000 people and found that women with low levels of vitamin C were more likely to get gallstones, according to Joel Simon, M.D., assistant professor of nutrition at the University of California at San Francisco. That's why it's important to add foods rich in vitamin C to your diet. Citrus fruit and juices are your best sources—a whole orange, for example, offers 70 milligrams of vitamin C.

Put away your diet books. When you are fasting, skipping meals, or severely restricting your calorie intake, you decrease the action of your gallbladder, which allows the bile to become oversaturated with cholesterol. The cholesterol settles into stones, and you become a gravel pit. So if you want to lose weight, instead of living on lettuce leaves and no-fat salad dressing, eat less at regular intervals, don't skip meals, and aim for a gradual, long-term weight goal.

Gingivitis:

Keep Those Dad-Blame Gums Healthy!

Unless somebody's whacked you right in the kisser, most of us have no excuse for holes in our jaws. If you live to be 100, do it smiling—with your 100-year-old choppers intact. Why lose 'em, when you can nip that possibility right in the . . . gum?

When inflamed gums begin to bleed, that's gingivitis—and it's a major cause of tooth loss. The process starts with plaque, that sticky film of bacteria, mucus, and food debris that forms constantly on your teeth. (Don't mind a little plaque? No problem—

Gum Paste

If you want to clear up a persistent case of gingivitis, try this inexpensive yet very effective gum paste. Shake about 1 teaspoon of baking soda into a small dish, and drizzle in just enough hydrogen peroxide to make a paste. Then work it gently under the gumline with your toothbrush. Leave the paste on for a few minutes, then rinse well.

NATURAL

Baking Soda

For Baking
Cleaning
& Deodorizing

Swish with Salt

Plain salt is a wonderful gum healer. Add ¼ teaspoon of salt to ¼ cup of warm water. Stir to dissolve, and use as a mouthwash two to three times daily.

leave it there, so it can mineralize into the hard substance called tartar. Then you can contemplate your decision while the dental hygienist is trying to knock the tartar off your teeth with a chisel.)

Most of the time, gingivitis is about poor dental hygiene, but it can also result from an injury to the gums, irritation from fillings and bridges, or *too* vigorous brushing and flossing. Diabetes can add to the risk, as can the use of birth-control pills. When the process starts, your gums may be red, swollen, and quick to bleed; but according to the American Dental Association (ADA), you can cure gingivitis at the early stage with good hygiene. Neglect it, however, and gingivitis can become periodontitis. That's when the gums and bone that support your teeth are seriously damaged, and teeth loosen, fall out, or, in the worst case, have to be removed.

Gingivitis can also lead to heart disease and stroke. Honest. Studies have found that people with periodontal problems risk letting bacteria seep into the bloodstream through the ruptured blood vessels in bleeding gums. And a massive amount of this bacteria can cause a thrombosis, a blood clot that could travel anywhere and cause a heart attack or stroke.

POWERFUL POTION

A MYRRHVALOUSLY SAGE MOUTHWASH

Myrrh (*Commiphora molmol*), sage (*Salvia officinalis*), and calendula (*Calendula officinalis*) tone and protect tissues against infection. Add 5 drops of tincture of *each* to a small amount of warm water, and swish around your mouth for several minutes two to three times a day.

O·D·D·B·A·L·L OINTMENT

Paint with Goldenseal

Goldenseal (*Hydrastis canadensis*) helps protect against infection, while strengthening the tissues of the gums and mouth. Use a clean, new paintbrush, and paint the gums with a tincture of goldenseal once or twice daily. (The tincture is generally available at health-food stores.) Goldenseal can irritate gums, so test first by just dabbing one spot on your gums with the brush. If no irritation shows the next day, go ahead, and paint away!

To minimize this danger, both the American Heart Association and the ADA not only advise a strict regimen of dental hygiene but also recommend that everyone with heart problems tell their dentists that they need to take antibiotics before any dental procedure—including simple cleaning.

Here's how to keep gingivitis from ever becoming a threat:

Spot the early warning signs. If you have chronic bad breath, tooth sensitivity to hot or cold, and red, shiny gums, you may have gingivitis. Left untreated, this progresses to chronic infection and bone degeneration. Watch for loose or shifting teeth, receding gums that leave the root exposed, gum pain, and inflammation and pockets or pus between teeth and gums. And get to your dentist to deal with them ASAP.

Keep your mouth clean. Conscientious dental care can stop bacteria buildup, gum swelling, and redness before they start. It's just as simple as you've been told: Brush at least twice a day and floss at least once daily. If you are prone to gingivitis, your dentist may also recommend that you do both right after every meal and also at bedtime.

Get a talking toothbrush. Brush your teeth for 2 minutes or more. Some electric toothbrushes are a great help with this because they have a built-in signal mechanism that reminds you to work on all four areas of your mouth for 30 seconds each, according to Stephen Markow, M.D. Try to cheat this type of Terrible Toothbrush by taking it out too early and you'll find yourself dealing with a vibrating machine that sprays toothpaste all over your bathroom.

Be an apple polisher. Apples contain compounds that inhibit the gum-destroying enzymes secreted by oral bacteria. So crunch an apple a day to help clean your mouth between brushings. If you don't like apples, look for apple extract at a health-food store. It provides the same protective action.

Keep your mouth well watered. Water stimulates the production of saliva that you need to fight excess mouth bacteria. Be sure to drink 8 to 10 glasses a day.

POWERFUL POTION

CHAMOMILE CLEANSER

Keep your gums in good health with chamomile tea. Infuse 2 teaspoons of dried chamomile in 1 cup of boiling water, and let the mixture steep for a good 10 minutes. Drink 1 cup after every meal, and let the chamomile do what it does best: kill germs and reduce your risk of gingivitis. **Caution:** People with ragweed allergies may be sensitive to chamomile.

Glaucoma:

Preserve Your Peepers

Because it usually has no warning symptoms, glaucoma is called the sneak thief of sight. "The tragedy is that 90 percent of the more than 80,000 Americans who are blind as a result of glaucoma did not have to lose their sight," says Robert Ritch, M.D., medical director of the Glaucoma Foundation. The good news? With regular eye examinations, even if you should develop glaucoma, you won't need to join their ranks. Caught early, glaucoma is treatable.

The simplest explanation is that glaucoma is like high blood pressure of the eye, according to Alex Eaton, M.D., of the Eye Centers of Florida in Fort Myers. Eye fluid that normally drains away as fast as it is secreted begins to build up—sometimes due to a faulty drainage channel between the back of the cornea and the iris. Drug treatment

POWERFUL POTION

SEE WITH C

Vitamin C is a powerful antioxidant that may help strengthen the vasculature of the eye. Try taking 1,000 milligrams of vitamin C with bioflavonoids two to three times daily.

usually helps reduce the pressure, and laser surgery can open a blocked channel or create a new one if necessary.

Who gets glaucoma? Anyone from babies to senior citizens. But the condition's more common in older folks and those with a family history of glaucoma. It's also more common in African Americans and Asian Americans, according to the Glaucoma Foundation. Here's how to preserve your peepers:

Get regular eye examinations. Dig out your day planner, call your ophthalmologist, and schedule a regular eye exam. If you're under 45, every 4 years is fine. But make an appointment for every 2 years if you are over 45, of African descent, have a family history of glaucoma, have diabetes, have had a previous eye injury, or have used cortisone steroid products.

Take your medication seriously. Glaucoma is usually treated with eyedrops, pills, surgery, or a combination of methods. Your eyesight's on the line, so it's vital to use your medications correctly. If you change your medication regimen without consulting your doctor, you could develop side effects or even go blind, warns the Glaucoma Foundation. Refill your prescriptions before they run out, so you don't miss any doses. Wait 15 minutes between drops so they are more effective. And *never* stop your medications just because you have no obvious symptoms. It can be tricky to apply eye drops properly, so ask your doctor for some hints.

FABULOUS FOLK REMEDY

Bilberry Tea Time

Bilberries (*Vaccinium myrtillis*) are high in vitamin C and rich in bioflavonoids, which may help reduce pressure in the eye. Include 1 to 3 cups of bilberry tea as part of your daily fluid intake. Steep 1 teaspoon of the herb in 1 cup of hot water for 15 minutes; then drink.

Hair Loss:

The Naked Truth

If you're a guy reading this, I'm about to do you a big favor. No matter how painful it may be to see that you're heading for cue-ball city, "comb-overs" are the ugliest, most pitiful thing ever invented. Period. Bar none. Any woman, on any planet, in any solar system, would rather rub, pat, or even kiss a nice naked scalp than have to sit across from you contemplating the pathetic strands of hair that start a few inches above your ear and wind up draped over the top of your head, totally defying gravity (and common sense). Believe me. The truth may hurt, but in this case, it's a kindness.

If you're a woman reading

Is It Something You Ate?

Not likely. Only about 1 percent of hair loss is related to nutrition. But in a few cases, an excess of vitamin A or a deficiency in iron or potassium can play a role in thinning hair. And if you frequently down raw egg whites, your body's supply of biotin, a nutrient needed for healthy hair growth, might be diminished.

this, I know it's harder. Hair loss is common and accepted in men. Heck, they can even grow a beard to compensate.

Unfortunately, at menopause, with diminishing estrogen, women's hair tends to thin. Sometimes hormone-replacement therapy helps, but there are other ways to compensate. Hair loss, or *alopecia,* can also be caused temporarily by chemotherapy, acute fever, a thyroid disorder, tuberculosis, and even pregnancy. But in these cases, once the underlying physical cause is corrected, the hair grows in again.

If you're getting thin up top, check with your doctor to rule out any serious cause like thyroid disease or a hormonal imbalance. Then consider the following strategies:

Be brave, be bald. If you no longer have a full head of hair, why not shave off what little is left? Bald is sexy. Think of Yul Brynner and Telly Savalas's *Kojak.* Why, these days, even women

POWERFUL POTION

A STIMULATING HAIR TONIC

Elder (*Sambucus canadensis*), nettles (*Urtica dioica*), prickly ash (*Xanthoxylum clava-herculis*), and yarrow (*Achillea millefolium*) are nutrient-rich herbs that help increase circulation—necessary for healthy hair growth. Steep 1 heaping teaspoon any of these herbs in 1 pint of hot water. Drink, warm, throughout the day.

FABULOUS FOLK REMEDY

Meddle with Nettles

An herbal vinegar rinse helps maintain a healthy scalp and encourages hair growth. Simmer 1 ounce of nettles in 1 cup of apple cider vinegar for 15 minutes. Strain, and store in a cool, dark place. After shampooing, mix 1/4 cup of the herbal vinegar in 1 pint of warm water and use as a rinse. Just remember to wear gloves when handling fresh nettle to avoid their stinging hairs.

Kink It Up a Notch

One handy way to disguise thinning hair is to get a perm for fullness. Curls cover more real estate than straight lines of hair do, and gentle mussing also offers some camouflage.

are making a statement with their naked pates: consider pop singers Sinead O'Connor and Joan Jett. So if you're feeling bold, reach for the razor.

Count heads. Want to estimate your chances? Men have more permanent hair loss than women. It's hormonal, and it usually runs in families. If you're wondering about your risk, just survey family members on both sides. If naked scalps pop up in those family photos, start thinking through how you'll want to handle that inheritance. Your options range from "bald is beautiful" to hair transplants and toupees. (Fortunately, they no longer look like weasels taking naps on your head.)

Reach for Rogaine. Rogaine is a hair treatment that has been approved by the U.S. Food and Drug Administrations (FDA) for use by both men and women. Read the directions carefully before you rub it into your scalp. And ask your doctor if it's safe for you—especially if you have medical conditions that require continuous use of

O·D·D·B·A·L·L OINTMENT

Reach for Rosemary

Scalp massage may be done—gently—to enhance circulation and encourage hair growth. Mix 4 to 6 drops of rosemary oil (*Rosemarinus officinalis*) in 1 tablespoon of olive oil. Gently massage into your scalp. For a deepening effect, cover your hair with a shower cap, and wrap a hot, wet towel around your head. Leave it on for 30 minutes; then shampoo.

medications. Rogaine is not for everyone.

Shampoo. There are so many volume-izing shampoos available that it's quite obvious that those of us who are Baby Boomers are trying to avoid as many bad hair days as possible. While these shampoos won't grow more hair, they will plump up your hair strands. Use these shampoos daily. Blow dry or shake out your hair, and it will seem much fuller than it is.

Color me full. Use hair color to reduce the see-through scalp look. If your hair color is close to your skin color, your scalp will be less noticeable. But if you color your hair at home, use only the semi-permanent dyes. These are not harsh, but they will plump up your hair shaft so that it looks thicker. Avoid permanent dyes. Since they don't wash out, they create a color line between natural and dyed hair that seems to make thinning hair more obvious.

POWERFUL POTION

SAW PALMETTO

Baldness. It's a guy thing—and so is saw palmetto. Some herbalists believe saw palmetto can treat baldness or at least slow down hair loss for men. It seems that saw palmetto contains an ingredient that reduces dihydrotestosterone (DHT) levels, which contribute to male-pattern hair loss.

If you'd like to try saw palmetto, buy a tincture at the health-food store. Drop 2 milliliters into a glass of water or juice, and take it up to three times a day.

Hangover:

Hair of the Dog Revisited

Some people still believe a Bloody Mary is a legitimate remedy for a hangover. The morning-after thinking seems to be that a little tomato juice early in the day has to be healthy; the Tabasco sauce proves I've still got my, er, potency; and maybe more alcohol will numb this terrible pounding in my head.

True, tomato juice is a good idea. It will help restore the fluids that the alcohol has sucked out of you. But Tabasco doesn't do anything except remind your taste buds that they're still alive. As for alcohol, well, skip the splash of vodka. It disrupts your body chemistry. It irritates your stomach lining. It dilates your blood vessels. And it's a diuretic, so it dehydrates you, which is how it created that throbbing headache. There are better ways to deal with your

Your Hangover Menu

Ease your poor self to the kitchen, where you can find the cure for what ails you.

For starters, drink lots of fluid. Lemon balm tea is delicious and will help ease your headache and lift your sagging spirits. Put 2 teaspoons of dried lemon balm leaves in 1 cup of boiling water. Let it steep and cool. Strain the herbs, and drink up. Another good choice is ginger ale (or ginger tea), which will help calm your stomach.

For the main course, load up on carbs. Try a slice of good rye bread with caraway seeds; the seeds combat nausea and indigestion. How about two or three ginger snaps? The ginger will soothe your stomach. Or dig into some strawberry shortcake. The strawberries will lessen that pounding in your skull.

To finish, eat some lean protein. Protein will help your brain cells regenerate. Good picks include a slice or two of cooked turkey breast; a hard-boiled egg, which is easy to digest and packed with protein; and a nice, cool glass of skim milk.

headache, queasiness, thirst, and befuddlement. Here are some tips:

Water your brain. Your most urgent need is to rehydrate your body, so keep guzzling the H_2O. No matter how much fruit juice, branch water, or ginger ale you may have mixed it with, alcohol is a potent diuretic which dries you out. Your brain is

FABULOUS FOLK REMEDY

Pucker Up!

A little lemon squeezed or sliced into a glass of water may help prevent a hangover. Drink a glass before bed and first thing the next morning.

mostly water, and it gets peeved when you make it thirsty. That pounding headache after a night of stacking swizzle sticks is no more and no less than your brain's cry for water.

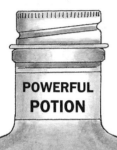

POWERFUL POTION

BITTERS FEEL BETTER

Bitters may help your liver metabolize alcohol. Make some by mixing equal parts of dandelion root (*Taraxacum officinalis*), gentian (*Gentiana lutea*), milk thistle (*Silybum marianum*), and peppermint (*Mentha piperita*). Steep 1 heaping teaspoon of the mixture in 1 cup of hot water for 20 minutes; then sip slowly before bed and again first thing in the morning. **Caution:** Dandelion is rich in potassium and shouldn't be taken with potassium tablets.

IT'S AN EMERGENCY!

If your hangover includes unusual symptoms such as fever, trembling, or nausea, get help immediately. You could have a serious problem caused by the alcohol or an inadvertent interaction with medication, which can also cause a hangover.

Pig out. Once you've rehydrated your sorry cells, your next mandate is to munch on carbohydrate-rich foods. These are the easiest to digest when your stomach is not up to any hard labor. Have a big muffin or a plate of leftover party goodies.

Start perking. If your stomach isn't too queasy, down a cup of coffee to help your headache. Choose the full-test kind with plenty of caffeine.

Say cheese. Wine and cheese are traditionally served together for good reason. The cheese absorbs some of the alcohol, so it doesn't go from your stomach right to your brain.

BEAR MOUNTAIN COFFEE

Headache:

Get Your Head
Out of the Vise

POWERFUL POTION

WILLOW WORKS

Willow bark contains salicin, which metabolizes in the body like aspirin, its synthetic sister. Chew some fresh willow twigs to ease the pain of a headache. Or, if there's no willow tree nearby, try the more powerful tea or tincture (30 drops of tincture every 4 to 6 hours).

Did you know there are his and hers headaches? Yep. Migraines affect mostly women, and cluster headaches seem to be a guy thing. All the rest, like tension headaches, are equal-opportunity pain producers. That's plumb fascinating—unless your head's an anvil, and your headache's the blacksmith's sledgehammer.

Like most women, migraines are seriously misunderstood. While men do get migraines, women have more attacks and more painful ones. The peak ages for the occurrence of migraines is between 35 and 45 years, and these headaches are tough to diagnose, since they come with a bewildering mix of symptoms. Along with the knee-buckling pain of the headache, you may be battling nausea, hypersensitivity to light and sound, and numbing exhaustion. Then throw in a little blurred vision or dizziness, for good measure.

Unlike migraines, the cluster headache mostly hits guys aged 25 to 50 years. A cluster headache starts fast, with excruciating pain in or around one eye, and may also bring redness, tearing, a drooping or puffy eyelid, and a stuffy or runny nose. The episodic type strikes once or several times every day at around the same time, lasting 15 minutes or several hours. Then it disappears for months or even years. The chronic cluster headache is the same torment, but full-time, unfortunately.

Many doctors and even people who get migraines do not distinguish between migraines and other headaches, according to Seymour Diamond, M.D., director of the Diamond Headache Clinic and of Chicago's Columbus Hospital Inpatient Headache Unit. The confusion's understandable. A migraine is a complex brain disorder that can be triggered by anything from diet and hormones to

FABULOUS FOLK REMEDY

Mash a Migraine

Feverfew (*Tanacetum parthenium*) is an herb used since the Middle Ages as a headache remedy, and its renewed popularity is supported by scientific research.

For prevention of headaches, chew one fresh leaf a day.

When a headache is starting up, prepare a tea of feverfew, lemon balm (*Melissa officinalis*), and gingerroot by using 1 teaspoon of dried herb per 1 cup of hot water and steeping for 10 minutes. Drink up to 3 cups daily. **Caution:** Feverfew may cause mouth irritation in sensitive individuals. It is also a uterine stimulant and should not be taken during pregnancy.

changes in the weather, seasons, or even sleep patterns. The trigger causes blood vessels in the brain to constrict and then relax, and their distortions prompt the pain.

Although it won't make you psychic, some migraines start with an "aura"—a show of lights or spots or another unexplained sensation, such as tingling, feeling cold, a food craving, mood change, a sudden burst of energy, or frequent yawning. Another type (aura-free) usually starts with pulsating pain on one side of the head and lasts from 4 to 72 hours. These can worsen when you're moving around—not that you're likely to when you're nauseated or vomiting—since both light and sound can cause you more pain.

Here are some ways to get some relief:

Needle your pain. The National Institutes of Health has released a lengthy list of conditions for which acupuncture is effective, including headaches. To treat headaches, the acupuncture needles remain in place for about 20 minutes. If you don't know a local acupuncturist, ask your doctor for a

POWERFUL POTION

EVENING PRIMROSE OIL

The night-blooming herb evening primrose contains phenylalanine, one of the best natural sources of pain relief. The powerful medicine in this herb is found in the seeds, specifically, in the seeds' oil. Because the seeds are tiny and the oil almost impossible to extract, you'll save yourself another headache by simply purchasing it at the health-food store. Look for evening primrose oil capsules. The recommended daily dose is 1,000 to 2,000 milligrams, or three to six capsules.

recommendation. All practitioners should be able to offer proof of their training; make sure they use only disposable needles.

Try the caffeine-and-aspirin fix. The combination of 130 milligrams of caffeine (that's about $1\frac{1}{2}$ cups of coffee) and two aspirins relieves a headache 40 percent better than does the pain reliever alone, according to the National Headache Foundation. In addition to starting your motor in the mornings, caffeine also helps your body absorb medications. The full effects are felt in 30 minutes and last 3 to 5 hours. Some headache remedies already contain caffeine, so be sure to read the ingredients—you may need to take fewer pain relievers if you take them with coffee.

But don't get too much jolt from your java. The average American drinks 2 to 3 cups of coffee a day—and that's okay. According to the World Health Organization and the American Psychiatric Association, caffeine is not addictive or habit-forming in the same way that other drugs are.

Try prescription prevention. One approach to frequent migraines is to prevent their start with ongoing medication. Talk to your doctor about the new drugs available to treat migraines, including antidepressants, beta-blockers, calcium-channel blockers, and serotonin antagonists.

IT'S AN EMERGENCY!

Sometimes, a headache can be due to some underlying disease process, such as a brain tumor or meningitis. Sudden, intense or chronic and worsening head pain should always send you skittering to the emergency room.

Don't let the cure kill you. If you prefer to treat each episode by taking medication prescribed by your doctor and using it when you need it, be sure you really take it—there's no sense being a martyr. But try not to give in when an extra dose is tempting, and stop taking the medication as soon as you can. Taking too much medicine can give you yet another pain in the brain, called a rebound headache.

Quit smoking. If you're hooked on nicotine, the next time you're flattened by a migraine or cluster headache, say these words to yourself: "Smoking triggers my headaches and makes them harder to treat." Repeat this mantra until you feel well enough to get to your doctor's office—then ask for help in quitting. There are many new stop-smoking aids these days. Even if you've tried and failed before, you can do it.

Don't feed your migraine. Many people with migraines find their attacks are connected to what they eat—starting 1 to 24 hours after a meal. Trigger foods include alcoholic beverages, particularly red wines and beer; aged cheeses; smoked fish; sour cream; yogurt; and, alas, chocolate, even though some people crave it just before an

POWERFUL POTION

AN EXOTIC ELIXER

For tension headaches, combine gentle pain- and stress-relieving herbs for fast relief. Try equal parts of tinctures of ginger (*Zingiber officinale*), jamaican dogwood (*Piscidia erythrina*), kava (*Piper methysticum*), and wood betony (*Stachys betonica*). Take 15 to 20 drops of the mixture every 30 minutes for relief of acute pain, up to four times in 24 hours. **Caution:** Kava has recently been linked with liver toxicity. Check with your doctor before using it.

It's All in the Family

While a migraine headache can affect anyone, two groups stand out: women and children who have a parent who is also affected by migraines. Migraines are more a result of genetics than anything else—70 percent of migraine patients have a family history of the disease. If both your parents had migraines, you've got a 75 percent chance of having them, too.

attack. Food additives and preservatives such as monosodium glutamate (MSG) and sodium nitrate (often found in luncheon meats) are known triggers, as are sweeteners containing aspartame. Caffeine and junk food can add to the problem.

To figure out if food's fueling your headaches, keep a simple diary. Write down what you eat and when as well as when your headaches occur. You'll spot the connections. And try to eat regularly, three times a day—that may also help fend off migraines.

Manage stress. A stressful situation can trigger a migraine immediately afterward—it's called a "let-down" migraine. If you are living a migraine lifestyle, you need to take stress seriously. Take up regular aerobic exercise, such as walking, swimming, or bicycling. Whichever activity 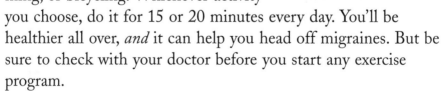 you choose, do it for 15 or 20 minutes every day. You'll be healthier all over, *and* it can help you head off migraines. But be sure to check with your doctor before you start any exercise program.

Treat your feet. Reflexology is a type of massage therapy in which pressure is applied to places on the feet that are believed to influence other parts of the body. Find a reflexology practi-

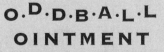

tioner and give the treatment a try—it may just be the answer to your desperate migraine prayers. In a Danish study, regular reflexology treatments helped 81 percent of people who got migraines find relief. And 20 percent were even able to go off their pain medication.

Treat sinus conditions. Sinusitis, which is basically an infection and inflammation of the sinus cavities in your head or face, can often cause a headache. The holes through which fluids drain out of your sinuses become clogged and create a vacuum. It is exquisitely painful. If you're prone to this, check

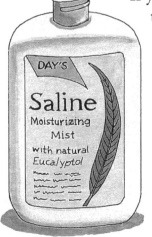

with your doctor. Antibiotics are frequently needed to clear the infection, but decongestants—saline sprays, nose gels with eucalyptus, and eating spicy foods—are the only thing that will unstuff your sinuses.

O·D·D·B·A·L·L OINTMENT

Level Pain with Lavender

A drop or two of essential oil of lavender (*Lavendula officinalis*) massaged into the temples can help relieve a headache. For sensitive skin, apply a thin layer of vegetable oil or lotion before using the essential oil. Better yet, massage the lavender into the tender pad of muscle between your thumb and index finger—an acupuncture point for headaches.

Heartburn:

You Are What—and How— You Eat

You've seen those TV commercials where guys get up in the middle of the night because they ate too many hot peppers, right? They can't sleep because they have heartburn. Of course, they take some over-the-counter antacid to ease the pain so they can sleep.

And once in a while, that's fine. But long-term use of antacids can alter calcium metabolism, cause diarrhea, and increase magnesium levels, which can damage the kidneys in those prone to kidney disease. That's why heartburn *prevention* is better than a medicine cabinet full of home remedies. If you feel the need to take antacids for more than 3 weeks, see your doctor to make sure the

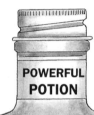

POWERFUL POTION

LICORICE

Licorice root (*Glycyrrhiza glabra*) soothes stomach fires and increases circulation for healing at the same time. Use chewable tablets of deglycyrrhizinated licorice, which have had the hypertension-causing component of licorice root removed. Chew 2 to 4 tablets before meals, or use as directed.

Slippery Elm to the Rescue

Tame heartburn quickly with slippery elm lozenges. You can buy them at the health food store or make up your own. For you adventurous souls, here's how to make them: Preheat the oven to 250°F. In a small bowl, mix ¼ cup of slippery elm powder with 3 tablespoons of honey. Form it into a nonsticky dough. Then add 4 drops of vanilla extract. On a cutting board dusted with flour, roll the dough into a long, thin shape. Cut the roll into bite-size pieces, and put them on a baking sheet. Allow them to bake for 1 hour. Cool completely, and store in an airtight container—ready to pop into your mouth when your tummy is troubling you.

problem is simple heartburn. Then resolve to do the following:

FABULOUS FOLK REMEDY

Mellow Meadowsweet

Meadowsweet (*Filipendula ulmaria*) is a digestive herb that protects and soothes the stomach lining while reducing excess acidity. Sip a cup of meadowsweet tea between meals. To prepare, steep 1 heaping teaspoon in 1 cup of hot water for 15 minutes.

Get chew trained. Sit down and relax; then chew your food thoroughly. This increases your saliva production and makes the entire digestive process work more effectively. So don't eat and run or gulp your food. Your mommy was right—it's a lousy way to treat your tummy.

Don't lie down on dinner. Restrain yourself from flopping down on the couch after you've just indulged in a too-big, too-heavy meal. Bending over after overeating can also result in heartburn. So stay upright and walk off the calories—and the heartburn with some exercise.

Don't eat and head for bed. Wait 2 or 3 hours after eating a meal to go to bed. This gives your food a chance to digest, so it won't cause you discomfort when you lie down.

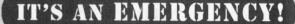

IT'S AN EMERGENCY!

The pain you believe is heartburn could be something more serious, like gallbladder inflammation or even a heart attack. Amateurs can't tell the difference. So if you have chest pain, particularly if it radiates into either arm or the jaw or is accompanied by nausea, fever, or chills, call an ambulance—and let the paramedics figure out the cause.

Skip the Starbucks. Coffee (decaf as well as caffeinated) promotes stomach acid production. And so do tea and cola drinks. The amount and acidity of the stomach acid you produce varies with each individual, but in most cases, cutting back on coffee, tea and colas can help prevent heartburn—and it won't hurt your smile, either (all three drinks can yellow your teeth).

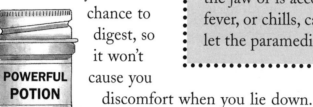

POWERFUL POTION

HEAVENLY ANGELICA TEA

Say a quick prayer of thanks for the lovely herb angelica (*Angelica archangelica*), which has the power to cool your heartburn. This herb can be made into a tea (it tastes a bit like celery) by putting 1 teaspoon of the dried herb (or 3 teaspoons of fresh, crushed leaves) in 1 cup of boiling water. Steep for about 10 minutes, strain out the herb, and enjoy 1 cup after meals.

Hemorrhoids:

Varicose Veins Where You Can't See Them

Hemorrhoids can be a real pain-in-the-you-know-what! Nothing more or less than varicose veins in the anus or rectum, hemorrhoids can be caused by pressures of pregnancy, chronic constipation, obesity, and, rarely, an obstruction in the lower intestine or a rectal tumor.

How do you know if you've got a hemorrhoid? Hemorrhoids announce themselves with intermittent bleeding during bowel movements, itching, and sometimes acute pain.

Whether and how to treat them simply depends on how

FABULOUS FOLK REMEDY

Horseradish Poultice

Whoa, Dobbin! It's time to mount an attack on those itchy, burny hemorrhoids with a homemade horseradish poultice, which can speed up the healing process by drawing blood to the area. Apply a thin layer of fresh, grated horseradish to a wet cloth, and place it on the hemorrhoids for 5 to 10 minutes. You can protect your skin by applying olive oil to the area first.

severe they are. For the more painful variety, your doctor is your best bet. He or she can offer chemical injections to control bleeding and shrink the swollen veins or, if necessary, surgery to remove them. For garden-variety hemorrhoids, here's how to cope at home:

Take a long warm bath. When you soak in warm water, not only do you relax but you let your blood vessels relax, too. When a tight sphincter muscle prevents blood from flowing freely in the veins, blood gets stopped up and causes hemorrhoids. The warm soak relaxes the anal sphincter muscle.

Cool it down. Soak a washcloth in cold water, wring it out, and hold it against the affected area until the cloth warms. Don't rub. Rinse the washcloth out, chill it in cold water, and apply it again. Repeat until the pain and itching stop.

Chill out. Sit on a bag of ice. A large plastic bag filled with crushed ice and covered with a towel may not suit as a long-term seat, but it can numb the pain and swelling for a while and help you feel more comfortable.

Baby yourself. The pain and itch of hemorrhoids can make a

O·D·D·B·A·L·L OINTMENT

Put a Potato Poultice Where?

To reduce pain and swelling, place a potato poultice on your external hemorrhoids overnight. Grate 1 to 2 tablespoons of raw potato, wrap in cheesecloth, chill, and apply.

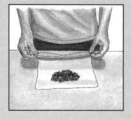

baby out of anybody. So even if you're a big bruiser, be bold and venture into the baby aisle for some baby wipes. They're softer than any toilet paper and help you avoid irritating an already uncomfortable area. And while you're there, take a look at Desitin, an over-the-counter remedy for diaper rash. It contains zinc oxide, which can sometimes help relieve hemorrhoid itch.

Use external remedies. There are a few drugstore standbys that can help ease the itch of a hemorrhoid. Aside from zinc oxide ointment, you might want to consider Preparation H, which is made from petrolatum and mineral oil. In a pinch, moisten a cotton ball with witch hazel, and dab it onto the swollen vein to help relieve the pain and itch.

Try an inside job. Your drugstore also carries suppositories, such as Anusol, that melt just inside your anus to provide a protective coating. Be sure to read the package instructions before you insert the suppository. This medication may interfere with other drugs you take, so ask your doctor before you use it.

Dunk into a doughnut. Cush your tush on a special

FABULOUS FOLK REMEDY

Ye Olde Witch Hazel

Witch hazel (*Hammemelis virginia*) is well known for its astringency. Its drawing action reduces swelling and eases the discomfort of itching. To make your own infusion, put 1 heaping teaspoon in 1 cup of hot water, and steep for 15 minutes, or buy a bottle of distilled witch hazel. Soak a clean cloth in the solution, and apply three to four times a day.

Another method is to tuck a fresh witch hazel leaf in the sore spot and, literally, sit tight. Replace the leaf a couple of times a day.

cushion made just for people with hemorrhoids. Known popularly as doughnut cushions, their strategically cut-out design prevents pressure on the hemorrhoids when you're sitting in the car or at your desk. The doughnut shape not only relieves pain but also helps the hemorrhoids to heal. Look in a health-products catalog or ask your pharmacist where you can find one.

Stop straining. Let your bowels move in their own sweet time, without pushing things along. Sitting on the toilet for long periods of time puts pressure on hemorrhoids and only compounds the problem. You can also make things move more easily by drinking at least eight glasses of water a day and by adding fiber to your diet.

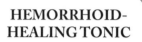

POWERFUL POTION

HEMORRHOID-HEALING TONIC

Yarrow (*Achillea millefolium*), horsechestnut (*Aesculus hippocastanum*), butcher's broom (*Ruscus aculeatus*), and rose hips (*Rosa canina*) are tonics for the venous system. Taken over time, these herbs can help strengthen your blood vessels and may relieve hemorrhoids. Mix equal parts of *each* herb; then measure 1 heaping teaspoon of the mixture into 1 cup of hot water and steep for 10 minutes. Drink 2 to 3 cups per day.

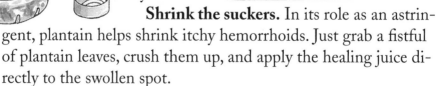

Shrink the suckers. In its role as an astringent, plantain helps shrink itchy hemorrhoids. Just grab a fistful of plantain leaves, crush them up, and apply the healing juice directly to the swollen spot.

Hiatal Hernia:

A Hiccup in Your Diaphragm

Here's a happy story—if you're like most people with a hiatal hernia, you don't even realize it, because most of the time, you have no symptoms to show for it. In fact, about one-quarter of folks over 50 are walking around with one.

What is it? First, a (very) short anatomy lesson: Your diaphragm is a broad, thin muscle that separates your chest cavity and abdominal cavity. The hiatus is the opening in the diaphragm where the esophagus

IT'S AN EMERGENCY!

Call your doctor right away if you have pain, shortness of breath, sweating, or nausea along with the sensation that food stops beneath your breastbone. Also, seek emergency medical care if you vomit blood, have a temperature over 100°F, or your symptoms don't improve within 1 hour after home treatment.

POWERFUL POTION

MARSHMALLOW TO THE MAX

A soothing tea of slippery herbs eases the discomfort of a hiatal hernia and minimizes symptoms of reflux. Make a cold infusion of marshmallow root tea by soaking 2 tablespoons of the herb in 1 quart of cold water overnight. Strain, and drink, cool, throughout the day.

passes through. When this opening weakens or herniates, it lets acid flow backward from the stomach into the esophagus—and lets the stomach protrude into the gap.

Symptoms are usually mild. However, because a hernia allows food and acid to back up into your esophagus, it can cause heartburn, indigestion (a burning sensation in the area of the heart and behind the breastbone), and—jolliest of all—lots of belching. Usually, these kick in about 1 hour after you eat.

In some cases, when the hernia is large enough to allow one-third of the stomach to poke through, the pressure it places on the lungs or diaphragm can make breathing difficult. But only 1 in 20 people need surgery because of severe symptoms. A hernia-repair operation pulls the stomach back down into your abdomen, reduces the size of the opening in your diaphragm, and/or reconstructs the weak sphincter.

Here's how you can handle the belching and discomfort that may accompany a hiatal hernia:

Understand the medications. Talk to your doctor about the best way to control any symptoms you may have. It's okay to experiment a little with antacids under your doctor's supervision. Normally, you should take antacids 1 hour before meals and at bedtime, but some people find they're more helpful 1 to 2 hours after meals. Try it both ways to see what works for you. Also, there are drugs available that hasten gastric emptying, so ask your doctor about the best medication plan for you before you start on a regular antacid routine.

Eat smart. Eat four or five small meals a day instead of three solid squares. There'll be less crowding in your esophagus and stomach, and less work for your digestive system. Eat slowly (bolting your food's rude anyway and doesn't help the acid situation). And don't eat anything for at least 2 hours before bedtime to avoid nighttime heartburn or reflux.

Don't relax. Avoid eating or drinking things that relax your diaphragm muscle, including alcohol. So if you're bothered by nighttime heartburn, skip the wine with dinner or any alcohol at night. Alas, you'll need to skip the after-dinner, chocolate-coated mints, too, since chocolate and peppermint also relax the hiatal sphincter muscle. You'll want to avoid any antacids that contain peppermint for the same reason.

Sleep slanted. Grab two bricks. Don't brain anybody, but raise the head of your bed 4 to 6 inches by sticking one under each of the bed's head-side legs. This will allow gravity to keep food down where it belongs (and keep creeping stomach acid away from your hernia).

Stay loose. Don't wear tight pantyhose, girdles, belts, or

FABULOUS FOLK REMEDY

Look, Ma, No Hands!

Osteopaths and craniosacral practitioners use visceral manipulation to maneuver the stomach back into position, but you can do a similar technique on your own with no hands! First thing in the morning, drink three glasses of water on an empty stomach. Now raise yourself on your toes, and drop down on your heels. Repeat 12 times. The weight of the water in your stomach will help put your organs back into place!

pants. Avoid anything that binds or constricts your middle section. (It won't hurt you to reduce the size of that midsection, either.)

Don't strain. When you're answering the call of nature, let bowel movements and urination happen at their own pace. Be wary of lifting, too, which can really strain a hernia. See **Constipation** for tips on adding more fiber—especially fruit—to your daily diet, as well as fluids and exercise.

Don't lift with your abs. Lifting heavy objects by tightening your abdominal muscles can sometimes cause a hiatal hernia or make it worse. So if you must lift, remember the classic advice to let your leg muscles do the work.

Boycott the bubblies. When the drink tray comes around or you're standing in front of the fridge, make sure to choose a noncarbonated beverage. The bubbles will increase belching and add to your discomfort.

Avoid foods that linger. Fatty foods stay in the stomach longer and can cause indigestion. And they're not good for you anyway, so now's the time to get serious about a healthy low-fat, high-fiber diet. Your diaphragm will thank you, and you'll soon enjoy looking in the mirror again.

Curb the coffee. You may crave your daily jolt of java, but keep it to a minimum. Coffee increases the production of stomach acid, and this only aggravates a hiatal hernia. You might try a soothing cup of herbal tea, instead.

High Blood Pressure:

Keeping the Lid On

Your nice new garden hose. All smooth and flexible, warm from the sun. Coils and uncoils easily, does its job. But what happens if you neglect it, leave it out year-round to suffer the weather? Yup, after a season or two it hardens, stiffens, doesn't work very well—and may eventually spring a leak.

In a way, your arteries are like that. The "tension" in hypertension is about them. Your arteries must continually contract and relax to ac-commodate the powerful force of blood pumping into your heart—

FABULOUS FOLK REMEDY

Limey, Mate!

Lime blossoms (*Tilea europea*) may be effective when the cause of your high blood pressure is associated with tension and stress. Add a few lime blossoms to the Berry Good Tonic (see page 246), or simply toss 1 heaping teaspoon of blossoms into 1 cup of hot water, and steep for 15 minutes. Drink 1 to 3 cups per day.

Yes, Please Have a Banana

Have a banana today! Potassium prevents thickening of the artery walls and works in conjunction with sodium, an electrolyte, to regulate your body's fluid levels. Those fluid levels are important because an excessively high volume of fluid in your arteries can elevate your blood pressure. Bananas are particularly high in potassium, so reach for one every day to keep healthy potassium levels in your body. Also enjoy other good potassium sources, including apples, string beans, peas, beans, and skim milk.

60 to 70 times a minute, and that's while you are resting. When the blood is moving at too high a pressure, it literally wears out the arteries. And down the line, untreated hypertension can also damage the heart. Your heart gets bigger as it works harder to pump; eventually, it can become more inefficient. Kidneys and eyes take a beating, too, and a stroke can damage your brain.

Yet these dire consequences are unnecessary. Although it's dangerous, high blood pressure is also highly treatable. But because it sneaks up without symptoms, once your doctor says you have it, you've got to make a commitment not to go into denial. Just do what's necessary to keep it under control.

It's hard to pinpoint precise causes for hypertension, but excess body weight, smoking, a salty diet, high-fat foods, and stress all contribute. Yet sometimes the condition strikes nonsmokers who exercise and are not overweight. Over age 50, it's more common in women but more deadly in men.

If you've been diagnosed with high blood pressure, you need

to be under a doctor's care. But there's also lot you can do on your own to keep it under control. Here's how to get started:

Get inside the numbers. The first step toward controlling your blood pressure is to understand the numbers used to define it. Pressure is expressed as two numbers, one over the other. The upper number (or systolic pressure) measures the pressure during the contraction of the heart as it pumps blood into arteries. The lower number (or diastolic pressure) measures the pressure as the heart relaxes between beats. Blood pressure varies within a normal range during waking hours and should be around 120/80 millimeters of mercury (mm Hg). When it stays above 140/90 mm Hg for a period of time, it is considered high, can damage the surface of blood vessels, and can lead to cholesterol being deposited on artery walls.

Follow your doctor's orders. High blood pressure is frequently controlled with medication. Some medications reduce the force of the heart's contraction, while others widen the blood vessels or decrease the volume of blood in circulation. You may be tempted not to take your medications once they've been prescribed because you note a side effect, you want to save money, or you just feel good. Resist the impulse. In-

POWERFUL POTION

PASSIONFLOWER TEA

Passionflower is one of Mother Nature's best tranquilizers. When you need to be rescued from anxiety or stress, try a cup of passionflower tea. Simply steep 1 or 2 teaspoons of the dried herb in 1 cup of boiling water. Wait about 20 minutes, strain, and then drink.

Learn to Relieve Stress

If you are easily stressed, your body repeatedly pumps adrenaline into your bloodstream, causing a rise in blood pressure. Take an honest look at your stress level, and take control. You can commit yourself to lowering the stress in your life. Regular exercise, yoga, and meditation are good places to begin.

stead, talk to your doctor. He or she may be able to prescribe a cheaper drug or one without the side effect that troubles you. And feeling good is no sign at all that your blood pressure has gone down. Remember—this condition is frequently without symptoms.

Stash the salt. Reducing salt may help people with hypertension—not just those especially sensitive to salt, a Harvard Medical School study showed. That's why doctors suggest you use less than 1,500 milligrams of salt a day. Bear in mind that just 1 teaspoon of salt contains about 2,400 milligrams of sodium.

Watch out for hidden salt. Many packaged, prepared, and junk foods are loaded with sodium—some are as much as 85 percent sodium! Always read labels before you buy lunch meats, soups, canned soups and food, dried packaged meals, frozen dinners, and other prepared foods. There are healthy, low-sodium alternatives. And avoid fast foods altogether, except for an occasional salad (be sure to tote your own bottle of low-sodium dressing).

Visit the produce and dairy aisles. A diet low in salt but high in fruits, vegetables, and low-fat dairy products can lower blood pressure as much as medication can, according to research. So load up your shopping cart and stock your fridge with a variety of these products.

Got fruit? Eat lots every day. The fiber in fruit apparently works even better than the fiber from vegetables and grains to lower systolic blood pres-

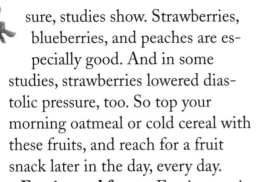

sure, studies show. Strawberries, blueberries, and peaches are especially good. And in some studies, strawberries lowered diastolic pressure, too. So top your morning oatmeal or cold cereal with these fruits, and reach for a fruit snack later in the day, every day.

Forgive and forget. Forgiveness is not only good for your soul but also good for your body. A study led by Kathleen Lawler, Ph.D., a psychologist at the University of Tennessee, tracked blood pressure and heart rate as people talked about betrayals in their lives. When some participants reported forgiving a grievance, their blood pressure numbers returned to normal. However, those who held a grudge kept their readings high. And across the board, men were more likely to forgive than women.

If you find it hard to forgive, remind yourself that the word does *not* mean excuse, forget, or condone. It simply means that you release *yourself* from the anger and resentment you've been holding, literally, in your heart.

Bring it down with biofeedback. Train your body to respond differently to stimuli that would ordinarily bring a spike in blood pressure. Many

FABULOUS FOLK REMEDY

Cuppa Kava

In the Pacific Islands, the herb kava has always played a vital role in special ceremonies and has served as a welcoming potion for visiting dignitaries. Even today, people flock to non-alcoholic kava bars (or *nakamals*, as they're called) to help them unwind after a hard day's work. The spotlight ingredient that delivers the punch in this herb is known as kava-lactone. It provides pain-relieving, muscle-relaxing, and mood-mellowing effects. In fact, herbalists consider kava to be the number one antianxiety herb.

To enjoy the calming effects of kava, grate 1 to 2 teaspoons of dried kava root into 1 cup of boiling water. Cover; then let steep for a good hour. Strain, and sip. You can try up to 2 cups a day. **Caution:** Kava has recently been linked to liver toxicity. Check with your doctor before using it—especially if you're taking antidepressant or antianxiety medication.

people have been able to cut their blood pressure medication in half or eliminate it altogether with this technique, according to the Association for Applied Psychophysiology and Biofeedback. So ask your doctor to refer you to a skilled therapist. It takes 4 to 6 weeks of biofeedback training to bring blood pressure down. The technique is not hard to learn; but for best results, you must commit yourself to using it in conjunction with careful monitoring, a proper diet, and exercise.

Get off the couch. We're not naming names, here, but many people with hypertension are couch potatoes. Even moderate exercise will help—as long as you do it for 30 minutes four to five times a week. Check with your doctor before you start. Then pick a regular exercise program you will enjoy and stick with it. (Even if you don't like it at first, you'll soon grow to love feeling fit.)

Cut down on alcohol. Limit daily consumption to one 12-ounce beer, one 4-ounce glass of wine, or one drink made with 1.5 ounces of hard alcohol. More than that can send your blood pressure moving up the scale.

Avoid things that bump it up. Blood pressure can increase with the continuous use of oral contraceptives, steroids, antacids with sodium, decongestants, over-the-counter appetite suppressants, and nonsteroidal anti-inflammatory drugs. Avoid them when you can, and talk to your doctor about the alternatives when you can't.

POWERFUL POTION

A BERRY GOOD TONIC

Hawthorn berries (*Cratae-gus* spp.) are widely used for their gentle hypotensive effects. But combining them with other antispasmodic herbs and relaxants can augment their effect. Try a mixture of equal parts of hawthorn, motherwort (*Leonurus cardiaca*), passionflower (*Passiflora incarnata*), and skullcap (*Scutellaria lateriflora*). Steep 1 heaping teaspoon of the mixture in 1 cup of hot water for 15 minutes. Strain, and drink 2 to 3 cups daily.

Be positive. High blood pressure is nothing to feel depressed about. It is a condition that can be controlled and managed with lifestyle, a doctor's care, and medical treatment.

Hang out with animals. The four-legged kind, that is. Some studies have shown that having pets to care for and love lowers high blood pressure. A cat purrs, and you purr. Or a dog looks into your eyes, and you melt. Stay away from them if you're not an animal lover. But if you are, visit your local humane society shelter and pick up a small creature that will give you as much or more than you give it.

> # Licorice: The Real Candy Ain't Dandy
>
> Here's an instance where the artificial is better than the real thing. Natural licorice can raise blood pressure and wash potassium from the body, according to an Icelandic study. It's found in some herbal teas, dark beers, and candy. So, if your blood pressure is a little iffy, read labels, and make sure the licorice taste is made with artificial flavoring.

Manage anger. Both aggressive, let-it-all-hang-out folks and the quiet types, who repress their anger, are likely to send their blood pressure soaring, according to Nancy Snyderman, M.D. If you tend to respond to negative events by acting like Clara Clam or Rick the Raging Bull, pick up a copy of *LifeSkills* by Duke University psychiatrist Redford Williams, M.D. By following his simple anger management techniques, you'll not only lower your blood pressure but also change your life.

High Cholesterol:

The Good, the Bad, and the Healthy

If you're math-phobic, cholesterol is not your favorite subject. I mean, do we have to do algebra to figure out what's going on in our arteries? Fortunately, it's not as complicated as it may seem. Here's the whole deal—in an eggshell: Your body needs cholesterol. Surprised? This waxy substance exists in all your tissues to insulate nerve fibers, protect cell surfaces, and serve as a building block for hormones. Your liver manufactures some, and the rest comes from your diet, especially from the saturated fat in animal products, including eggs, meat, and dairy foods.

Microscopic fat and protein molecules, called lipoproteins, move cholesterol through your circulatory system. They vary in size and density, which is why they wear the labels they do: Low-density lipoprotein (LDL) carries cholesterol into the bloodstream for your body to use, whereas the high-density lipoprotein (HDL) transports the excess back to the liver for disposal. Problems begin when too much cholesterol enters your blood, and the liver can't carry enough away. And the biggest problem is when the stuff collects like sludge in your arteries. It's hard for your heart to do its job when its main vessels are clogged.

Confused? Here's your first shortcut. Just think of the two types of cholesterol as "healthy" for HDL (so high numbers of HDL are great) and "lousy" for LDL (you want low readings here). Remember, it's the HDL that gets rid of the excess—that's why you want plenty of it. Likewise, if you've got too much LDL, you're getting more cholesterol than your body (and your arteries) can handle.

The U.S. Food and Drug Administration (FDA) put the kibosh on a movement to make cholesterol-lowering drugs available without prescription. They thought people might not stick

It's All in the Way You Brew It

Apparently, the rumors about coffee raising cholesterol levels are not true, and I'm not saying that just because I love the stuff. The cholesterol connection comes from the coffee-brewing method. When coffee's unfiltered, as when it's made with a French press, it can add as many as 20 points to your cholesterol tally. Scientists believe that two compounds in coffee—cafestol and kahweol—are to blame. But brewing through paper or gold-plated filters is said to remove these troublemakers. So if you prefer the French press method, just strain your brewed coffee through a filter before you drink it.

BEAR MOUNTAIN COFFEE

FABULOUS FOLK REMEDY

A Little Lemon, Please

Living in the toxic world that we do can overburden our liver and compromise its ability to metabolize fats and cholesterol. Perk it up a bit by squeezing a lemon into your daily water ration. The lemon juice helps prod your digestive system, including your liver, encouraging it to go to work.

with the regular testing that goes hand in hand with using such drugs. Yet at least 53 million Americans have high cholesterol, and only a small fraction us who have the worst levels are using prescription medication. Many don't even realize they have high cholesterol; others have no insurance coverage for treatment. The FDA was also concerned that people simply don't understand high cholesterol well enough to self-medicate. Let's learn, then. Here are some ways to keep your cholesterol in check:

Know how to score. According to the American Heart Association, the most important cholesterol number is the ratio you get when you divide the HDL into the total. If your total cholesterol is 220 and your HDL is 50, for example, your ratio would be 4 to 1. Your goal is to keep the ratio below 5 to 1—the best is 3.5 to 1. Okay? So when you get your numbers back from your cholesterol screening test, whip out your calculator, and do the math. (Or just ask your doctor to give you a copy of your cholesterol report, and keep it handy to track your progress.) Schedule your first screening test at age 20, then get a follow-up every 5 years.

Avoid the deadly spread. Saturated fat, the kind that stays solid even at room temperature, does the same thing inside your arteries. But even worse are the hydrogenated oils or trans-fats used in margarine, according to Walter Willet, M.D., chairman of the nutrition department at the Harvard School of Public Health. Manufacturers force hydrogen to react with oil, which is then said to be "hydrogenated." Technically, it is unsaturated (that's how they get away with it via FDA restrictions), but these fats look and act just like saturated fats. A study comparing equal amounts of margarine, which is made from these hydrogenated oils, with soybean oil showed that margarine raised cholesterol levels 14 points, increasing heart attack risk by *10 percent!* So in addition to ditching the saturated fats found in meats and dairy products, give up your old-style margarine, and try the new, more healthful spreads, like Benecol. They contain plant esters that actually lower cholesterol.

Slow down on fast food. Hydrogenated oils and trans-fats are widely used in fast food (especially French fries) and most commercially prepared snacks (like cookies), according to Dr. Willet. Forget the fries on your next lunch break, and get into the habit of reading labels on cookies and other snack foods.

POWERFUL POTION

GET GARLIC

Garlic is the real deal in lowering cholesterol, dropping levels by up to 15 percent according to many scientific studies. To keep your arteries free and clear, try a glass of garlic juice once a day. Follow it up by chewing a big sprig of fresh parsley, so you don't asphyxiate all of your friends!

Another idea: Peel and chop a clove or two, let it rest on the cutting board for at least 10 minutes; then slip it into everything from soups and stews to salads and poultry dishes. Letting the clove rest allows the cholesterol-lowering compounds to form.

Magic Bean Cuisine

At least one fairy tale has come true! Just ask Jack. He'll tell you that beans really *do* have magical properties. They contain soluble fiber that not only lowers cholesterol but also may make your arteries more flexible, according to a study presented at a 1999 American Heart Association meeting.

If you're concerned about high cholesterol—and who isn't?—look for ways to incorporate beans into your daily diet—and watch your cholesterol level hit the floor!

✔ Have a bean burrito for lunch.

✔ Snack on bean dip and crackers.

✔ Toss some garbanzos into your salad.

✔ Learn to love bean soup.

✔ Replace sour cream with soft tofu.

Appreciate the Mediterraneans. Scores of studies and many doctors agree that the heart-healthiest diet is the one Mediterranean populations enjoy. Mostly vegetables and fruit, beans, fish, nuts, and plenty of olive oil, Mediterranean meals have a positive effect on both cholesterol levels and blood pressure. Add generous amounts of vegetables, peas, beans, fish, and whole grains to your low-fat diet, and you'll lower both your total and your LDL cholesterol by twice as much as people who eat ordinary low-fat meals, according to a study presented at the American Heart Association.

And go nuts. The Mediterranean diet's good for the heart, but substituting a handful of walnuts (8 to 11) a day for some of the oil in that diet could be even better. Walnuts can lower cholesterol even more than olive oil, according to a study reported in the *Annals of Internal Medicine.* These nuts lowered the risk of coronary heart disease by 11 percent, reported lead researcher Emilio Ros, M.D., whose study was done in conjunction with Loma Linda University in California. Furthermore, the Hospital Clinic Provincial de Barcelona noted that walnuts incorporated into the Mediterranean diet reduced bad cholesterol by almost 6 percent more than did the base Mediterranean diet.

Eat your oatmeal. Make it a daily habit to eat a breakfast with lots of soluble fiber. Oatmeal's a great source. Savor a bowl every day, and you'll lower your cholesterol, according to more than 40 scientific studies. Not only is it rich in a type of fiber called beta-glucan but oatmeal also fills you up, according to Joseph Keenan, M.D., of the University of Minnesota Medical School.

Get the basics on barley. You're not likely to find this one in Starbucks—at least not yet. But according to at least one study comparing muffins made with hulled barley to ordinary, low-fiber ones made from refined wheat, the barley muffins were cholesterol-flattening champs. They reduced artery-clogging LDL cholesterol by 12 percent. Overall, changes like this can produce around a 20 percent reduction in the risk of developing heart disease. Hulled barley is available at natural-foods stores.

Ditch the sticks. Along with all of its other terrible consequences, smoking raises cholesterol levels by increasing the stickiness of blood platelets, which makes clotting in narrowed arteries more likely. It also reduces the blood's capacity to carry oxygen and damages the lining of coronary arteries, most likely by contributing to the formation of plaque. Consider this for motivation: When you quit, your risk of heart disease drops rapidly, as does your cholesterol. If you haven't tried in a while, see your doctor for help.

Eat more often. It may seem surprising, but the more often you eat, the lower your cholesterol may be. In a study of men and women between the ages of 50 and 89, those who ate four or more meals a day lowered their cholesterol by 2.5 percent compared to the people who ate only once or twice a day.

Pass the pectin. It binds up cholesterol, preventing absorption in the blood. Good sources include apples, grapefruit, carrots, prunes, and cabbage.

FABULOUS FOLK REMEDY

The Artful Artichoke

The globe artichoke (*Cynara scolymus*) has been used in traditional European medicine for liver complaints since Roman times. With its liver-protective, cholesterol-reducing, and appetite-stimulating actions, the artichoke is an excellent all-around digestive herb—especially if you have trouble digesting fat and often feel bloated or nauseous after rich meals. Simply add the plant to your diet—just skip the buttery dipping sauce!—or take it as a dried extract (2 grams, three times a day). **Caution:** People with gallbladder disease should consult with their healthcare providers before eating artichokes. If you are allergic to artichokes, skip this remedy (even the extract part) altogether.

Hives:

How to Ditch the Itch

True, hives aren't pretty. But if you've got a crop of those big red blotches, chances are you're too busy going nuts over the itching to stare in the mirror anyway. When you do get a look, however, don't panic. They're temporary.

Hives are usually an allergic reaction to food or medications, but they can also result from touching a plant such as stinging nettle or from an insect sting. They can erupt on any part of the body—even in the mouth. But they're usually on the skin, and, boy, are they visible! In some cases, the red wheals may be as large as 1 inch in diameter. Most hives develop within hours of contact with a trigger substance,

---

FABULOUS FOLK REMEDY

Soak in Oats

Nothing beats the discomfort of hives like a warm (not hot) oatmeal bath. Scoop 1 cup of oats into a sock, and hang it under the faucet while you run the water for your bath. Squeeze the sock a few times to extract the milky oat juice; then slip into some blessed relief.

but sometimes they appear days later, particularly if you're reacting to a medication. One way to tell is that a drug allergy usually starts around the head and face and spreads downward.

In folks who are extra-sensitive, extreme heat or cold or even the ice in a drink may cause hives. If you have hives, call your doctor. Here's how to reduce the stress of having hives and how to get rid of them—fast:

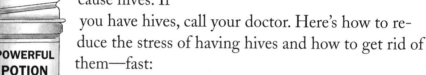

IT'S AN EMERGENCY!

If, in addition to the hives, you have any swelling in your throat or difficulty breathing, speaking, or swallowing, call 911 or your community's emergency response number immediately. You could be showing signs of anaphylaxis—a severe allergic reaction that can be fatal.

POWERFUL POTION

COOL MINT

You may find some temporary relief from those hot, itchy hives by dabbing them with cool mint tea. Stir 1 teaspoon of dried or fresh leaves into 1 cup of boiling water and simmer for 10 minutes. Strain out the herbs. After the tea has cooled, rub it on your skin as a healing lotion.

Attack with antihistamines. Hives can fade within minutes or last for days or even weeks. But you can fight back. Start with the first line of defense—take an over-the-counter antihistamine such as Benadryl. In most cases, it will ease the reaction. A topical anesthetic ointment or lotion may also provide relief. If the problem persists, ask your doctor whether a prescription antihistamine might prevent additional eruptions.

Find out who dunnit. When hives first hit, try to remember everything you've recently eaten and any medications you've just taken. If you can identify the trigger early, especially if you suspect a medication, you can avoid a more serious recurrence. Drawing a blank? Keep a daily food diary until you're sure whether or not something in your diet might be triggering the hives.

Avoid the known culprits. The risk of hives increases with foods high in niacin, which is believed to inhibit histamine release. The most common foods that cause this reaction are niacin-rich shellfish, nuts, and berries, but you may also be sensitive to poultry, seeds, cereals, and breads. Boycott these foods for a while to see if niacin may be your trigger. Likewise, if

O·D·D·B·A·L·L OINTMENT

Cold Salve for Hot Hives

Chickweed (*Stellaria media*) salve soothes itchy, burny hives in no time. For extra relief, keep the salve in the fridge, and dab it on cold. Another way to use chickweed is to make a strong infusion of the herb by steeping a handful of fresh chickweed in 2 cups of hot water for 15 minutes. Strain into a spray bottle, chill, and spritz on the hives to relieve the itch.

Say Ta-Ta to Tartrazine

Tartrazine? Who eats *tartrazine*? You may, but you probably know it better as the food dye Yellow Number 5. Reading food labels can help you avoid this common cause of hives. This not-so-mellow yellow is found in cheeses, artificial fruit drinks, and often in the coatings of vitamins or candy.

you're allergic to aspirin, try eliminating foods that contain salicylate, the active ingredient in aspirin. These include apricots, berries, grapes, raisins and other dried fruit, and tea. Also beware of foods that are processed with vinegar, such as pickles, which cause hives in some people.

Hot Flashes:

Unplug Those Power Surges

Bet you never thought you'd grow up to be a flasher. But here you are, hot flashing through the day and night. While a few lucky women sail through menopause with nary a bead of sweat, others go straight through Dante's inferno. And it's all it's reputed to be!

One thing that makes a hot flash so uncomfortable is its suddenness. It isn't like gradually adapting to the heat of August. It's more like, out of the blue, you're tossed into a blast furnace. You want to tear off your clothes or stick your head under a cold water faucet—immediately! (That can be a little awkward if you're not in your favorite armchair, but in a meeting at work!)

While a hot flash lasts only a few seconds, it leaves your entire body

---

FABULOUS FOLK REMEDY

Red Clover

Red clover contains isso-flavones, naturally occurring substances that may reduce hot flashes. To make your own: Put 3 teaspoons of dried clover flowers in 1 cup of boiling water, and let it steep, covered, for 10 minutes. Strain out the blossoms, and voilà! A cup of isoflavone tea!

bathed in sweat. The usual cause is the changing hormone levels that affect every woman at midlife. But other factors can contribute to hot flashes, too, including smoking, psychological stress, a history of premenstrual syndrome, alcohol, caffeine, spicy foods, and a tendency toward flushing early in life.

For most women, however, hot flashes are a garden-variety sign that your body is moving into menopause, and your changing hormone levels have temporarily thrown your body's thermostat out of whack. Here's how to cool off:

Dress like an onion. That is, dress in layers of clothing, and you'll feel more comfortable. Just peel off a layer or two when you feel hot, and put them back on when you are cold. Also, wear silk or cotton underwear—these fabrics breathe and won't trap the heat as much as synthetics do.

Try cool cream. Ask your pharmacist about over-the-counter menopause creams that relieve skin flushing and hot flashes. Some contain cooling ingredients such as menthol. Just rub on the cream when your body temperature begins to rise for a breezy skin sensation.

Spray away the flames. Try one of the menthol cooling sprays that come in palm-size canisters. Tote one in your purse for instant heat relief. Or for a less expensive option, carry your own spritzer bottle filled

POWERFUL POTION

HOT FLASH TONIC

Traditional herbs with hormone-balancing activities may help reduce the frequency and severity of hot flashes. Combine the following herbs in equal parts: dong quai (*Angelica sinensis*), chastetree berry (*Vitex agnus-castus*), black cohosh (*Cimicifuga racemosa*), and motherwort (*Leonurus cardiaca*). Steep 1 heaping teaspoon of the mixture in 1 cup of hot water for 15 minutes. Drink 2 cups of cooled tea daily for 2 months or longer.

with water. Just spray it over your face and neck when you feel the heat coming. You might add a dash of lemon or lime juice for a citrus sensation.

Turn down the heat with E. Vitamin E often helps relieve the severity and frequency of hot flashes and other menopause symptoms, according to Lila Nachtigall, M.D., who advises starting with 400 International Units (IU) twice a day. If you already take a multivitamin, be sure to note how much vitamin E it contains, and figure that into your total vitamin E intake. Although no one knows exactly how vitamin E reduces hot flashes, it does produce remarkable results for many women with moderate symptoms.

Why supplement? Dietary sources of vitamin E are so high in fat and calories that you'd need to eat 1 pound of sunflower seeds or 2 quarts of corn oil (8,000 calories!) to equal 400 IU. But be sure to discuss your vitamin regime with your doctor, as vitamin E is also a blood thinner. This can create problems for people who take blood-thinning medications or supplements, such as daily aspirin or garlic.

FABULOUS FOLK REMEDY

Cool Down with Alfalfa

Alfalfa (*Medicago sativa*) contains plant sterols, making it an ideal choice for hot flashes. Steep 1 teaspoon in 1 cup of hot water. Strain, and drink 1 cup of the cooled tea daily.

Light at the End of the Tunnel

Is there good news about hot flashes? You bet! For many women, they can be very mild or nonexistent, and for all women, they do end. Less than half the women in the Massachusetts Women's Health Study reported having hot flashes or night sweats. Those who did reported they occurred mostly at the beginning of perimenopause, reached a peak at menopause, and then diminished.

Put plants on your plate. If you eat more fruits and vegetables, you'll have fewer blasts from your internal furnace. The relief is caused by naturally occurring plant sterols (called phytoestrogens), which are not as powerful as human estrogens but have a similar effect, according to Cornell University researchers. Phytoestrogens are found in apples, alfalfa sprouts, split peas, spinach, and especially soybean products.

Go easy on ginseng. This root has been used for centuries as a folk medicine to relieve hot flashes and other "women's troubles"—it happens to be a potent source of plant estrogen. If you take it for hot flashes and other symptoms, in essence you're taking estrogen-replacement therapy. Ginseng may be natural, but it is still estrogen and affects your body in the same way that hormone pills, patches, or creams do. Furthermore, with ginseng, you are taking estrogen without the progesterone most doctors add to a woman's hormone prescription. This is called "unopposed" estrogen; and when taken continually or in high doses, it can stimulate overgrowth of the uterine lining, or hyperplasia. Because you have no way of knowing how much phytoestrogen you are getting with ginseng, you will never know if you are overdosing, according to Dr. Nachtigall. Despite its stellar rep-

Natural Native Medicine

Black Cohosh

Native Americans have long used the herb black cohosh to treat menopause symptoms—often combining it with other herbs to quell hot flashes. German studies found the herb worked as well as estrogen for night sweats and sleep disruption, and a study conducted at the University of Bridgeport showed it to be safe and effective. Black cohosh is usually taken in capsules or as a tincture. **Caution:** Because it may produce estrogen-like actions, black cohosh isn't recommended during pregnancy.

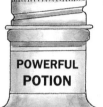

POWERFUL POTION

PARSLEY POWER

Hot flashes are just one problem associated with menopause. Bloating is another—and parsley is the key to getting rid of all that extra fluid that accumulates and makes you look like Wanda the Whale. To experience the benefits, simply add parsley leaves to your salads or parsley seeds to your soups. And, of course, *eat your garnish!*

utation, don't take ginseng without talking with your doctor about hormone-replacement first.

Keep moving. Vigorous exercise may ease your way through menopause. According to a University of Illinois study, women who spent the most time dancing or playing tennis experienced fewer hot flashes, night sweats, and mood swings than women who led a less active life.

Use sensible solutions. Don't make a hot flash hotter with hot drinks, spicy foods, or alcohol. Instead, sip cold drinks and take cool showers. These will ease the flames, as will a fan or air-conditioning and low humidity.

Talk to your doctor about HRT. Doctors are moving toward a consensus that hormone-replacement therapy (HRT) has been oversold. Although it's great at relieving hot flashes, it has no positive affect on heart health and is certainly not the only way to prevent osteoporosis. But in some women, principally those who have had their ovaries surgically removed, HRT may be the way to go. The bottom line? Ask your doctor to look into the latest research on your behalf. Then decide if HRT is right for you.

Insomnia:

The ABCs of
Getting Some Zs

We know, we know—counting the dad-blamed sheep doesn't work. And neither do drugs. Or vitamins. No, for the true insomniac—the person who either can't stay asleep through the night or wakes up way before the birds—there's no one single strategy that will send her off to the land of Nod in the blink of an eye. Instead, most insomniacs find that tinkering a little here and there with their sleep cycles is what finally tricks them into behaving. Here's how to get started:

Knock yourself out. Physical activity during the day will help you sleep better at night. Exercise reduces stress and induces sleep by depleting chemicals like epinephrine, which stimulate the body. Exercise also helps you sleep longer and fall asleep faster, according to Abby King, Ph.D., of Stanford University School of Medicine, who is researching the relationship between exercise and sleep. Her study showed that exercise, even a brisk walk before dinner, made a big difference.

Set your brain clock. Sleep is malleable, like a muscle, and within limits can be trained and refined, according to Claudio Stampi, M.D., director of the Chronobiology Research Institute in Newton, Massachusetts. So repeat the same sleep pattern every day to set your brain clock to a good schedule. Your body will adapt to the regularity and get ready for sleep, with glands and hormones functioning and by-products breaking down. Stay as regular as you can and don't skimp on sleep, and you will be able to feel great in the morning.

Reset your snooze button. If you fall asleep at 8:00 P.M. and wake up at 4:00 A.M. instead of 6:00 A.M., your sleep cycle is off. Spend more time outdoors during the day. That way, daylight can help your internal clock counteract its tendency to fall asleep earlier in the evening and wake you up earlier in the morning.

Pay attention to aches and pains. The real reason older people sometimes sleep less is that they have more medical conditions, like arthritis, that keep them awake. So don't be a stiff-upper-lipper when it comes to pain. Talk to your doctor—and do something about it.

Know your type. A morning person goes to sleep relatively early in evening, wakes up early, and is most effective doing complex tasks in the

Natural Native Medicine

Dream Spirits Pillow

Native American healers invented a sleep-enhancing "dream spirits" pillow to ease one into dreamland. To make your own, put equal amounts of dried leaves of catnip, rabbit tobacco, mint, and sage into a small calico or plain cotton pillowcase. You can also add some rosemary leaves, lavender, or mugwort. Then sew it shut. This aromatic, sedative pillow is said to make dreams more memorable, and its effects are even more noticeable in hot, humid weather.

morning, rather than in the evening. An evening person goes to bed later, gets up later, and is slower coming to full horsepower. He or she does better at complex tasks in the evening rather than in the morning. If insomnia is a major part of your life, odds are good that you're fighting your natural sleep type. Just decide which type you are and readjust your daily priorities so that complex tasks are scheduled for the proper time slot. Sleep will soon follow.

Darken your room. Your body needs darkness to trigger its sleep cycle. So if you have a big streetlight shining in the window, or if you have to sleep during the day because you're on night shift, close the blinds or pull opaque drapes across your window so the light won't get through.

Block out night noises. Whatever sounds make your body relax and your mind still, make a tape of them, and play it just as you've turned out your lights.

Wind down with rituals. The best way to get to sleep more quickly is to establish and follow bedtime routines, according to neurologist Dr. Stampi. These rituals have a big influence on your ability to get to sleep and to wake up in a regular pattern. Try reading a book, breathing deeply, or sipping a cup of herbal tea. They all can work, in the same way that shaving, a morning face wash, or having a cup of coffee help you accelerate in the morning.

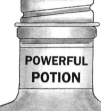

POWERFUL POTION

CATNIP PROMOTES CATNAPS

Catnip (*Nepeta cateria*) may turn your lazy feline into a rowdy cat, but it has the opposite effect on us humans. A little catnip tea after dinner might be just the ticket for winding down after a long day. Steep 1 teaspoon in 1 cup of hot water for 10 minutes. Strain, and enjoy! **Note:** Secure your stash of catnip out of reach of all cats!

Time your tubs. If you take a warm bath 1 or 2 hours before you go to sleep, it could help you sleep by relaxing you. But if you take it just before you jump into the sack, it could stimulate you and actually keep you more awake than ever. So time your tub for at least 1 hour before you hit the hay.

Hold the high test. I cannot have coffee after 3:00 P.M. Even coffee ice cream keeps me awake all night. Alas, this began only in middle age. If you find no other reason for your sleeplessness, consider your coffee habit. Keep the high test for the morning, and switch to decaf in the afternoon or evening. See if it makes a difference.

Change tea time to bedtime. Some Native American healers brew a summer meadow relaxing tea to help them sleep. Try one of the commercial herbal teas that are marketed for bedtime use, such as chamomile or Sleepy Time.

Make your bed heavenly. Be as comfortable as possible for the third of your life you spend in bed. A good mattress and pillow help you enjoy your stay. Use a feather bed under your sheet for a floating-on-a-cloud feeling. And treat yourself to high-quality smooth sheets and covers that will caress you rather than make you itch or sneeze.

Why Sleep?

Sleep restores energy to the brain's nerve cells, according to Andrew A. Monjan, Ph.D., chief of the National Institute on Aging's Neuropsychology of Aging branch. So while you're asleep, your brain is recharging. This is why you feel so much brighter and smarter in the morning—even without that first jolt of java. It's also why you shouldn't be let loose on the planet after a sleepless night.

And make your bedroom serene. If your bedroom is cluttered, dusty, cramped, and/or poorly ventilated, you may not even want to be there. And who is in the room next to you? A teenager who plays hip-hop into the night? Arrange your bedroom so that it is restful and serene. (Think Japanese garden.) If you have a noisy neighbor on the other side of the wall, install some soundproof paneling.

Wake up your libido. If you can't sleep, you might as well have sex. Seriously, if sex puts you to sleep, be glad. Sex enhances sleep. After getting worked up sexually, your body goes quite naturally into a state of total relaxation. If your significant other is sound asleep, make some romantic moves to get him or her in the mood. Turn on the sexual vibrations, and you'll unwind all the others.

Fake it. No, not the orgasm, the sleep. Use guided imagery, a form of self-hypnosis, to help yourself sleep. Listen to a meditation tape or use a progressive muscle relaxation exercise to get deeply relaxed; then picture yourself comfortably asleep. While you're at it, imagine that you're in a more comfortable bed, maybe in a luxury hotel or on a mountaintop or in a gently rocking

POWERFUL POTION

STINKY TEA

Valerian, an herb more commonly known as heliotrope, is a mild sedative that smells like stinky socks. A few drops in a cup of bedtime tea is reputed to help you sleep. Research shows valerian root depresses the central nervous system and relaxes smooth muscle tissue. It can be used as a tea or taken as a pill or tincture. Valerian doesn't result in a hangover or dependence, but it isn't advisable if you have asthma or you use sleeping pills or alcohol. Other sleep-promoting teas to try are chamomile, hops, lemon balm, and peppermint.

sailboat. Visualize every possible detail of the scene to increase the suggestion's power. Do this nightly for several weeks, and you'll soon be able to fall asleep more easily.

Evict the buzz-saw operator. I lived for years with a husband whose snoring kept me awake. Waking him up and telling him he was snoring failed to change the situation. Use earplugs if this is your problem.

Get a purring security blanket. Many people sleep with their pets, and some say it's like a security blanket. They know that should anything go wrong during the night while they are asleep, the dog or cat will alert them. This makes them relax when they go to bed and primes them for sleep.

Stop trying. Striving to sleep only makes the problem worse, so if you haven't fallen asleep after a little while, get up and distract yourself. Sit in another room, and read or do some paperwork.

Check your medications. Drugs that interfere with sleep include beta-blockers for high blood pressure, thyroid medications, bronchodilators and corticosteroids for asthma, sinus and nasal decongestants, and antidepressants. If you're taking any of these, ask your pharmacist whether a change in medication may help ease your insomnia.

FABULOUS FOLK REMEDY

Poppy Power!

Poppies are known for their soporific effects, and the good news is that you don't have to travel to Oz to find them. The common California poppy (*Eschscholzia california*) is a gentle sleep inducer and can be made into a tea on its own or added to any of your favorite bedtime herbs. Steep 1 heaping teaspoon in 1 cup of hot water for 15 minutes. Strain, and sip.

Intermittent Claudication:

Leg Cramps Gone Mad

If you've ever had a nighttime leg cramp, you probably stumbled out of bed to walk the floor for 15 minutes or so while giving your dog a demonstration of your shocking midnight vocabulary. These occasional leg cramps are normal and nothing to worry about. But if your legs cramp up during the day when you're already walking around, the pain could indicate a more serious condition called intermittent claudication.

Best described as hardening of the arteries in the leg, intermittent claudication causes

---

FABULOUS FOLK REMEDY

Garlic to the Rescue!

Garlic (*Allium sativum*) is both a clot buster and cholesterol reducer. Its heating properties also make it a great circulatory tonic, because it gets the blood moving to where it needs to be. Eat one raw clove per day to help alleviate intermittent claudication.

Minty Leg Wraps

To stimulate circulation in your legs, exercise your blood vessels with cold herbal wraps of yarrow (*Achillea millefolium*) and peppermint (*Mentha piperita*). Make a strong infusion by steeping 2 tablespoons of *each* herb in 2 cups of hot water, covered, for 15 minutes. Strain, and chill. Meanwhile, prepare several lengths of gauze, muslin, or cheesecloth. When the infusion is thoroughly chilled, saturate the cloths, wrap them around your lower legs, and relax—with your legs elevated—for 20 minutes. Do this daily for several weeks.

cramping and heaviness in your legs and buttocks when you walk or exercise moderately. The blood can't circulate freely because fatty deposits have blocked a major artery in your upper leg. And the resulting pain can be severe enough to make you limp. Intermittent claudication isn't life threatening, but you can sometimes be immobilized by the sudden pain.

Although you can do plenty to help the condition, if you suspect that you have intermittent claudication, be sure to see your doctor for treatment. The new drug cilostazol (Pletal) may help relieve the pain, but it isn't appropriate for everyone. In extreme cases, surgery is needed to bypass or clean out the diseased artery. In the meantime, however, here are some things you can try:

Rule out arthritis. Arthritis can cause leg pain, too. So how can you tell whether arthritis or intermittent claudication is causing your limp? If you have arthritis, you limp when you begin to walk, and with continued walking—as your muscles and joints loosen up—your limp tends to go away. With intermittent claudication, you're fine when you start out, but the pain develops after you've walked for a while.

Cease and desist. It doesn't take a doctor to figure out that if you stop walking, you'll stop limping. And the pain of intermittent claudication in your lower leg that causes you to limp will subside after a period of rest. So when your legs begin to hurt, sit down for a bit and give them a break.

Get with the program. Although walking can cause the pain in your legs, no one with intermittent claudication should become a couch potato. In fact, a gradual and moderate walking program is what most doctors recommend to fix the problem. Ask your doctor for exercise guidelines that are tailored to your particular condition; then add regular walking to your routine.

Lay off the lard. Follow a heart-healthy lifestyle, and cut back on dietary fats. Too much fat clogs all your arteries—including those that lead to your legs. So while you're taking your daily constitutional, march yourself over to your local farmer's market for some fresh fruits and veggies. Eat lots of them, and don't forget

POWERFUL POTION

HAWTHORN HELPER

Hawthorn (*Crataegus* spp.), lime blossoms (*Tilia europea*), and gingerroot (*Zingiber officinale*) are recognized for their ability to reduce the stickiness of blood platelets and enhance circulation. Use them together, or choose just one. To do the former, mix the dried herbs in equal parts; then add 1 heaping teaspoon of the mix to 1 cup of hot water, and steep for 15 to 20 minutes. You can drink 2 to 3 cups of this tea per day.

the whole grains and low-fat meats or fish, which will also help keep your arteries flowing freely.

Give up the cigarettes. Seems like I say this in almost every section of this book, but it's true—smoking is a health hazard. It's not just lung cancer you need to worry about, but heart disease and myriad other afflictions. For instance, smoking constricts your blood vessels, hampering blood flow. And if you have intermittent claudication, your blood vessels can't handle anything that makes circulation that much more difficult. So help out your vessels by stamping out your habit.

Ponder your poundage. Get on the bathroom scale, please. Uh, oh! Your limping will only get worse if you don't shed some of those unnecessary pounds.

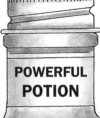

POWERFUL POTION

CIRCULATION-BUILDING TONIC

Ginkgo biloba is most noted for the way it can boost brain function by improving circulation to and within the brain. And that same benefit—improved circulation—may help people with intermittent claudication.

The most efficient way to take ginkgo is in tincture form or in capsules. For the tincture, the standard dose for adults is 30 to 50 drops in a glass of water or juice, up to three times a day. For the capsules, the daily dose is 120 to 240 milligrams. **Caution:** If you are on blood-thinning medications, however, don't take ginkgo without checking with your healthcare provider first.

Irritable Bowel Syndrome:

Bust Those Belly Spasms

If your bowel is irritable, you're well within your rights to be irritable, too. It's no fun when your body produces painful belly spasms and unpredictable bouts of diarrhea and constipation.

Irritable bowel syndrome (IBS), sometimes called spastic colon, is a stressful condition—and to add to the aggravation, stress makes it worse. Many people with IBS are so desperate for relief that they bounce back and forth from gastroenterologists to nutritionists to energy healers.

"Research suggests that IBS stems from a physiologic abnormality," notes Lin Chang, M.D., co-director of the Neuroenteric Disease Program at the University of California at Los Angeles Medical School. The nerves lining the colons of people with IBS may be abnormally sensitive. And, as a result, the nerves controlling the muscles in the gut may overreact to stimuli like gas or the passage of food or fluid from a meal. The resulting spasms inappropriately speed or slow the passage of stool through the colon, triggering a painful cycle of diarrhea and constipation.

Many people with IBS don't enjoy going out to dinner, because symptoms usually occur after a meal and are relieved only by a bowel movement. Worrying about being near a bathroom when you need it just ups the level of stress, which, along with menstruation and dairy products or fatty foods, can make IBS symptoms worse.

A recent large, national IBS survey focused on women, who represent 70 percent of the people who suffer from IBS. Nearly 40 percent of the women surveyed reported experiencing abdominal pain that they described as intolerable without some kind of relief.

Yet, despite the frustrations it involves, IBS is a benign condition that comes and goes. Episodes may be triggered by eating a spicy hot meal or very cold food or during times of emotional upset or depression. Most doctors advise lifestyle changes to eliminate the triggers that bring on the bouts. And, although medications can quell muscle contractions, the best remedies for IBS may well be relaxation techniques to counter stress and diet

---

FABULOUS FOLK REMEDY

Slippery Soother

When mixed with water, slippery elm (*Ulmus fulva*) powder makes a drink that will soothe your irritated gut from end to end. This is a good remedy to take first thing in the morning and last thing at night to help your tissues heal 24 hours a day. Pour 1 cup of warm water over 1 teaspoon of slippery elm powder. Stir briskly, and drink immediately.

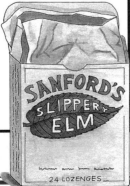

modification to soothe your gut. Here's how to feel better fast:

Keep a trigger diary. Write down what you eat every day and how your body seems to respond. Also note periods of stress and other known IBS triggers. If you're a woman, pay special attention to when you have an episode during your menstrual cycle. Look for any patterns. Then use the diary to help avoid the triggers that bring on a bout.

Try a tummy rub. Chronic conditions like IBS can create a vicious circle when flare-ups are greeted with increased stress, tension, and anger toward a body that isn't behaving the way it's supposed to. A good exercise for breaking this pattern and focusing on healing your gut is to give yourself a 10- to 15-minute abdominal massage every day. Using ¼ teaspoon lobelia (*Lobelia inflata*) oil or catnip (*Nepeta cateria*) tincture to every 1 tablespoon of massage oil (any vegetable oil will do) and beginning at your belly button, massage in small, gentle, clockwise circles until you've covered your entire abdomen. Visualize your intestines relaxing and returning to their normal, healthy state.

Check your medications. Jot down a list of all the medications you take, including over-the-counter supplements, and ask your doctor if they are contributing to your gut pain in any way. Your doctor may be able to adjust your prescriptions or suggest alternate medications that won't aggravate your IBS.

Graze, don't gorge. Eat small meals often. When you give your digestive system smaller amounts of food to process, it may relieve some of the strain.

Zap fat. Cut back on fatty foods, which are harder to digest and more likely to cause discomfort than low-fat foods.

Ditch the gut busters. Avoid beans and other gas-producing foods; ice-cold foods, which can cause spasms; and excessive alcohol, which can irritate your colon.

Balance the bugs. Consider trying milk-free acidophilus tablets (also found in live yogurt cultures) to balance the bacteria in your intestines. You can also take capsules of peppermint oil three times a day, between meals, to calm your digestive tract.

Cut the caffeine. Either eliminate or strictly limit the amount of caffeine you consume. Whether it comes in coffee or your favorite soda, caffeine is a bowel stimulant.

Choose noncarbonated drinks. Reach for noncarbonated drinks, such as fruit juice or water. Even the bubbles in carbonated drinks can cause problems for people with IBS.

Get moving! Exercise is critical for counteracting stress and preventing constipation—provided you choose a form of exercise that you enjoy. In other words, don't pick an aerobics class run by a drill sergeant in Spandex when you'd really prefer a solitary, low-key swim. Check with your doctor to make sure you're in good shape; then start out slowly. Many experts suggest you begin with two 10-minute walks a day before slowly increasing your time until you're up to one 45-minute session a day. Once you're in shape, you can move on to other forms of exercise.

Breathe deeply when you're stressed. Studies show that meditation (which involves controlled breathing) can lower the levels of stress hormones in your body and reduce anxiety and pain. But deep breathing can be soothing on its own, says Emeran Mayer, M.B., a gastroenterologist and IBS specialist at the University of California at Los Angeles. At least half of his patients who adjusted their diets and practiced deep breathing cut the severity of their symptoms. Instead of breathing shallowly from your chest, inhale deeply until you feel your abdomen expand; then slowly exhale. Repeat three more times. Why is this so effective? When your diaphragm moves, it lowers your body's stress response.

Drink lots of water. Plenty of fluid keeps your digestive system in great working condition and helps prevent constipation.

Soothe the pain. If your abdominal discomfort is not relieved by moving your bowels, lie down and get some rest. If the pain persists, place a hot water bottle against your abdomen.

Try muscle relaxants. Low doses of some muscle relaxants and antidepressants relax the bowel muscles and bring temporary relief of symptoms. Ask your doctor which drugs might help you forestall your IBS attacks.

POWERFUL POTION

CRAMP BUSTER

Peppermint (*Mentha piperita*) oil, taken in capsules between meals, is a powerful spasm and pain reliever. If capsules aren't available, try using peppermint leaves to make tea. Steep 1 heaping teaspoon of leaves in 1 cup of hot water, covered, for 10 to 15 minutes. Strain, and drink 3 cups daily between meals.

Itchy Skin:

When You Feel Like a Prickly Pear

Our skin may be silkily sensuous when we're born, but it doesn't take long for its miles of nerves to discover their capacity to send our brains an aggravating signal: the itch—that prickly sensation triggered by everything from bugs and poison ivy to antibiotics, cold air, and even your home's overheated dry air.

Sometimes, itchy skin can be a sign of a serious infection or illness, such as diabetes or anemia, so if you can find no reason for the itch, see your doctor. Otherwise, here's how to get your birthday suit feeling its brand-new best again:

Chill out. Take a cold shower when the itch gets the

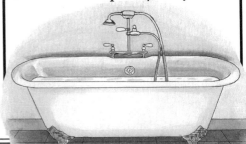

FABULOUS FOLK REMEDY

Cider and Barley Bath

Add 1 cup of apple cider vinegar and 1 cup of barley flour to a tepid bath to relieve itching and restore the proper pH of your skin. Don't worry, the vinegar smell will dissipate quickly!

best of you. While a hot bath stimulates itching, cold water and ice reduce blood circulation, thus reducing swelling and inflammation. If you can't take that much cold water all at once, put some ice packs on the itchy areas until they chill out.

Take a dip in the ocean. Sea water can kill fungi, dry up poison ivy blisters, and relieve almost any skin condition. And it's readily available—even to landlubbers: Just convert your tub to your very own ocean by adding salt to your bath water. Use sea salt if you think it will feel more authentic, although it's a bit pricey just to soak in. The recipe is 2 tablespoons of salt for every 1 pint of water, but filling the tub a pint at a time can be tedious. Try salting the water to taste: Dip a finger into the mix and if it's just slightly tangy, it's probably okay. Soak for 5 to 10 minutes at a time.

Roll in oats. Save the rolled oats for breakfast. Instead try a commercial brand of finely milled or "colloidal" oatmeal, such as Aveeno, that's designed to soothe itchy skin by relieving various types of contact dermatitis, such as prickly heat and eczema. Just throw a few handfuls into the tub, and your bath water will instantly become silky and comforting. Soak for at least 20 minutes

---

O·D·D·B·A·L·L OINTMENT

Chickweed Salve

Chickweed (*Stellaria media*) salve is a favorite for relieving whatever itches. To make your own, chop cleaned leaves, place them in a glass jar, and add enough olive oil to cover the leaves completely. Break open a capsule of vitamin E, and add the liquid to the jar. Cap the jar, and let it sit in a sunny window for 1 week, turning the jar end to end several times, once a day. Strain, and pour the oil into a clean bottle. For the best results, store in the refrigerator, and apply to itchy areas as needed.

O·D·D·B·A·L·L OINTMENT

Baking Soda Soother

Baking soda has a major reputation as an itch fighter. If your skin is especially irritated, try shaking some baking soda into your hand and rubbing it right onto your damp skin when you get out of the bath or shower. The light, pasty film that forms will soothe your skin for hours.

to let the tiny particles thoroughly penetrate the pores of your skin.

Get the starch out. Cornstarch is another reliable itch reliever. Dust this satiny powder right onto your body, or add it to your bath water for soothing itch relief.

Water your air. If you're itching and twitching your way through winter, your home's indoor heat may be sucking all the moisture from your skin. Ask an electrician about installing a central humidifier to keep a healthier moisture balance in the air. Or, for a temporary and cost-free alternative, place pans of water near heating units or forced-air registers. Just remember to refill them regularly.

Fish for winter itch relief. If your wintertime itch is due to the dryness of the weather and heated indoor air, help protect your skin by eating foods rich in omega-3 fatty acids, such as cold-water fish (salmon, mackerel, and sardines), nuts (almonds and walnuts), and seeds (sesame, flax, and sunflower). You should be getting at least one serving a day.

Lactose Intolerance:

Got Milk? No Way!

If you can't digest milk, join the club. Except for those of northern European ancestry, approximately 9 out of 10 people lose their ability to digest milk and milk products by age 20.

Turns out, once our ancestors were weaned, they never got milk again, so the necessary enzyme to digest it—lactase—got programmed out of existence. And without lactase, milk can't be metabolized without the discomfort of gas and cramps—the symptoms of

Non-Dairy Treasure Troves of Calcium

Here are some non-dairy foods that are high in calcium:

- ✔ Canned salmon with bones
- ✔ Cooked dried beans
- ✔ Tofu made with calcium sulfate
- ✔ Collard greens
- ✔ Chicken stock made with bones
- ✔ Soy milk

lactose intolerance. (Note: These symptoms are similar to those of other conditions, such as irritable bowel syndrome and colitis. So when these discomforts occur after eating any and all dairy products, ask your doctor for the simple blood test that can diagnose the problem correctly.)

Fortunately, most people with lactose intolerance can drink up to a pint of milk or eat an ice cream cone without discomfort. For the rest of us—well, here's some help to work it out:

Drop some enzyme. Lactaid, one of several other over-the-counter products, does the work of natural lactase. Just drop a caplet in a glass of milk; then guzzle the moo juice. Follow the directions on the package to take it before eating cheese, sour cream, and other high-lactose foods. Your bones will benefit from the calcium, and you can enjoy your favorite Ben and Jerry's without the bloating aftereffects.

Ferret out the fillers. Many foods con-

POWERFUL POTION

MARSHMALLOW TEA

Marshmallow (*Althea officinalis*) tea soothes inflamed tissues and helps heal the lining of the gut. Make a cold infusion by soaking 2 tablespoons of marshmallow root in 1 quart of cold water overnight. Strain, and drink throughout the day.

Some Really Cheesy Ideas

Who says you can't have a grilled cheese sandwich? There is now a lactose-free cheese that melts just like real American cheese. Pop it under the broiler, and you'll have a melted cheese sandwich. Or a tuna-cheese melt. Or a baked potato topped with cheese. Look for this lactose-free yummy in the dairy case.

tain milk solids as filler. If you're especially sensitive to lactose, these can cause you discomfort if you ingest enough, so read food labels carefully, and search out lactose-free products instead.

Don't do dairy solo. Have a cookie with your glass of milk, or ham up your cheese. Studies have found that eating other foods with a dairy product increases the likelihood that the lactose can sneak into your body without bothering your gut.

Send in the second string. Because milk is such a rich source of calcium and vitamin D—major dietary bone builders—you need to find those nutrients elsewhere. Eat plenty of dark green leafy vegetables, sardines, salmon, and almonds for calcium. And add fatty fish like salmon and herring to your diet, too. If you're still coming up short on these bone basics, ask your doctor if you should take calcium supplements.

Shop for fakes. Shop around until you find as many lactose-free products as you can. There is now a yogurt with added lactase, for instance. While all stores may not carry everything, you may find many of these products in health-food stores.

Get some great recipes. Check out the Web (for example, www.lactaid.com). You'll find many recipes and menu ideas to help enjoy dairy-free living.

FABULOUS FOLK REMEDY

Sour Power

Traditional nomadic peoples who continued to use dairy products as a food source beyond infancy cultured their milk products to make them more easily digestible. If you are lactose intolerant, you may be able to handle fermented dairy products (such as yogurt and kefir) and, perhaps, even goat's or sheep's milk cheeses. If your lactose intolerance is severe, however, it's best to omit milk from your diet completely.

Laryngitis:

Give Your Pipes a Rest

W as that you or Marlene Dietrich shrieking your lungs out at the football game? If you're in the hollering habit, you've probably found that after a few hours of smoking, drinking, talking above a noisy crowd, or even singing loudly—you're suddenly sounding sexy!

That husky voice, that throaty sound—it may be fun at first. But when laryngitis (or an inflammation of the mucous lining of the larynx that affects your breathing as well as your voice) goes all the way, best your swollen vocal chords can manage is a croaky ribbit. You go from marvelous Marlene to a frog on a log—and that's not so much fun after all!

While laryngitis can result from an infection (in which case you might also have a

---

Thyme the Pot

An herbal steam can help soothe respiratory passages and alleviate laryngitis pain. Place 3 to 4 drops of essential oil of thyme in a pot of hot, steaming water. Bend over the pot—taking care not to get a steam burn!— and tent your head with a towel. Breathe in deeply.

fever) or exposure to industrial fumes, most cases are from the ordinary abuse of your voice box, and there are warning signs (a dry cough, a tickling sensation in the throat, hoarseness, and a need to clear your throat continuously). So you can often evict that frog from your throat before it settles in. If the laryngitis doesn't go away in a few days, call your doctor. If it's been 1 week without improvement, you could have a bacterial infection or a serious disorder, like tuberculosis or cancer. In the meantime, however, try these tips to relieve it:

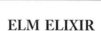

POWERFUL POTION

ELM ELIXIR

Slippery elm (*Ulmus fulva*) is used by professional singers and speakers to recover their voices and keep their laryngeal tissues in tip-top shape. Steep 1 heaping teaspoon of the dried herb in 1 cup of hot water for 15 minutes. Strain, add honey and lemon if desired, and drink 3 to 4 cups per day.

Be mute. The most effective treatment is silence. Don't use your voice at all—not even for whispering. Trying to express yourself in squeaks and croaks just aggravates your inflamed vocal cords, actually causing them to bang together and slow your recovery.

Create a greenhouse effect. If you've got an extreme case of laryngitis, try resting in a warm room with high humidity for a day or two. Use a humidifier if necessary, and let your worn-out throat soak up some moisture while you sleep.

Get serious about smoke. The most serious cause of laryngitis is long-term smoking. If you haven't been convinced by now that smoking is a major health risk, let the damage to your delicate vocal cords motivate you. Look into all the aids to help you quit—from prescription medications to nicotine gum to group therapy.

That's a Wrap!

A carrot neck wrap may ease inflammation and help you recover more quickly. Grate a carrot onto a length of cheesecloth. Fold the cloth in half lengthwise, and moisten with warm water. Wrap it around your neck, and then wrap a warm towel on top. Keep in place for 20 to 30 minutes. For extra heat, sprinkle some cayenne pepper on the grated carrot.

Ask your doctor to help you find the right method for you.

Suppress a cough. The more you cough, the more you irritate your sensitive larynx. When your cough is dry and unproductive, use cough suppressant medications to keep your larynx from further harm.

Gargle galore. A red sage tea gargle can ease the mucous membranes of your larynx and boost your immune system. Pour 1 cup of warm water over 1 teaspoon of red sage, and steep for 10 minutes. Strain; then gargle.

Wear a muffler. Place a warm, wet cloth compress on your neck for 2 to 3 minutes. Then replace it with a cold one. Keep a wool scarf around your neck to keep the cold compress in place for 30 minutes.

Try tepid tea. Drink lots of water, but keep it tepid—not too hot or too cold, either of which might further inflame your vocal chords. Or enjoy a few cups of tepid tea with lemon and honey, which is very soothing for your larynx.

Swallow with caution. When your throat is under siege with laryngitis, be wary of what you put down it. Avoid very spicy foods, hot soups and beverages, and any other edible irritant.

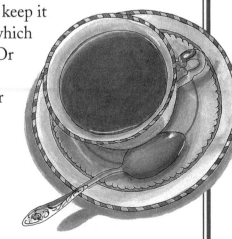

Leaky Bladder:

No Laughing Matter

Age brings its insults, that's for sure. But some problems crop up that too many of us accept as inevitable, when, in fact, we can do a lot to fix them. Incontinence is one of those problems, and it hits mostly women. In fact, many women give up favorite activities and stop socializing, because they're afraid of leaking if they sneeze or laugh. Part of the problem is that women often don't ask for help. One study showed that it typically took 10 years from the first symptom for a woman to ask her doctor what to do about it. And that's a shame, because there's a lot you can do to address the problem—part of which is physiological.

FABULOUS FOLK REMEDY

Muscle-Toning Tonic

Skullcap (*Scutellaria lateriflora*) relieves nervous tension, which may help restore adequate sphincter tone in the muscle that controls the bladder opening. Steep 1 teaspoon in 1 cup of hot water for 10 minutes. Drink 1 to 3 cups daily.

Women have a shorter urethra—the tube through which the urine flows—than men do, so it is more prone to leak in women than in men. Excess weight, estrogen depletion (after menopause or a hysterectomy, for instance), stroke, and diabetes can all add to the problem, as can nerve damage, infection, some medications, and even too much caffeine.

Finally, a woman's pelvic floor muscles can weaken after she gives birth to several children, allowing the pelvic organs to slip out of place and weakening the bladder neck. Sneezing, coughing, and heavy lifting put pressure on the abdomen, and the bladder neck opens because it is too weak to stay shut, explains Lila Wallis, M.D., a specialist in women's health based in New York City.

In extreme cases, surgery can restore the pelvic floor muscles and connective tissues that support the bladder. An artificial urinary sphincter can be inserted to compress the urethra and prevent involuntary urination. But in the great majority of cases, nothing so dire is needed to get your trustworthy bladder back. Try these leak-proofing tips to get back into your old routine:

Do some detective work. Don't be afraid to talk candidly with your doctor about urinary incontinence. Together, with the help of a few diagnostic tests for bladder function, you can figure out what's causing it.

Take notes. Keep a daily record of when and how often you leak urine, how often you urinate voluntarily, how

POWERFUL POTION

HEALTHY H$_2$O

Always drink plenty of fluids to keep your entire urinary tract in good working order. People often believe if they drink less, the urge to urinate will be lessened. This is not true. Dehydration irritates your bladder and makes the condition worse.

evian
Natural Spring Water

often you feel like urinating, and what seems to cause the leaking. Share these notes with your doctor if you can't determine the cause of the trouble on your own.

Research your medicine. Sometimes, medications cause incontinence. Diuretics and blood pressure drugs can weaken the urethra and allow urine leakage. Antihistamines and decongestants may also cause you to retain urine, creating a situation in which overflow incontinence may occur. Some antidepressants and narcotics can also cause this reaction. Keep a record of medications you take, and see if you notice any connection. Then consult your doctor about your suspicions.

Ditch the diuretics. Is it something you ate? Or drank? Pay attention to your daily intake of food and drink. Incontinence can sometimes be managed with changes in diet. Some foods irritate the bladder, so if you avoid them, you are bothered less. Try boycotting caffeinated and carbonated drinks, alcohol, citrus fruits and juices, spicy foods, and artificial sweeteners to see if this eliminates the problem.

Get regular. Severe constipation can also cause you to retain urine by compressing the bladder outlet. A healthy, high-fiber diet can prevent things from compacting down below. See **Constipation** for remedies.

Tighten up. If your doctor believes your leaky bladder is due to weak pelvic floor muscles, you may be able to correct the problem with simple exercises known as Kegels. Here's how to do them: While you're on the toilet, stop and start the flow of urine. This action will help you locate the pelvic floor muscle. Once you've learned exactly where this muscle is, you can squeeze it shut and open it anywhere, not just on the toilet. Repeat your Kegels several times a day, perhaps while you're sitting at your desk or watching television.

Don't lose your marbles. Insert a small weight, such as a clean marble, into your vagina, and squeeze your muscles around it. Hold for a count of four, then relax. Repeat 10 times, several times a day. For an alternative exercise, ask your doctor about using vaginal weights, which are shaped like tampons. These can be worn for 20 to 30 minutes at a time.

Lower the impact. Running and high-impact aerobics can cause leakage, which is hard to control during bouncing. If this is a frequent problem for you, try swimming or bicycling instead. These activities require less impact and create fewer leakages.

Retrain your bladder. Try to wait a bit longer before you urinate, even when you feel some urgency. You can briefly stop the feeling by contracting the pelvic floor muscles. Each time you do this, you are increasing the time between urinating, which trains your bladder to wait.

Try biofeedback. This simple and painless technique, usually performed in a hospital or office setting, can help you retrain your bladder. A sensor is placed in your vagina or rectum, and another electrode sensor is put on your stomach. These sensors read the signals given when you contract or relax your pelvic floor muscles, and you can view the signals on a video screen. By watching the monitor you learn what your muscles are doing and thus can begin to control them. In a study at the University of Alabama, medication alone reduced women's episodes of incontinence by 68.5 percent. But the women who used biofeedback and exercise without drugs reduced the episodes by 81 percent. If you'd like to give it a try, ask your doctor to refer you to a biofeedback specialist.

Get shocked. In electrical stimulation therapy, a tiny amount of painless electric current is sent to the pelvic floor muscles and your bladder to help the muscles contract so they can get stronger. This is especially helpful if you have very weak pelvic floor muscles. Ask your doctor if this type of therapy would help you.

Check out collagen implants. When all else fails, implants of collagen, a natural protein, can be injected near the bladder neck to bulk up your urethral tissue, narrowing the urethral opening so that the muscle has a smaller space to open and close. Several injections create a seal that prevents leaks. Talk with your doctor about this procedure. It may require more than one treatment and need to be repeated in a few years.

Don't depend on Depends. Many women seem willing to accept the advice of an aging film actress who used to hawk disposable adult diapers on television. Such absorbent products are a stop gap—a temporary measure, not a life sentence. If you do opt to use them, however, be sure to change them frequently. You can also use special deodorant products to reduce any telltale odors until you can change the pad.

Go hot and cold. Sitz baths increase circulation to the pelvic organs and may help tone and strengthen tissues. Simply prepare a warm bath—this can be done in the tub—and immerse yourself up to your belly button. After soaking for 5 minutes, get out of the tub, and apply a cold, wet towel like a diaper. Leave the towel on for 5 minutes. This may be repeated two to three times in a session. The greater the contrast between the hot and cold, the greater the tonifying effects. The hot phase should be warm enough so that you don't become chilled during the cold phase. Modify the temperatures to your comfort level.

POWERFUL POTION

IRRITABLE BLADDER BOOSTER

When a nervous bladder is the source of the leaky tendency, an infusion of kava (*Piper methysticum*) may help reduce bladder irritability. Steep 1 teaspoon of the herb in 1 cup of hot water for 15 minutes. Drink 1 to 3 cups per day. **Caution:** Kava has recently been linked with liver toxicity. Check with your doctor before using—especially if you're taking antidepressant or antianxiety medication.

Macular Degeneration:

The Eyes Don't Have to Have It

You know the old joke: How many people does it take to change a light bulb? Well here's a question that's no joke: How often are you changing your light bulbs and replacing them with higher-wattage bulbs? A major symptom of age-related macular degeneration (AMD) is the need for a brighter light in your reading lamp.

AMD causes blurred vision, which usually begins as difficulty reading fine print. The condition tends to be mild in

---

the early stages, but with the passage of time, it can lead to a severe reduction in vision. This gradual loss of central vision is caused by the degeneration of the macula, a tiny bull's-eye point at the center of the retina. By age 65, approximately 15 percent of us will suffer some macular degeneration; and by age 75, the prevalence more than doubles to nearly 33 percent.

"We don't yet know how large a part genetics plays in the development of AMD, because there are so many more potent risk factors, such as environment and diet," says Alex Eaton, M.D., an ophthalmologist and retina specialist in Fort Myers, Florida. Siblings—and especially twins—of people who have macular degeneration are at a higher risk than the general population. The good news is that even if you come from a family with AMD, you are not likely to develop the disease—if you reduce your other risks, says Dr. Eaton.

POWERFUL POTION

ANTIOXIDANT ACTIVITY ENHANCER

Increasing the microcirculation of the eyes and enhancing antioxidant activities may help prevent the onset and slow the progression of macular degeneration. Make an infusion of ginkgo (*Ginkgo biloba*) and bilberry (*Vaccinium myrtillis*), using 1 heaping teaspoon of *each* steeped for 15 minutes in hot water. Strain, and drink 2 to 3 cups daily. **Caution:** Do not take ginkgo if you are on blood-thinning medications without checking with your healthcare provider first.

PICTURE THIS NEW THERAPY

A less common, but more damaging form of AMD is choroidal neovascularization (CNV). Abnormal blood vessels grow under the retina, much like the roots of a tree growing under and lifting up a sidewalk. These abnormal vessels may also leak fluid or bleed. The longer this goes on, the more central vi-

Hit the Greens!

Do you ski? Sail? Surfboard? In-line skate? If you're trying to avoid macular degeneration, you might want to trade in your sporting equipment for a set of golf clubs. Golf, you see, is easier on the eyes. A golf course reflects far less sunlight into your eyes than the ski slopes or the open sea, and sunlight is so powerful that even reflected rays can damage your unprotected eye. Bottom line: Always protect your eyes with the proper shades, because even if you think you are not looking at the sun, the sun's rays are still reflecting up at you.

sion is lost. Laser treatment can halt the progress of CNV, but it also forms a scar that creates a permanent blind spot in the field of vision. Photodynamic therapy, in which the abnormal vessels are closed off to prevent retinal scanning, is a new treatment that can halt the progress of this condition. The technique, which needs to be repeated about three times a year, was approved by the U.S. Food and Drug Administration in 2000.

SOME SMART (AND EASY) WAYS TO PREVENT AMD

While macular degeneration is a serious disease that needs a doctor's attention, there are many ways to prevent it or catch it in the early—and treatable—stage. Here's how:

Get chummy with your ophthalmologist. Get regular eye checkups—at least once a year—so your doctor can detect any symptoms of AMD, such as the appearance of drusen, which are spots on the retina that are visible during an eye exam. Drusen don't do much damage, but they may cause changes in vision, such as the distortion of straight lines. A telephone pole may appear bent, for example. If you have several relatives who have macular degeneration, begin getting retinal examinations when you are age 40.

Watch out for health problems. Be aware of how other medical conditions may affect your vision. For example, hypertension and diabetes each increase your risk for macular damage and loss of vision, according to Dr. Eaton. Hypertension, often related to hardening of the arteries, affects the blood flow throughout your body—including your eyes. Diabetes sometimes leads to diabetic retinopathy, a condition that can interfere with proper metabolism of oxygen in the retina. Talk with your eye doctor as well as your medical doctor about keeping such conditions under control—and AMD at bay.

Limit your exposure to harsh sunlight. Wear proper sunglasses, and a brimmed hat, and avoid the sun at the peak hours of 10:00 A.M. to 2:00 P.M. Also, make sure your sunglasses provide 100 percent protection from ultraviolet light. Buy the darkest possible lens color. Brown and tan offer the best balance of

POWERFUL POTION

A DOWN-UNDER CHOWDER

An Australian study found that omega-3 fatty acids, might help reduce the risk of macular degeneration. Study participants who ate fresh or frozen fish one to three times a month had about half the risk of macular degeneration than those who ate fish less often. To make a basic chowder, place 2 white potatoes, cubed; 2 large carrots, sliced; 1 onion, diced; seafood seasoning (Old Bay is good); and at least 1 pound of fish into a pot. Cover with water, and add 1 more inch. Bring the water to a boil; then simmer until the veggies are done and the fish is opaque.

comfort and protection, with gray and green second best.

Eat more antioxidants. Antioxidants counteract the oxidative wear and tear going on in your body and are especially important for your macula, says Dr. Eaton. Because the macula contains a protective pigment made up of antioxidants, you need to replenish the pigment with antioxidants found in food and supplements to offset the breakdown. If you don't, years of oxidative stress left unchecked can result in the formation of drusen. The best antioxidants are foods rich in vitamins A, C, and E, but ask your doctor if you should take vitamin supplements to add to your protection.

Try nature's sunglasses. Eat plenty of green leafy vegetables like kale, spinach, and chard for lutein. Your macula contains pigment made up in part of lutein. This pigment helps filter out the light implicated in macular degeneration and also fights oxidation. A study by the National Eye Institute found foods rich in lutein and zeaxanthin were associated with reduced risk of AMD, so lutein supplements are popping up all over the place. But their long-term effectiveness hasn't been proven yet.

Chamomile Compresses Help

Warm compresses made with an infusion of chamomile (*Matricaria recutita*) or eyebright (*Euphrasia officinalis*) may help relieve eye strain from macular degeneration. Steep 1 teaspoon of the herb in 1 cup of hot water, covered, for 10 to 15 minutes. Strain, and saturate a clean cloth or gauze pad with the cooled solution. Cover your eyes, and rest for 20 minutes.

Eyes-Right Guide to Vitamins

Just in case you weren't paying attention, here are some of the best sources of the vitamins you need to help prevent macular degeneration:

Vitamin A: carrots, squash, cantaloupe, and oranges

Vitamin C: citrus fruits and juices, berries, melons, peppers, broccoli, and potatoes

Vitamin E: vegetable oils, eggs, nuts and seeds, fortified cereals, and wheat germ

Learn to love orange food. Carrots are good for your eyes and so are other orange and yellow vegetables and fruits. They are all rich sources of beta-carotene, the plant-based building block for vitamin A. So add some carrots, squash, and pumpkin to your menu, along with plenty of greens.

Don't say cheese. Avoid those bacon cheeseburgers and other high-fat foods. Just as fat can clog the arteries of your heart, it can also clog those that go to your eyes, reducing the flow of blood and nutrients to your retinas. In fact, studies reveal that many of the same factors that lead to atherosclerosis also contribute to the development of AMD. These include smoking, high blood pressure, and high cholesterol levels.

Kick the habit. Smoking increases your risk of developing macular degeneration two to six times, warns Dr. Eaton, both by depriving your retina of oxygen and by constricting your blood vessels, making it more difficult for nutrients to be carried through those vessels to your eyes. Get help today to overcome this addiction.

Menopause:

The Change Has Changed!

Tossing like a rototiller in soaked sheets all night long? Finding the Sahara where there used to be a sexy swamp? Feeling emotions that make premenstrual syndrome look like a Perky Mood for Sure? Aaarrrgghh!

Plenty of women sail through menopause, but most experience at least a few of the most common symptoms of changing hormone levels, such as hot flashes, vaginal dryness, and mood swings. Yet, until we let menopause out of the closet a few years back, not many women knew to expect these symptoms, much less how to handle them. Women were in the

Dress Like an Onion

Here's a good way to cope with hot flashes: Dress in layers, so you can always remove some of your clothing to feel less heat, suggests Lila Wallis, M.D., a New York City–based specialist in women's health. With enough layers to remove and replace, you can more easily adapt to your body's erratic thermostat.

dark, with little useful knowledge. The good news is that menopause is easy to manage if you're armed with accurate information.

That's because the occasional flushes, sweats, and palpitations associated with menopause can occur for 6 years before actual menopause begins. This time is known as perimenopause, during which there is either a gradual decline of estrogen or a stretch of hormonal ups and downs more precipitous than the daily NASDAQ report!

ESTROGEN: NOT FOR EVERYONE

A friend of mine was advised to start hormone-replacement therapy (HRT), despite the fact that she had few of the pesky symptoms associated with menopause. When she asked why, her doctor said, "Oh, my wife takes this and likes it."

Hello! Not all women are the same. Each woman faces different risks and has different individual requirements. And, therefore, the decisions about treatment must be made on an individual basis according to each

---

FABULOUS FOLK REMEDY

Pick the Wonder Weed

Red clover (*Trifolium pratense*) is a weed found growing wild in many fields and along roadsides. Known as a blood purifier, it is used in many tonic and restorative teas. It also has a history as a woman's herb and has been acknowledged more recently for its plant sterol content and gentle estrogenic effects. Red clover may be taken as a tea (1 teaspoon per 1 cup of hot water, steeped for 10 to 15 minutes)—drink 1 cup twice daily—or in a commercial preparation called Promensil. **Caution:** Breast cancer survivors should not use it.

woman's health, lifestyle, and risk factors, emphasizes Lila Wallis, M.D., a New York City specialist in women's health. There is no "one size fits all" when it comes to taking HRT.

Recently, the Women's Health Network, a national consortium of women's health professionals and advocates, evaluated the latest research on HRT. They found that, despite the drug-company hype blanketing the airwaves, HRT was not necessary to prevent osteoporosis.

What's more, for women with heart disease, it actually increased the risk of a heart attack for 2 years after they began taking the drug. A few months later, the American Heart Association came out with a statement that backs this up.

Given these considerations, whether or not to replace hormones can be a tricky question. But here are some ways to make the decision easier:

See an internist. If you are like many women who consider their gynecologist their main medicine man or woman, you may want to branch out as menopause approaches. An internist is better trained to appraise the effects of menopause on the total woman than is a gynecologist, who is trained mostly in surgery, says Dr. Wallis. And a woman facing menopause has to consider her heart, bones, and immune system and her likelihood of developing cancer.

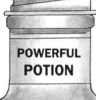

POWERFUL
POTION

GINSENG FOR NIGHT SWEATS

American ginseng (not Siberian or Korean) is considered a cooling herb that can be used to tame the nighttime sweats of menopause. You can chew ginseng root or brew it into a tea. For the best results, try a standardized extract—100 milligrams, two times a day. **Caution:** Ginseng can raise your blood pressure. So if you are taking medicine for high blood pressure, check with your health-care provider before using it.

Trust Yourself

Did you know that hormone levels can affect your thinking and memory? Well, they can and often do. Fortunately, our brains are capable of adapting to changing hormone levels, so don't make a big deal out of a temporary memory lapse or two as hormone levels fluctuate. The last thing we want to do is add fuel to that tired male fantasy that women can't be trusted with power in high office because their hormones make them irrational or forgetful.

Get a comprehensive physical exam. Before you make any decisions about taking HRT, schedule a thorough physical exam that includes an investigation of your own and your family's health history. Ask your doctor to check your cholesterol level and thyroid function and to arrange for an electrocardiogram, mammogram, a bone density measurement, and a chest x-ray, says Dr. Wallis.

Evaluate your risk. Figure out your risk factors for heart disease, osteoporosis, and cancer. Work with your doctor and talk about your personal history and family health history. If you have a family history of heart disease or breast or ovarian cancer, for example, HRT may significantly increase your risk of developing those diseases yourself. The point is to consider your total risk profile. Talk with your doctor, and decide how you can use menopause as a time to build your health.

NAVIGATING THE SEAS OF CHANGE

Whether you decide to replace hormones or not, there are ways to get through both menopause and those up-and-down months that precede it with little difficulty:

Consider the alternatives. If you are in your early 50s with moderate symptoms, vitamin E and primrose oil can be very effective at lessening hot flashes, according to Orli Etigen, M.D., director of the Center for Women's Healthcare and vice chairman of the Department of Medicine at the Weill Cornell Medical College in New York. If you'd like to try them, check with your doctor for the amount that's right for you.

For mood swings, Dr. Etigen also usually recommends B vitamins, especially vitamin B_6. For a woman in her late 40s, about 2,000 milligrams of calcium may also help mood swings, Dr. Etigen says. So ask your doctor if these remedies would be effective and safe for you.

Check out black cohosh. This herb has become a best-selling menopause remedy. It is sold in health-food stores as tinctures, syrup, or dried root for tea. It is also marketed as Remifemin, a menopausal supplement that has been clinically tested in Europe and the United States, and was shown to significantly improve hot flashes and other menopausal symptoms in 6 to 8 weeks, says Dr. Etigen. In one study, 80 percent of women rated it good to very good in reducing menopausal symptoms.

Does Your Doctor Pass the Test?

Find out if your doctor is up to date on menopause. The North American Menopause Society (NAMS), a nonprofit education organization for women and their doctors, offers study guides and exams nationwide to qualify healthcare providers as either "menopause clinicians" or "menopause educators." The next time you visit your doctor, check out all those framed diplomas on the wall.

Chaste Berries

Modest, pure, and unsullied, the chasteberry is often called the menopause herb, because it is used to alleviate many symptoms of hormonal imbalance, such as hot flashes, mood swings, and vaginal dryness. Try it as a tincture—$\frac{1}{2}$ teaspoon, one to two times a day—*after* you get the okay from your healthcare provider.

Apparently, black cohosh does not have estrogenic effects on breast tissue or on the lining of the uterus, but more long-term research is needed to be sure. The German regulatory agency (the equivalent of the U.S. Food and Drug Administration) recommends a dose of 40 milligram a day, or one 20 milligram tablet, twice a day, for no longer than 6 months. Be aware there may be side effects, such as occasional abdominal pain, dizziness, and headaches.

Try soy. Soybeans contain plant sterols, which have an affinity for estrogen receptor sites. This means that they have a slight estrogenic effect in your body and can help reduce the symptoms of perimenopause. In addition, soy products—such as tofu, soy protein, tempeh, and edamame—can give you a low-fat, high-protein boost that may be just the thing for relieving hot flashes.

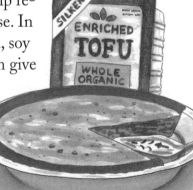

Menstrual Conditions:

Cure Cramps and Other Periodic Pains

Remember the calendar codes? When we Boomers were young, there were more strange, recurring hieroglyphics on girls' calendars than they found in Tutkankhamen's tomb. "My friend visits" (that was a subtle one), a big round solid dot (uncannily resembling a large period), and even "Feed the gerbils" (true story! a college freshman's inspiration—and not a gerbil cage in the room).

When some of us were

teenagers, we used to call our monthly period "the curse." It didn't have anything to do with mummies or ancient tombs, but sometimes, the people living with us thought we were cursed. Normally happy-go-lucky and mostly sweet, some of us would turn, overnight, into snarling wolverines.

But most of us had good reason. More than half of menstruating women have cramps and low back pain. The discomfort may begin before any bleeding, may peak in the next few hours, and then usually stops in a day or two. The intensity of the pain varies among women and can even vary for the same woman from one period to the next.

Prostaglandins (the hormones released during menstration) increase the contraction of uterine muscles. If they contract too strongly, the flow of blood (and oxygen) to those muscles is temporarily decreased, causing cramps. Cramps sometimes come with a headache and gastrointestinal symptoms—not to mention fatigue, if you aren't getting enough iron! Here's what you can do to fight cramps:

POWERFUL POTION

THE LADIES' TONIC

Chastetree berry (*Vitex agnus-castus*) and black cohosh (*Cimicifuga racemosa*) have a normalizing effect on hormonal balance and may be useful when taken together for menstrual difficulties. Blend with two other traditional woman's herbs—partridge berry (*Mitchella repens*) and lady's-mantle (*Alchemilla vulgaris*)—for a tea that will support you all through the month. Mix equal parts of *each* herb together; then add 1 teaspoon of the mixture to 1 cup of hot water, and steep for 10 minutes. Strain, and drink 1 to 2 cups per day.

When a Cramp Is Not Just a Cramp

Certain cramps may signal a serious medical problem, such as endometriosis or fibroid tumors, that has nothing to do with menstruation. See your doctor when:

✔ Menstrual cramps do not disappear after your period begins.

✔ The pain is on one side only, rather than over the entire abdomen.

✔ There is no relief with aspirin or other anti-inflammatory remedies.

Eat right and exercise. Before using over-the-counter drugs to relieve menstrual discomfort, try diet and exercise, suggests Lila Wallis, M.D., a specialist in women's health based in New York City. Cut back on sweets, which just make you more hungry and bloated. Opt for complex carbohydrates, such as fresh fruits and vegetables. And exercise to stretch your muscles—and, as a bonus, lift a nasty mood.

Take the right stuff. Aspirin and other nonsteroidal anti-inflammatory drugs (NSAIDs), such as acetaminophen and ibuprofen, block the production of prostaglandins, which cause uterine contractions. In fact, Tylenol has developed a new medication just for menstrual pain and bloating, says Mary Ellen Mortensen, M.D., executive director of medical affairs at McNeil Consumer Healthcare. Take the standard dose of two caplets every 4 to 6 hours, but no more than eight caplets in 24 hours, says Dr. Mortensen.

Eat from the sea. Antiprostaglandins are also abundant in seafood. So add a daily serving of oil-rich fish like mackerel, sardines, salmon, or cod to help reduce your symptoms.

PMS IS REAL AND TREATABLE

In the few days before menstruation begins, many women get more than a few cramps or bloating. They get depressed, irritated—even angry. They get, in a nifty little acronym, PMS (or, premenstrual syndrome). And while scientists have proved that PMS is physiological, not psychological, in origin, there are some things you can do to ease the symptoms:

Boost your endorphins. Don't just sit around and suffer. Studies show that women who exercise regularly are less likely to have PMS, possibly because exercise increases oxygen to the muscles and boosts the amount of serotonin and other uplifting brain chemicals, called endorphins, in the blood. So don't wait

Make a Flower Spritz

Make your own flower water to spritz on your skin during the day for a fragrant lift. Made from essential oils that relieve the pain and stress associated with menstration, flower water can be used whenever the need arises. Add 10 drops *each* of essential oils of lavender (*Lavendula officinalis*), clary sage (*Salvia sclarea*), and roman chamomile (*Anthemis nobilis*) to 5 milliliters of isopropyl alcohol (available at most drugstores). Add to 100 milliliters of distilled water. Store in a glass spray bottle, and use liberally.

until the mood strikes you to start exercising. Include 20 minutes a day of regular exercise in your life. Even a simple after-dinner walk can go a long way toward preventing the aggravation of PMS.

Consider a new escape route. PMS Escape, an over-the-counter treatment, is made of complex carbohydrates, vitamins, and minerals. Studies show it reduces craving for sweets and eases anger and depression, says Dr. Wallis. But most nonprescription tion PMS remedies contain a mild diuretic and a mild sedative, she notes. The diuretic helps reduce bloating, but it can also deplete potassium. So if you use this type of remedy, restore potassium levels by adding an orange, banana, or other potassium-rich food to your diet every day.

Mind your minerals—especially calcium and magnesium. Calcium was voted by women as one of the top treatments for PMS, because it can soothe cramps, low back pain, bloating, food cravings, and mood swings all at once, says Mary Hardy, M.D.,

Natural Native Medicine

The Tummy Touch

Historically, many Native American women used abdominal massage to relieve cramps and bloating. Some women would sprinkle a pinch of sage, tobacco, or sacred pollen on the abdomen while singing sacred songs to soothe away the pain. Today, there are a variety of herbal oils, such as evening primrose, that you can use with massage.

medical director of the Cedars-Sinai Integrative Medicine Medical Group in New York City. Try taking 1,000 milligrams a day. Magnesium helps, too, but you might want to go easy on the stuff (stick with 200 milligrams, one to two times per day), because too much can give you diarrhea.

End the day with evening primrose oil. Named for a North American yellow wildflower that opens in the evening, evening primrose flowers produce seeds that are rich in essential fatty acids. The seeds help the body make prostaglandin E, which has anti-inflammatory properties. Take 2 to 3 grams a day of the oil in capsules, recommends Orli Etigen, M.D., director of the Center for Women's Healthcare and vice chairman of the Department of Medicine at Weill Cornell Medical Center in New York City. Just make sure the label says "standardized to 8 percent gamma-linolenic acid," which means you're getting an adequate amount of the active ingredient. Keep evening primrose oil refrigerated to prevent it from becoming rancid.

Midlife Crisis:

It's Renewal Time!

Even though plenty of folks have been mocked for doing a double-take (or even a backflip) in midlife, the good news is that it's usually not a real crisis at all. Midlife brings changes—sometimes big ones. But they're usually for the better. For example, when the kids grow up and move out, you may find your energy levels suddenly surge. Not to mention that the whole notion of life's midpoint has moved back a few decades. Remember when 30 was considered middle-aged? Then 40? Then 50? A survey at Harvard revealed that most people are happiest in their 50s. So, if you're determined to have a midlife crisis, better wait until you retire!

This suggestion isn't as unrealistic as you think. The average human life span nearly doubled in the twentieth century, and experts believe that by the middle of the twenty-first century, we will live well into our 100s. Even today, the biggest increase in population is among people over 100, according to the U.S. Census Bureau.

MIDLIFE RENEWAL

Midlife is a time to trade in those "same-old, same-old" activities for something different. One woman I know took up rowing. She started at age 50 and went from being a person who hated getting up early and doing any kind of exercise to someone who has found new joy in her life on the river at 5:30 every morning. Another friend invited several long-time buddies who are the same age to participate in a week-long Outward Bound program to see if they still had "the right stuff." And guess what? They did! Here's how to change your crisis into a fountain of opportunity:

Take stock of your life. Our life patterns are more diverse today. The empty-nest blues have vanished. Most parents I know can't wait for their kids to get on with their lives, so they can stop trying to be Super Parents and have more time to pursue other interests. In fact, studies show that women over age 35

The Midlife Crises Myth

Because the core years between 40 and 60 had rarely been studied, two dozen scholars at Harvard Medical School in Boston looked at the midlife crises of 15,000 people beginning in 1989. The result? They found that a crisis is no more common at midlife than at any other age. Yes, we all go through a midlife transition during which we reevaluate who we are, where we've been, and where we're going. But by midlife, most of us have moved past the anxiety and uncertainty of our youth and are ready to bloom—which is why midlife is actually the happiest time of all.

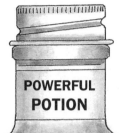

POWERFUL POTION

DISCOVER YOUR ROOTS

Roots are what ground us in reality and hold us to our center. To help give yourself some solid ground to stand on, be sure to include some roots in your diet, too—especially burdock (*Arctium lappa*) and beets. If you're really feeling like your feet are not on the ground, make a tea of burdock and dandelion (*Taraxacum officinalis*) by simmering 1 heaping teaspoon of dried root (¹⁄₂ teaspoon of *each*) in 1 cup of water for 20 minutes. Strain, and drink 1 to 2 cups daily. **Caution:** Dandelion is rich in potassium and shouldn't be taken with potassium tablets.

are more fulfilled than ever. Only one in four feels that the world is closing in at midlife. Instead, it's opening up.

If you're feeling less than excited about your life at midlife, take a look at where you've been and where you'd like to go. Reevaluate your work, social activities, and family life, and take a moment to see where your time goes—and where you want it to go.

Pause for second thoughts. Many people never bother to "think." We simply tote around the ideas we learned when we were young, never giving them a first thought, let alone a second.

Yet nothing ages you faster. So take a second, third, or even a fourth look at how you think about things—and get your brain in gear by going back to school. Take a course in gardening, art, photography, even a foreign language. In many states, midlifers can attend college classes for free or at a significant discount.

Figure out where you want to go from here. Think about the greater meaning of your life. Up until now, you've probably been so busy with the day-to-day realities of life that you've had little time to explore a higher plane of existence. Then mortality rears its head, and many people find themselves thinking about the legacy they'd like to leave behind, says Joni Johnston, Psy.D., a San Diego psychologist. She suggests that a midlife review may be the process by which people not only evaluate the first half of their lives but also figure out the pleasures of the second.

Solve your identity puzzle. Typically, it isn't until we hit middle age that it becomes more urgent to know exactly who we are and where we came from. This isn't really an identity crisis, so let's call it an identity puzzle. We simply want to find out who and why we are. To begin, check out the Ellis Island Web site, which provides information about families that immigrated from the Old World. Or surf the Mormons' expanded family history archives. Or, better yet, do a Web search on your own name and see where it leads.

Get health savvy. Midlife can be a crisis if you don't take care of your health, so get serious about routine checkups and screenings. If your health is deteriorating in any way, you can stop it before it's too late.

Change your career. Do you get up every day so filled with love for your job that you can't wait to get there? Or are you harboring a desire to be a cruise director and sail the globe? Perhaps you'd like to do something more meaningful, such as teach little children. It isn't too late, and medical science has learned that when we start to learn something new—at any age—our brain goes into high gear and is more efficient than ever. With our expanded life span, many people are changing careers in their middle years. You probably already know an office worker who became a schoolteacher or a retired cop who is now a disk jockey. Add your name to that midlife list.

Get back in touch with your faith. The church, synagogue, or mosque you left when you graduated high school is still there waiting for you to grow up. So is God. And, trust me—both will welcome you home with open arms.

Mouse Shoulder:

Avoid the Trap

Here's another reason to resent Bill Gates. Not only has he made us totally dependent on his computer software (and himself obscenely rich in the process) but his mouse-driven invention is literally giving us a pain—or several pains. As many as 80 percent of workers nationwide are now reporting some kind of physical problem related to the use of computers, say researchers at San Francisco State University.

The Bureau of Labor Statistics says injuries from repeated, stressful motions of all kinds cost us $20 billion a year in workers' compensation

O·D·D·B·A·L·L OINTMENT

Creamed Comfort

For quick pain relief at work, use capsaicin cream three or four times during the day. For deeper effects, use an oil-based ointment, or make your own by adding 3 to 4 drops of cayenne pepper (*Capsicum minimum*) tincture to 1 teaspoon of olive oil.

claims. The average computer work injury costs $29,000 in medical bills and rehab. Makes you wonder what would happen if we began suing the computer companies for health-related damages in the same way we are finally suing the tobacco companies for cigarette-related injuries.

Mouse shoulder is an injury that comes from prolonged bracing and elevation of your shoulder to accommodate a mouse that is usually in an inappropriate place. Short-range movements of the mouse also force you to tense your muscles, thus reducing blood flow to them. These tight muscles can also pinch your nerves and send pain down your arms into your hands. Here's some ways keep your mouse under control:

Take a micro-break. The muscle tension begins within the first minute of sitting down at the keyboard, but most of us are not aware of it until much later. So every few minutes, whether you feel tense or not, drop your shoulders, and stretch your arms, shoulders, upper back, and neck.

Take a macro-break. Quickie breaks do help, but you also need longer breaks to prevent serious problems, says Lawrence Schleiffer, Ph.D., an ergonomist and professor at the University of Maryland and a former fellow at the National Institute of Occupational Safety and Health (NIOSH). He recom-

POWERFUL POTION

HOT TODDY

Turmeric (*Curcuma longa*), an ingredient in curry, is a potent anti-inflammatory. Stir 1/2 teaspoon of turmeric into a glass of water, and drink twice daily. Unlike non-steroidal anti-inflammatory drugs, such as ibuprofen and acetaminophen, turmeric is safe to use long term.

Soothing Shoulder Pack

Mullein (*Verbascum thapsus*) packs can be used to ease local inflammation of the shoulder. Blanche three to four mullein leaves in boiling water for 1 to 2 minutes. Remove the leaves from the water, and have a friend or spouse apply them to your painful shoulder. The leaves should be hot, but not hot enough to burn you. Have your helper cover them with a hot, moist towel, and then place a dry towel on top. Leave the hot pack on for 20 minutes. Remove; then apply an ice pack for 5 minutes.

mends taking a couple of 5-minute breaks and one 15-minute break each morning and each afternoon.

Keep it close to your chest. If your mouse is close to your body, there is much less strain on your arm and shoulder. So keep your arm by your side and your wrist straight and parallel to the desk.

Armrest your mouse. One way to keep you mouse close is to look for a device that allows you to strap it to the arm of your chair.

Fire your mouse. If you do word processing with a mouse, you use it about 30 percent of the time. Doesn't sound like much, but because the mouse is at the side of the keyboard, you must reach out to use it. And this motion puts twice as much stress on your neck, arm, and shoulder muscles than using a trackball or pointing device mounted in the center of a keyboard.

Be a switch hitter. If you use your mouse a lot, try manning it with your opposite hand once in a while. Switch hitting, so to speak, spreads out the stress and gives your primary arm a break. Or, get a split keyboard that allows you to use both hands more efficiently, and use the mouse in the center, between the two

The Luck of the Lefties

In some weird form of reverse discrimination, left-handers have an advantage when using a mouse. The little rodent can be held closer to the body of lefties, because the number pad, which extends the keyboard, is on the right side of the keyboard, not the left.

But all you righties don't despair. You can convert that square of numbers into a landing pad for your mouse. The next time you're in one of those office-supply superstores, look for a product that covers the number pad and converts it into a mouse pad. Or replace your standard keyboard with one that has no number pad on the right.

halves. These keyboards are expensive and can be hard to find, but your hands will be in a more natural position.

Make your mouse a drag queen. Visit your computer control panel, and adjust the speed of your mouse. You can adjust the time interval for double clicking, use the click function to lock the drag control, and select the proper buttons for right- and left-hand use. While you're at it, clean the mouse and the mouse pad, too, so you can move smoothly.

Use keyboard shortcuts. You wouldn't even have to touch your mouse—if you knew all the keyboard shortcuts for moving the cursor around. Mine your instruction book for shortuts, then tape a handy list of them to the side of your monitor.

Muscle Aches, Spasms, and Cramps:

Chill Out!

Are you a weekend warrior who's got something to prove? A go-for-it gardener who even dreams in green? Or an out-of-shape Boomer who's suddenly serious at the gym? If any of these descriptions rings a bell, then you probably already suffer more than your fair share of muscle aches, spasms, or cramps.

Lucky for us, most muscle aches get better by themselves in 48 hours with rest. But some aches and pains persist. And because they do, they may be symptoms of a systemic illness, such as the flu or Rocky Mountain spotted fever. For that reason, if the aches don't ease after 48 hours, or if you also have symptoms such as a fever or headache, you should call your doctor. And never brush off unexplained arm or chest pain as a muscle cramp.

It could signal a heart attack, so get medical attention immediately to be on the safe side. Otherwise, here's how to ease most muscle misery:

Give it a rest. If your muscles ache because you played 6 hours of softball after a winter on the couch, head back to its soft embrace for a day or two. Bedrest, followed by gradual exercise, will improve most muscle aches, says David Borenstein, M.D., a Washington, D.C.– based rheumatologist.

Hit all the hot spots—with cold. A cold pack can ease the pain of muscle aches, but use it for just 15 to 20 minutes at a time. The effects of cold last longer than heat because your body takes longer to warm up than it does to cool off.

Use your slush fund. To make an ice pack that molds to your contours, fill a zipper-locking plastic bag with a mixture of one part rubbing alcohol to four parts water. Put that bag into a second bag to ensure it doesn't leak.

Soak that ache. Applying heat can also soothe sore muscles. While relief from heat won't last as long as cold, it does help for 1 hour or more. Moist heat penetrates more deeply than dry heat, so stand in a hot shower, soak in a tub, or use

> ### FABULOUS FOLK REMEDY
>
> # Hot Vinegar Pack
>
> Try a hot vinegar pack for sore muscles. Heat equal parts of water and vinegar, soak a towel in the mix, and wring it out. Apply the towel as a hot compress to the sore area, leaving it in place for 5 minutes. Then follow with a cold compress (a wrung-out towel that's been soaked in cold or ice water until it's well chilled). Repeat the cycle three times, ending with the cold compress. Then cover the area warmly, and rest.

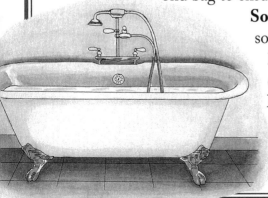

a hot compress—rewetting it several times with hot water when it cools. Whatever heat source you choose—heating pad, microwave heat packs, or a hot compress—leave it on the sore muscle for no more than 20 to 30 minutes at a time. And let your muscles cool down for 1 to 1½ hours before you reapply heat.

Drink lots of water. Physical exertion depletes fluids and minerals, which can create cramps, especially if you're overheated. To avoid heat cramps (and, later on, heat exhaustion or stroke) in the first place, drink at least 1 cup of water before you exercise and another every 15 minutes during the activity.

Energize your electrolytes. Your muscles move in response to nerve signals. They receive these signals via electrolytes, which are the minerals that surround your muscle cells. An imbalance in these minerals can interrupt the flow of signals and cause cramps. So give your body what it needs by including adequate chloride, sodium, potassium, calcium,

POWERFUL
POTION

SALUBRIOUS
EPSOM SALTS

If you think your internal electrolytes may be out of whack and causing leg cramps, soak in a tub of "external" electrolytes—Epsom (or magnesium) salts combined with kosher salt and a bit of potassium. Just dissolve 2 cups of Epsom salts, 2 cups of kosher salt, and 2 tablespoons of potassium crystals (available at most health-food stores) in a warm bath. Slip in when you're feeling whipped or when your legs feel achy.

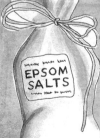

EPSOM
SALTS

and magnesium in your diet. Chloride and sodium are found in table salt and prepared foods. You'll find plenty of potassium in vegetables and fruit—especially bananas, citrus fruit, and dried fruit. Calcium, of course, comes in dairy products. Try to get 1,200 milligrams of calcium a day (1,500 milligrams after menopause). You also need 280 milligrams of magnesium daily, so pile leafy greens, whole grains, and beans on your plate. If you believe you need a supplement, ask your doctor which one would be appropriate for you.

Keep on your toes. Here's a simple way to stretch your calf muscles and relieve a cramp there: Stand with the balls of your feet on the edge of a step, and lower your heels.

WHEN IT HURTS ALL OVER

If you ache all over and your muscles are always stiff, you may have a mysterious condition known as fibromyalgia. Although it's difficult to pin down a diagnosis, deep aching pain and sometimes a burning sensation may overtake your entire body and be especially prominent in

---

O·D·D·B·A·L·L OINTMENT

Comfrey Comfort Rub

Fill a 12-ounce glass jar with freshly chopped comfrey (*Symphytum officinale*) leaves, and cover completely with castor oil and the contents of one vitamin E capsule. Steep in a sunny window for 1 week, shaking the jar once or twice daily. Strain, and store in a clean glass bottle. Add 15 drops of essential oils of juniper (*Juniperus communis*) and wintergreen (*Gaultheria procumbens*). Rub into sore muscles as needed. To prolong the life of your oils, always store them in a cool place or in the fridge.

your arms and legs. Fibromyalgia can also make you sensitive to weather changes.

Although it can feel like arthritis, fibromyalgia isn't a joint disease. It's a chronic pain condition with no known cause or cure. Current research suggests that sufferers may have an abnormally sensitive central nervous system.

There is no way to confirm a diagnosis of fibromyalgia, but the American College of Rheumatology established this general guideline: widespread aching for at least 3 months in a minimum of 11 areas of the body that are abnormally tender when you press on them lightly. Sound familiar? Run your suspicions by your doctor. You may be able to relieve your symptoms through exercise and medication.

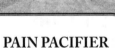

PAIN PACIFIER

Combine herbal anti-inflammatories and pain relievers to alleviate discomfort and help you sleep. Mix equal parts of passionflower (*Passiflora incarnata*), ginger (*Zingiber officianale*), Jamaican dogwood (*Piscidia erythrina*), and meadowsweet (*Filipendula ulmaria*). Toss 1 heaping teaspoon into 1 cup of hot water. Sip 1 or 2 cups throughout the day and another before bedtime.

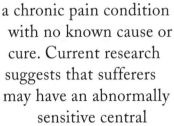

FABULOUS FOLK REMEDY

Apple Cider Liniment

Make your own liniment to relieve painful muscles. Combine ½ ounce of powdered cramp bark (*Viburnum opulus*) and 1 cup of apple cider vinegar. Add a pinch of cayenne pepper (*Capsicum minimus*), and let stand for 1 week in a cool, dark place. Shake well every day; then decant, and store in a clean, glass bottle. Apply to sore muscles as a rub or soak a clean cloth in the liniment, and place it on the aching area.

Nails:

The Mirror of Your Health

I wanted to look nice for my new boyfriend. Is that a crime? So what if I was about to be wheeled into the operating room? Mr. Wonderful was coming to visit me after my surgery. So there I sat, painting my nails scarlet, when the nurse came to get me.

"Where do you think you're going, to a party?" she asked, laughing. Then she ordered me to take off the polish and went to find some remover. Needless to say, my blushing cheeks matched my nails.

Taking pity, she patiently explained that the anesthesiologist needed to see my bare fingernails to be sure I was getting enough oxygen while I was unconscious. Otherwise, in those days, he had no way of checking.

FABULOUS FOLK REMEDY

Lemon Scrub

Clean up dingy, tired-looking nails with a lemon scrub. Cut a fresh lemon in half, and dig your fingers into the juicy flesh. Just make sure that your fingers don't have cuts or scrapes on them, or you'll be in for a stinging surprise!

What Lurks beneath the Talon Long?

Germs, that's what. Not long ago, a hospital study of practical nurses caring for infants revealed that nurses with very long nails were carrying harmful bacteria into the nursery. All kinds of bacteria and mold were imbedded under their nails! So here's a tip: If you must play Dragon Lady, wear gloves when you are cooking or caring for someone.

FORGET YOUR PALM—READ YOUR NAILS

While your eyes may be the mirror of your soul, your fingernails can be a portal to knowledge about your basic health, says Lila Wallis, M.D., a pioneer in the field of women's health.

Take a look at your own nails. Are they pitted? Split? Ridged? These conditions all can be caused by a variety of health problems. For example, psoriasis, a chronic skin condition, can cause nails to be pitted. An underactive thyroid or skin allergies can cause nails to split. Malnutrition forms horizontal bands, and iron deficiency creates soft, spoon-shaped nails. Discolored nails could indicate a fungal infection. And sometimes, just before menstruation, women's hormone levels affect their nails, too, by splitting and cracking them.

TIPS FOR GARDEN-LOVING PAWS

Nails are made of keratin, the same protein found in our hair and outer skin. Growth slows as we age; but until then, nails grow about $1/8$ inch a month. How do yours measure up? Yikes! If they look like my garden-loving paws, you'd better try the following:

Eat for your nails. Healthy nails are strong, smooth, and pale pink. To stay that way, they need lots of oxygen and nutrients. If you are not eating a well-balanced diet, the nutrients you do get will rush to meet your body's most important needs, and your nails will be short-changed. So be sure to include high-quality protein, whole grains, and plenty of fresh fruits and veggies in your diet. Your nails will thank you.

Give polish the brush-off. Wearing nail polish all the time can make your nails brittle. Give them some breathing time by periodically laying off the polish. Don't paste on false nails, either, because some of the adhesives can cause severe allergic reactions. And speaking of allergies, both polish and polish remover contain harsh chemicals—including formaldehyde resin—that can cause an allergic reaction on your eyelids and the sides of your neck, even though the substance is on your nails, says Dr. Wallis.

Don't cover the moon. When you do polish your nails, be sure you don't cover the white half moon at the base with polish. This is live tissue that needs air. As I learned on that long-ago day before surgery, the color of those moons provides a way to read whether oxygen is circulating to the tips of your fingers.

Start a glove collection. Buy latex or rubber gloves to protect your hands and nails when you do dishes or clean house. Constant immersion in water makes nails brittle. They swell when wet and shrink when dry, and this repeated change makes them vulnerable.

Keep your cuticles cute. Your cuticle acts as a gasket to keep bacteria and water from getting under the nail bed and inside your body. The best way to care for your cuticles is to push them back, away from your nail. If they stretch down onto your nail, they'll dry

O·D·D·B·A·L·L OINTMENT

Grapefruit Nail Paint

Fungal infections on or beneath the nail can be difficult to get rid of. Before trying more toxic therapies, begin a regimen of nail painting with grapefruit-seed extract. Paint only the affected nail one to two times a day, taking care not to apply the extract to the surrounding skin, which may become irritated. Give it about 6 weeks for best results.

Don't Hoof It!

Because gelatin is made from animal hooves, it was once assumed that if we ate it, our nails would grow stronger. But gelatin is an incomplete protein and lacks the sulfurous amino acids that give nails strength. Gelatin as a supplement has no value.

out and become a painful, pantyhose-catching hangnail. When you are in the bath or shower, push your cuticles back gently. They are soft then and will move easily. You can use a finger to do this or buy a special cuticle pumice stick, which is like an orange stick, but softer.

Shun the fungus among us. Fingernails and toenails are vulnerable to fungus infections that can cause discoloration and deformity. The best treatment is to keep your fingers and toes as clean and dry as possible.

See your doctor. If you are diabetic or have poor circulation, be very vigilant in caring for your toenails, because toe infections can spread to the bone. Have your toenails trimmed by a podiatrist, so you don't risk serious problems.

POWERFUL
POTION

MINERAL MAGIC

Calcium and magnesium are essential to nail health. Make your own herbal mineral potion by mixing together equal parts of nettles (*Urtica dioica*), horsetail (*Equisetum arvense*), and oats (*Avena sativa*). Steep 1 heaping teaspoon in 1 cup of hot water for 10 minutes, and drink 1 to 2 cups daily. **Caution:** Be sure to wear gloves when handling fresh nettles to avoid their stinging hairs.

Nausea:

Quelling the Queasies

My friend Jerry has an iron gut. Nothing can make him queasy—not even his nephew's diaper. But Jerry's apparently part of a rare breed. The rest of us can get queasy from a lot of things— anger, shock, or fear; a surge of hormones during pregnancy; a virus; eating bad food; motion; and smelling noxious odors.

If you're feeling queasy for no obvious reason, you need to get immediate medical help. Otherwise, give the follow- ing tips a try:

> **FABULOUS FOLK REMEDY**
>
> ## A Dilly of a Cure
>
> A homemade infusion of dill (*Anethum graveolens*) seeds can help calm an upset stomach and ease nausea. Steep 1 teaspoon of dill seeds in 1 cup of hot water, covered, for 15 minutes. Strain, and sip.

Let it be. For the first 12 hours after a bout of nausea, drink only clear liquids such as gin- ger ale, plain water, or soothing teas. Vomiting

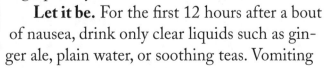

How to Prevent Motion Sickness

Turn green on curves in the car? Suffer from mal de mer on a boat? If so, these tips are for you:

Face forward. I always wondered why some people wouldn't ride backward on a train or a boat. I thought it was because they preferred to see where they were going rather than where they had been. Now I realize it's for balance. If you face forward when you travel, you're more likely to prevent motion sickness.

Carefully select your seat. Sit in the most stable section of a moving vehicle—midship on a boat, the middle of a bus, over the wings in a plane, the first car of a train, and the front seat of a car.

Don't read. Reading while in motion can make you queasy, so don't follow the trip's progress by staring at the map.

Keep the air smelling sweet. Crush some angelica leaves (*Doug-quai* in Chinese) in a sachet, and hang it in your car. Not only will the sachet help prevent motion sickness, but it will keep your car's air fresh, too!

Ban odors. The American Academy of Otolaryngology suggests avoiding strong odors before and during trips. At pit stops, for instance, make sure nobody gets in the car with a bag of fries or a double cheeseburger. And keep the fresh air flowing. If you are sealed up in a plane, make sure the air vent over your seat is working.

Book the QE2. Try a big ship cruise, rather than that romantic, bare-boat charter. The bigger the boat, the more stable it is in the water. You won't be tossed around as much unless you're sailing through a hurricane in the middle of the Bermuda Triangle!

and diarrhea cause your body to lose a lot of liquid, which it's important to replace.

Snap up some ginger. Ginger is widely used to remedy upset stomachs and nausea. You don't even have to chew on the root; simply make a tea by boiling a quarter-size piece of ginger in 1 cup of water for 5 minutes, says Gary Null, Ph.D., a well-known alternative healer. If you are pregnant, ask your doctor before you try this remedy.

Chew on some sagebrush. My friend Kay Whitefeather, a traditional healer of the Blackfoot tribe and teacher at the Red Mountain Health Resort in Utah, says that if you are in the Southwest, look for some native sagebrush in the desert, and chew on a leaf to ease symptoms of nausea.

Make a beeline for bee balm. Bee balm leaves contain a compound called thymol, which helps ease nausea, vomiting, and even embarrassing flatulence. Simply combine 1 teaspoon of dried bee balm leaves with 1 teaspoon of black or green tea leaves. Put 1 teaspoon of the mix into 1 cup of boiling water, and let it steep for 5 to 10 minutes. Strain,

POWERFUL
POTION

YUMMY TUMMY SOUP

Here's a healing remedy that originated with herbalist Martha Sarasula. Mix together two 12-ounce cans of vegetable broth or bouillon (or 2 cups of water with 3 packets of instant vegetable bouillon), 2 quarter-size pieces of gingerroot, 2 cloves of minced garlic, and ¼ cup of soy or tamari sauce. Bring it all to a boil, turn down the heat, and let it simmer for 30 minutes. Then sip it slowly by the spoonful.

and sip, sweetening the tea with 1 teaspoon of honey.

Stop and smell the lemons. If you're feeling queasy, forget about florabunda's rosy fragrance, and head for the fridge instead. Grab an uncut lemon, and scratch into the peel. Now sniff the clean, fresh citrus scent. That's what they do in India to handle nausea!

Soak and sniff. The volatile oils in peppermint (*Mentha piperita*) can help counteract nausea. Simply uncap a vial of essential oil of peppermint, and inhale it for a few seconds. If you're feeling up to a bath, add 4 to 6 drops to your tub, and slip in. Just remember to breathe deeply while you're soaking.

Rub your tummy. Our pets love a belly rub, and so will you. If your nausea is caused by anxiety, a gentle massage can sometimes calm that hyperactive nerve center.

POWERFUL POTION

STOMACH SETTLER

For nausea caused by stress and anxiety, sip a cup of meadowsweet (*Filipendula ulmaria*) tea to settle your stomach. Steep 1 heaping teaspoon of meadowsweet in 1 cup of hot water, covered, for 10 minutes. Strain, and sip slowly.

IT'S AN EMERGENCY!

If your nausea is accompanied by chest pain, sweating, or shortness of breath, call your doctor right away. These symptoms can indicate a heart attack.

Bring on the bland. When your appetite finally returns, scout around the kitchen for bland food. In fact, think of baby food. Consider eating easy-to-digest applesauce, a little plain rice, dry toast, or even a mild cooked vegetable.

Osteoporosis:

Keeping Up with Your Bones

After decades of chasing rug rats, lugging groceries, playing tennis, walking pooches, pounding the pavement, and especially drinking our milk, most of us have pretty sturdy skeletons. And bless those bones! We need them to hold us straight and tall for a lifetime. But our inner scaffolds are generally about as obvious to us as a coral reef is from the ocean's surface. That's why it's easy to overlook osteoporosis—the development of fragile, porous bones that can result in painful fractures.

Though we can't see, hear, or feel it coming, osteoporosis

Natural Native Medicine
Chicory Juice

Chicory is a plant that has helped Native Americans heal bones damaged by osteoporosis, according to Gary Null, Ph.D., a well-known advocate of alternative medicine. Elders, who drink lots of juice from cooked or raw chicory, say their bone fractures due to osteoporosis heal faster.

can happen to anyone. While men generally have larger, stronger bones and don't suffer a drop in bone mass the way women do after menopause, they're still at risk as their testosterone gradually declines. The good news? Osteoporosis is completely preventable. Here's how to help keep body and bone together:

Get hip to risk factors. Although there is a genetic component to osteoporosis, the two big risk factors for the disease are lack of weight-bearing exercise and not getting enough calcium to prevent your bones from becoming too porous. Smoking is also a major deterrent to healthy bones, as are certain drugs such as prednisone, which is frequently taken for asthma. Slender white and Asian women are generally at highest risk, and so are women who had an early menopause due to surgery or who have not gotten enough exercise during their lives. Among men, those who suffer from alcoholism are frequently headed straight for bone breakdown.

Check your density. Many women don't get bone-density tests until something happens—like a broken hip—and then it's too late to reverse the damage. This easy test—you simply stick your foot in a boot and read a magazine for a few minutes while a machine meas-

POWERFUL POTION

BONE SOUP

You've heard of stone soup? Well, bone soup is better! Pick up some soup bones at the meat counter and prepare some homemade soup. Any kind of bones will do—beef, chicken, ham, or whatever you prefer. Add vegetables, potatoes, and your favorite herbs and spices. But the magic ingredient is vinegar. Add some to the soup pot. It will dissolve a significant amount of calcium from the bones in the soup. Just 1 pint of soup can give you as much as 1,000 milligrams of calcium.

ures your bones—should first be conducted at the time of peri-menopause and then every year thereafter to monitor your bones for any changes in density.

If you have risk factors, such as small stature, lack of exercise, or years of smoking, ask your doctor to give you this test sooner rather than later. Likewise, if osteoporosis seems to run in your family, or if you've had an early, surgically induced menopause, ask your doctor for an all-body bone scan instead of just a heel scan.

Don't drink everyday. Alcoholism is a major cause of osteoporosis in men. Alcohol poisons the bone-forming cells called osteoblasts, says Sydney Lou Bonnick, M.D., director of the Institute for Women's Health at Texas Woman's University. So if you do drink, do so in moderation, and not every day. One drink a day for women and two for men is considered moderate.

SHAKE DEM BONES

When your bones are challenged, they rise to the occasion. If you lift weights, for example, your bones will become stronger so that you can lift even heavier weights. If you stamp your feet in a Riverdance, your bones will become dense enough to carry you on a tour through Ireland. Take advantage of this wonderful physical ability. Consider the following tips, and choose your challenge:

Hit the bricks. Just 60 seconds of running during a brisk walk is enough to shift your bones into a strengthening mode. Since you need to perform 30 to 45 minutes of weight-bearing exercise three times a week, and the American Academy of Orthopedic Surgeons says running ranks the highest for bone building, hit the pavement, and walk or run your way to better bones.

Stamp your feet. No, don't have a tantrum—but do take up step dancing or get out the castanets and try some flamenco. With every step you take, the striking of your heel on a hard surface creates stress on your skeleton. In response, your skeleton strengthens and renews itself, says Judith Andariese, R.N., director of the Osteoporosis Center at the Hospital for Special Surgery in New York City. Going down stairs is ideal, as is ballroom dancing—especially if you do it for 2 hours several times a week.

Dig for density. According to the *Journal of the American Geriatric Society*, moderate physical activity such as gardening reduces the risk of hip fracture from 20 to 60 percent. In fact, one study showed that women, who did some form of leisure activity for more than 3 hours a week, had about half as much chance of fracturing a hip as those who were sedentary.

Hoist a few. Regular strength training does more than just keep you fit: The pull of your muscles as you work out stimulates your bones to increase their density. In fact, in a landmark study, 20 sedentary, postmenopausal women attended two weekly supervised weight-lifting sessions of about 45 minutes each. In just 1 year, they gained an average of 1 percent in bone

---

O·D·D·B·A·L·L OINTMENT

Oil Your Spine

As osteoporosis progresses, the bones in your spine can begin pinching the nerves that run between them. St. John's wort (*Hypericum perforatum*) oil is specifically indicated for nerve pain. Massage a small amount of oil into any painful areas two to three times daily. The oil can be found at your local health-food store.

density, while the control group, who didn't lift weights, lost about 2 percent in bone density. What's more, members of the weight-lifting group were soon in-line skating, playing tennis, gardening, shoveling snow, and walking—doing things they hadn't done in years! If you don't have dumbbells, hoist a couple of heavy cans of food. Just be sure both cans are the same weight.

Hit the wall. Wall pushups are an easy way to strengthen the bones in your upper body. Put your hands flat on a wall, level with and about as far apart as your shoulders. Now take a step away from the wall. Lean into the wall, and then push your body away from it. Repeat several times, at least three times a week.

CALCIUM IS KEY

If you don't absorb enough calcium from what you eat, your body will take it from your bones, which you can think of as kind of like a savings bank for calcium. Any extra amount of that mineral is stored in the bones for safekeeping. When your body needs calcium to accomplish certain functions like cell regeneration, for instance, it searches for it. If you haven't consumed enough calcium, the body withdraws what it needs from its friendly, neighborhood bone bank.

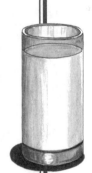

See why it's important to take in ample calcium? The daily adult requirement is 1,200 milligrams; 1,500 milligrams if you're a postmenopausal woman. Here are some of the best dairy sources: 1 glass of milk (300 milligrams), 1 ounce of Cheddar cheese (200 to 300 milligrams), and 1 cup of yogurt (275 to 325 milligrams).

Milk is generally fortified with vitamin D, which you need to help your body absorb calcium. Here are some additional ways to increase your calcium account:

Chew on some bones. No, not like a puppy. But try this: Eat a can of sardines or salmon with bones once or twice a week for a calcium boost. Just 3 ounces of canned salmon with bones has about 200 milligrams of calcium.

Put tofu on the table. Serve ½ cup of tofu made with calcium sulfate in salads and stir-fries to get 250 milligrams of calcium. As an added plus, tofu is rich in two major types of isoflavone, a compound that acts like a weak estrogen and may inhibit bone breakdown.

Avoid phosphorus-rich foods. Some foods, such as red meat, soft drinks, alcohol, caffeine, and phosphorus-rich foods, interfere with calcium absorption. Antacids with aluminum can also prevent absorption of calcium. So don't follow your tofu salad with a cup of high-test coffee or a large cola.

Get vitamin D. Your body needs vitamin D—which you can get via food, a supplement, or regular exposure to sunshine—to absorb calcium. Take 400 International Units (IU) of vitamin D each day if you are over age 50. If you are over age 70, you need 600 IU a day. The best food sources for vitamin D are salmon and tuna and some types of mushrooms.

Expose yourself. If you spend sufficient time outdoors, you may

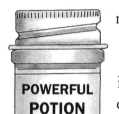

POWERFUL POTION

WILD ABOUT TEA

Nettles (*Urtica dioica*), horsetail (*Equisetum arvense*), oatstraw (*Avena sativa*), alfalfa (*Medicago sativa*), dandelion (*Taraxacum officinale*), chicory (*Cichorium intybus*), kelp (*Nereocystis luetkeana*) and bladderwrack (*Fucus vesiculosis*) can all be made into bone-boosting teas. Combine equal parts of two or more herbs; then steep 1 heaping tablespoon in 1 quart of hot water for 10 minutes. Strain, and sip. **Caution:** Dandelion is rich in potassium and should not be taken with potassium tablets. Also, be sure to wear gloves when you're handling fresh nettles to avoid their stinging hairs.

not need a vitamin supplement. However, after age 50, our bodies have more difficulty manufacturing vitamin D from sunlight and absorbing it from food. If you want to soak it up from the sun, expose your face and arms for 15 minutes before you put on any sunscreen. In northern climates, the sun's low angle from November to March prevents it from providing much of a benefit, so drink vitamin D–enriched milk during the winter months.

ADDITIONAL VITAMINS AND MINERALS

Medical scientists are beginning to understand that other nutrients—namely, potassium, vitamin C, and magnesium—are also important in preventing osteoporosis. Here's what they know so far:

Potassium is potent. The Framingham Heart Study found that women whose diets are rich in potassium have denser bones in their spines and hips than women with potassium-poor diets. Bananas and oranges are terrific sources of potassium.

Vitamin C is valuable. Vitamin C is an antioxidant that combats the aging process and appears to play a role in collagen production—the first step in bone formation. Eat plenty of fresh fruits and veggies to be sure you get enough.

There's magic in magnesium. The best sources of magnesium are potatoes, seeds, nuts, legumes, whole grains, and dark green vegetables. Ask your doctor about supplements if you don't think you are getting enough in your diet.

FABULOUS FOLK REMEDY

A Comfrey Compress

Comfrey (*Symphytum officinalis*) packs can be used over a fracture site to relieve swelling and inflammation. Blanche three to four leaves in boiling water, remove from the water, cool slightly, and apply to the affected area. Cover with a warm, moist towel with a dry towel on top. Keep in place until the leaves cool off.

Pain:

Don't Put Up with It—Control It

"Oh, my aching back," groans my neighbor Thelma as she heaves herself up from weeding her vegetable garden. She tells me that next year, she'll probably skip planting her tomatoes and peppers, even though she loves tending them and—even better—eating them. "It's the bending and kneeling at my age," she says. "It's killing me."

What a shame that Thelma just accepts the pain, along with her Social Security check, as part of her golden years. And it's a double shame that she plans to give up a satisfying, lifelong hobby.

Apparently, there are a lot of people like Thelma. A Gallup survey shows that most Americans resign themselves to pain—and accept it as a normal result of aging! Nearly all Americans say they experience pain, yet only about half of those polled have vis-

---

FABULOUS FOLK REMEDY

Bark at Your Pain

Cramp bark (*Viburnum opulus*) releases pain-causing spasms and promotes relaxation. Simmer 1 heaping teaspoon of crumbled bark in 1 cup of water for 10 minutes. Sip 1 or 2 cups daily.

Why Won't the Chicken Cross the Road?

Because that's where the doctor's office is! Men are less likely to see a doctor and will do so only when urged by others. Women, on the other hand, just do it. The Pain in America survey revealed that 38 percent of men will wait to consult a doctor until someone encourages them to get treatment for their pain. Only 27 percent of women demonstrate the same reluctance.

ited a doctor in the last 3 years for treatment—and nearly two thirds don't see a doctor until they can't stand the pain any longer. Personally, I don't understand it. And neither do most doctors.

"Pain is not a natural part of growing older and is not simply a fact of life," assures Jack Klippel, M.D., medical director of the Arthritis Foundation, one of the survey's sponsors. "There are things people can do to reduce their aches and pains. By talking to a healthcare provider about their pain, people can start taking control of their lives by controlling the pain."

Here's how to begin:

Paint a picture of your pain. Don't just say your leg hurts. Tell your doctor where the pain is centered and when it occurs. Describe the pain as sharp, stabbing, throbbing, radiating, or cramping. List any activities or time of day that make it feel better or worse. "Unlike a broken bone," says Dr. Klippel, "pain cannot be identified by a medical test or x-ray. So these patient–doctor conversations are important for helping healthcare providers better understand and treat pain."

Check out pain clinics. At a pain clinic, a group of pain-relief specialists will review your history and develop a treatment tailored just for you. It may involve medication, lifestyle changes, diet, exercise, and electrical stimulation. To locate a pain clinic, talk to your doctor, inquire at the local hospital, or visit the Web site of the American Academy of Pain Management (www.aapainmanage.org) for clinic listings.

Feel the burn, not the pain. Exercise is a great pain reliever. According to a recent study, people with chronic back pain felt relief after 25 minutes on a stationary bike. Other studies support the finding that aerobic exercise tames pain. Even a brisk walk around the block can make you feel better—provided the walk lasts at least 10 minutes.

Play a little night music. If your doctor prescribes medication, turn on the radio or plug in your Mozart CDs. People taking pain medicine experienced even more relief when they listened to music and relaxed, according to a study led by Marion Good, Ph.D., R.N., at the Bolton School of Nursing at Case Western Reserve University in Cleveland. The study focused on people recovering from major abdominal surgery, but researchers say it has major implications for managing other types of pain.

Say ohmmmmm. Just as women in childbirth have learned that focused breathing can help get them though labor pain, that same kind of focused breathing may also help with other pain. Deep breathing relaxes your muscles, increases oxygen to the cells, and encourages your body to produce endorphins—your body's own natural pain killers. Try this breathing exercise recommended by the National Cancer Institute:

Breathe in slowly and deeply. Then breathe out slowly. Be aware of your body relaxing, and feel the tension leave. Use a mantra to help you breathe rhythmically. Say, "In two three. Out two three." Or use the popular mantra from Transcendental Meditation—say, "Ohmmmmm."

Get needled. Acupuncture on a regular basis has helped some people fight pain. Doctors say that people seem to benefit when the needles are placed near the pain's location, rather than at the body points indicated on acupuncture charts. If you plan to try this alternative therapy, make sure the therapist is licensed and uses sterile, disposable needles.

Opt for Botox. If chronic back pain is your problem, Botox, the magic wrinkle remover made from a deadly toxin, may be an option. Volunteers with low back pain received Botox injections and felt better within 2 to 3 days, according to a study at the Louisiana State University Health Sciences Center. Botox kills nerve endings; and when they grow pack, the pain doesn't always come back with them. Ask your doctor about these injections, but get them only from a trained pain-management specialist.

Simplify, woman, simplify. You don't have to do it all, Supermom! Women are more likely than men to experience daily pain, according to

POWERFUL POTION

ROOT FOR RELAXATION

Anti-inflammatory herbs help relieve pain throughout the body and may be combined with antispasmodic herbs to increase relaxation. Combine equal parts of meadowsweet (*Filipendula ulmaria*), lemon balm (*Melissa officinalis*), prickly ash (*Xanthoxylum clava-herculis*), calendula (*Calendula officinalis*), and gingerroot (*Zingiber officinale*). Steep 1 heaping teaspoon of the mixture in 1 cup of hot water, covered, for 15 minutes. Drink 2 to 3 cups daily.

the Gallup survey. In fact, one in three women cite the trials of balancing work and family life as a significant cause of their pain. "Frequent pain for women often is associated with both physical and emotional factors and can affect many aspects of their lives," says Dr. Keppel. Stress makes you tighten your muscles for hours on end, and the result is pain! pain! pain! (See **Stress** for tips on reducing the stress in your life.)

Soak and sleep. For general pain, treat yourself to a bath-and-bed remedy. First, scoop ⅓ cup *each* of chamomile (*Matricaria recutita*), lavender (*Lavendula officinalis*), and lemon balm (*Melissa officinalis*) into a muslin bag. Toss the bag into the tub while you run hot water. Add 2 pounds of Epsom salts to the water, and agitate the water to dissolve the salts. Soak in the tub for 10 to 15 minutes, or until you break a healthy sweat.

Now, for the bed part. Get out of the tub, and, without drying off, wrap yourself up in an old sheet that's been saturated with cold water and wrung out. Then wrap up in one to two outer layers of wool blankets, and go to bed. This is best done at night, so you can simply go to sleep. The sheet should feel cold for only a few minutes and will then dry out. You can place a hot water bottle at your feet and put a hat on your head for extra heating. This can be repeated once a week for deep relaxation and pain relief. **Caution:** It is imperative to stay well hydrated during this treatment. Should you experience any dizziness or adverse symptoms, discontinue the treatment immediately.

Painful Intercourse:

Get on Top of Discomfort

Unfortunately, once you've had painful intercourse, you may always flinch at the thought of sex. And that sure puts the kibosh on romance, doesn't it? Contrary to popular belief, however, physical problems—not psychological ones—are usually the culprit when sexual intercourse hurts. It's also usually a woman's problem, not a man's—although a tight foreskin or a sore on the penis can make things uncomfortable for guys, too.

Frequent causes of women's pain are deep penetration during intercourse; a dry vagina; a yeast infection; a bad back; or a muscle spasm in the

Are You Allergic to Sex?

Allergy to semen can also cause painful intercourse. You can tell you're allergic if your pelvic area becomes red, and you experience a very intense burning sensation after your partner ejaculates. Even if you do, however, you don't have to give up on love. Simply ask your partner to use condoms to protect those sensitive membranes.

pubic area, back, or abdomen. Be sure to ask your doctor to help you figure out what's going on—and consider these feel-better tips on your own:

Become the dominant force in your sexual relationship. Pin your partner to the mattress, and stay on top. Deep thrust—or deep dyspareunia—is the most common cause of painful penetration. But if the woman sits astride the man during intercourse, she can control how deeply his penis can go. (Of course, there are lots of other pleasures in being on top...)

Put a finger on the problem. Here's an exercise that will be so much fun, you'll always come back for more—especially since it may help you relieve the pain of intercourse caused by vaginismus (involuntary spasms of the pubic muscles can make penetration painful and difficult). If your gynecologist has identified the source of your pain as vaginismus, then this exercise may help stretch your vagina and make you more capable of comfortable intercourse.

POWERFUL POTION

A VAGINAL WASH

For pain that occurs *after* intercourse, use a vaginal wash made from soothing, antimicrobial herbs. Combine equal parts of echinacea (*Echinacea* spp.), goldenseal (*Hydrastis canadensis*), and lavender (*Lavendula officinalis*). Steep 1 heaping teaspoon of the mix in 1 cup of hot water for 20 minutes. Strain, and pour into a peribottle (available at drugstores). Keep the bottle by your toilet, and after intercourse, wash your labia and vaginal entrance with this solution. If the irritation persists, use this wash throughout the day after every urination.

Are You Ready to Swing?

Your estrogen levels are lower right after childbirth. This can leave your vaginal tissues less flexible than they normally would be and cause painful intercourse. To tell when intercourse will once again be comfortable, gently rub your lower abdomen and vaginal area with your fingers. If you feel no pain, your body's ready to get back into the sexual swing of things.

First, ask your partner to refrain from actual intercourse. This way, you can remain relaxed. He should lubricate his fingers (with Astroglide or similar vaginal lubricant), and insert one finger into your vagina. Ask him to keep it there until you get accustomed to the feeling. Then have him do the same thing with two fingers and then three, until you feel secure and relaxed. Eventually, you should be able to participate in intercourse again.

Get flexible with estrogen. If your sex hormones are on permanent vacation because of menopause, ask your doctor for a prescription for vaginal estrogen cream. Just 1 gram of an estriol cream, three times a week, should help restore flexibility to vaginal tissue and may reduce any pain associated with intercourse.

Kill the pain. Take a painkiller before you get ready for sexual pleasure. It's rare, but it sometimes hap-

O·D·D·B·A·L·L OINTMENT

Vitamin E Night Therapy

If you live on Mars, and can't get to a doctor for a prescription hormone cream to encourage more vaginal flexibility, try this: Every night before bed, prick a vitamin E capsule with a pin, and insert the capsule into your vagina. Do this for 2 weeks; then continue to do so three times a week.

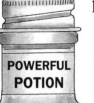

A MIGHTY FINE TEA

Studies in Germany show that echinacea tea can prevent yeast infections. However, you need to drink it regularly for it to be effective. Make a cup of the tea by putting ½ teaspoon of the herb in 1 cup of boiling water. Let it steep for about 10 minutes, strain, and then sip. Researchers found that the tea loses its effect after 8 weeks. So stop for 1 month; then start drinking it again.

pens that the uterine contractions from an orgasm can cause pain. (Talk about a body's mixed messages!) If that's happening to you, doctors at the Florida Hospital Family Practice in Orlando suggest taking some ibuprofen before intercourse to block the pain of these contractions.

Banish yeast infections. If you feel a burning sensation during intercourse—and notice a discharge that looks like cottage cheese—you may have a yeast infection. Try some of the over-the-counter remedies for yeast infections such as Monistat or Lotrimin. These remedies are widely available as pills, gels, and suppositories.

Enjoy an herbal bath. Warm sitz baths using an infusion of comfrey (*Symphytum officinalis*) and horsetail (*Equisetum arvense*) can help soothe inflamed tissues and, over time, make them less susceptible to irritation. Make a strong infusion by simmering 1 cup of comfrey root in 1 pint of water for 20 minutes. Remove from the heat, add 1 heaping tablespoon of horsetail, and steep for an additional 10 minutes. Strain, and pour into your bathtub. Then fill the tub with enough warm water to come up to the top of your pelvic bone. Soak for 20 minutes, three times weekly.

Pink Eye:

It's Not Just for Bunnies

The red eye is what we call the last night-flight out of Los Angeles, because that's how most of the passengers' eyes look when they arrive on the East Coast in the morning. Pink eye, on the other hand, has no such sophistication attached to it, although it is an apt description of what your eyes look like when the conjunctiva—the protective membrane covering the insides of your eyelids and the exposed whites of your eyes—is infected.

If your eyes are itchy, burning, and discharging some sticky goop, chances are, you've got pink eye. It usually begins in one eye and quickly spreads to the other. It can be caused by bacteria or

---

FABULOUS FOLK REMEDY

Strawberry Soother

Strawberry (*Fragaria vesca*) tea helps soothe inflamed eyes and fight infection. Steep 1 teaspoon of the leaves in 1 cup of hot water for 10 minutes. Strain, and cool. Use as a compress, or place in an eye cup, and rinse your eyes with it once or twice daily.

POWERFUL POTION

CHAMOMILE CURE

To make a soothing eye-wash from chamomile, steep 2 to 3 teaspoons in 1 pint of boiling water (or use a teabag) for 10 minutes. Let cool, and strain through a sterile cloth. Use an eye cup to rinse your eye with the solution two to three times daily until the problem is resolved. **Caution:** People with ragweed allergies may be sensitive to chamomile.

an allergy, but it's most commonly the result of a virus.

It's also very contagious—but not very serious. Once in a great while, however, a case of conjunctivitis can do some real damage. So if your pink eye doesn't clear up within 1 week, or if you have a fever or changes in vision along with it, call your doctor. Otherwise, here's how to soothe the garden-variety pink eye that troubles most of us:

Chill out. Ice-cold compresses can soothe your eyes. Simply place a damp washcloth that's been chilled in the freezer or just a cool, wet paper towel over your closed eyes for about 20 minutes. Stop for 30 to 60 minutes, then do it again. Apply cold as often as you feel the need, and keep the compress on for 10 minutes.

Stay out of the pool. Until your eyes have cleared up, don't go swimming! Not only can you spread conjunctivitis bacteria to others in the pool but the chlorinated water can also increase the irritation.

Keep your hands to yourself. While infected, avoid shaking hands; use disposable tissues that you discard yourself; and be sure to disinfect doorknobs, countertops, and telephones. Also, don't share towels or pillows.

Trash your mascara. Get rid of any mascara, eye liner, or eye shadow that you've used since you developed pink eye. They're harboring germs. Then, when your peepers are no longer pink, treat yourself to some new cosmetics.

Lose the contacts. Don't wear contacts while you have pink eye. Your eyes will feel worse with the lenses in, since the lenses will hold the germs close against your eyeball.

Pull down the shades. Wear sunglasses to protect your eyes from glare and irritation. You'll look cool, and you'll feel less self-conscious about your mascara-free peepers.

Make crocodile tears. Check your local drugstore for artificial tears and other soothing eye remedies. According to the American Academy of Family Physicians, these lubricating eye drops are especially helpful if your pink eye is from allergies, but they can also help reduce the swelling of the conjunctiva.

Attack your allergies. If your pink eye is allergy related, ask your doctor if you should take over-the-counter antihistamines, such as Benadryl, which can help reduce itching, swelling, and discomfort. If these drugs don't do the job, ask your doctor if prescription antihistamine eye drops are right for you.

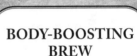

POWERFUL POTION

BODY-BOOSTING BREW

When pink eye is a recurrent complaint or particularly severe, support your whole body with infection-fighting herbs. Combine equal parts of echinacea (*Echinacea* spp.), eyebright (*Euphrasia officinalis*), calendula (*Calendula officinalis*), and cleavers (*Galium aparine*). Steep 1 teaspoon of the mixture in 1 cup of hot water for 10 minutes. Strain, and drink 2 to 3 cups daily.

Poison Ivy:

Getting Out of the Woods

I once got a nasty case of poison ivy from a gardening glove I had worn a whole year earlier to tug out some poison ivy vines. I also got it from my neighbor's cat, who, in rubbing up against my ankles, brought the oil of the plant to me on his coat.

But these are both pretty odd ways to get poison ivy. Most people simply blunder into the toxic plant because they don't recognize it, and they forget the old adage: Leaves of three, let it be!

DASH THAT RASH

If you've been exposed, you'll see a rash (first red patches, then blisters) in about 2 days. It will be most miserably itchy by about the

Kitchen-Counter Itch Stopper

Make a paste using one of the following combinations:

- ✔ Water and cornstarch
- ✔ Water and oatmeal
- ✔ Water and baking soda
- ✔ Water and Epsom salts
- ✔ Witch hazel and baking soda

Apply the paste to the rash to help stop the itch.

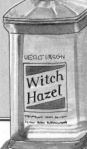

fifth day; then it will begin to fade. The rash is usually completely gone in 7 to 10 days.

If the rash lasts more than 2 weeks or shows signs of infection, have it checked by your doctor. It may not be poison ivy at all and could be something more serious. Also, have your doctor examine the rash if you get it near your eyes. Otherwise, the following tips will give you some relief:

Pop an antihistamine. Over-the-counter antihistamines, like Benadryl, will reduce the itch. Simply follow the package directions.

Bathe in baking soda. Dump ½ cup of baking soda into your bath water, and soak for a while.

Make a grindelia compress. Compresses soaked in a strong infusion of grindelia (*Grindelia camporum*) relieve itching and reduce inflammation. Steep 2 heaping teaspoons of grindelia in 1 cup of hot water for 15 minutes. Strain, and let cool. Apply to the affected area, continuing to wet the compress as it dries. Leave it on for an hour at a time, if you can.

Soothe with salve. After you pat yourself dry, apply calamine lotion or zinc oxide ointment. This treatment should help put those itchy nerve endings into a coma.

Patch your patches. Place sterile gauze patches over any patches of blisters to keep your skin clean and help absorb any fluid that runs from the blisters.

FABULOUS FOLK REMEDY

A Jewel of a Weed

Gardeners and hikers alike swear by the power of jewelweed to clear up poison ivy. Look for this plant, which is a wild type of impatiens, wherever poison ivy grows, because (isn't Mother Nature thoughtful?) they're usually found side by side. You'll recognize jewelweed by its bright yellow or orange flowers. Folk healers suggest you squeeze the juice from the stems or leaves, then swab it onto your skin.

Hit the C. Vitamin C may help reduce your reaction to poison ivy. Once you've been exposed, take 1,000 milligrams of vitamin C every 2 hours, up to 6,000 milligrams per day. The side effect of taking too much vitamin C is loose stools. Should this occur, simply lower the dose by 1,000 to 2,000 milligrams. Keep this up for 3 to 4 days. **Caution:** Those who have kidney disease should avoid vitamin C supplements.

HOW TO PREVENT THE ITCH IN THE FIRST PLACE

Yikes! Standing knee-deep in poison ivy? Here's what to do:

Hit the showers. Quick! Poison ivy penetrates the skin within 20 minutes. So if you're near home, head for the shower, and use plenty of strong soap and cool water, which closes your pores, possibly shutting out some of the ivy toxin.

Schlep your shower with you. Carry a small container of liquid soap and some bottled water in your backpack or picnic basket. You can use it to wash off poison ivy no matter how far you are from home.

Cream it away. A new poison ivy cream, called Zanfel, is said to wash the toxins off your skin in under a minute. It's pricey, but if you're seriously affected by poison ivy, it may be worth purchasing. Keep the cream in your daypack when you're hiking, and head for the nearest stream—or even a puddle—so you can wash away the toxins, as soon as possible.

O·D·D·B·A·L·L OINTMENT

Calendula Cream

Creams containing calendula (*Calendula officinalis*) or chickweed (*Stellaria media*) may ease the itching and discomfort of poison ivy. You can find them at your local natural-foods store.

Postnasal Drip:

Turning Off the Faucet

Adelaide, one of the dolls in the Broadway musical *Guys and Dolls,* developed a bout of postnasal drip from the stress of waiting for a marriage proposal. As she sang her lament, she snuffled, sniffed, and even snorted. You know the feeling.

Of course, most times, a postnasal drip has absolutely nothing to do with wedding vows. The usual causes, in fact, are the following: colds and flu, allergies, cold temperatures, chronic sinus problems, certain foods and spices, pregnancy or birth-control pills, and some high blood pressure medicines.

TOO MUCH OF A GOOD THING

That drag of a drip has everything to do with excess. Did you know the glands in your nose produce as much as 2 quarts of mucus a day? (Did you even know you have glands in your nose!?!)

O·D·D·B·A·L·L OINTMENT

Natural Nasal Balm

Make your own nasal balm: Place ¼ cup petroleum jelly in a small saucepan, and warm it until it melts. Remove it from the heat, and stir in 10 drops *each* of peppermint essential oil, eucalyptus essential oil, and thyme essential oil. When the balm has reached room temperature, pour it into a clean jar for storage. Apply a small amount to your nostrils one to three times daily. The petroleum jelly prevents the essential oils from being absorbed into the skin, so that you can inhale the volatile oils for a prolonged period.

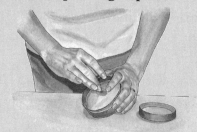

The American Association of Otolaryngology says that this amount of mucus production is perfectly normal. In fact, we need that much to moisten and cleanse our nasal membranes, trap dust and other foreign matter, fight infection, and humidify the air we breathe.

Normally, we swallow all this mucus without even noticing it. But when you begin to feel it accumulating in your throat or running from the back of your nose, you are experiencing postnasal drip.

A correct diagnosis of the exact cause requires a detailed examination of your ears, nose, and throat. If your postnasal drip is caused by medications or a medical condition, then you need your doctor's advice. But for the everyday kind of drip, here's what you can do:

Think thin. You might logically reason that if you want to dry up the drip, you ought to cut back on liquids. But just the opposite is true. You need to drink lots of water—at least eight glasses a day—to thin mucus.

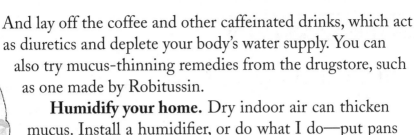

And lay off the coffee and other caffeinated drinks, which act as diuretics and deplete your body's water supply. You can also try mucus-thinning remedies from the drugstore, such as one made by Robitussin.

Humidify your home. Dry indoor air can thicken mucus. Install a humidifier, or do what I do—put pans of water atop your radiators. Worried about spillage? Check your local hardware store for little trays that hang from radiators.

Douche your nose. You can simply wash away that irritating, thickened mucus with a nasal douche or a Water Pik with a nasal nozzle. Simply make a solution of 1 teaspoon of baking soda or salt to 1 pint of warm water. Then use it to irrigate your nose two to four times a day. If this treatment seems too elaborate, try using a simple saline nasal spray to moisten your nose often, suggests the American Association of Otolaryngologists.

Attack your allergies. Ask your doctor for a prescription for one of the newer antihistamines that won't put you to sleep. And while you're at it, find out whether you should avoid milk and milk products, which can thicken mucus. On your own, you might want to make an effort to avoid everything you're

POWERFUL POTION

DRIP-STOPPER TONIC

Attack that drip with an herb combo that reduces congestion, strengthens mucous membranes, and supports immunity. Simply combine equal parts of eyebright (*Euphrasia officinalis*), golden rod (*Solidago virgauria*), calendula (*Calendula officinalis*), and elder (*Sambucus canadensis*). Steep 1 teaspoon of the mixture in 1 cup of hot water for 10 to 15 minutes, then strain. Sip 1 to 3 cups daily.

Steam Sniffing Solution

Sniffing steam is a great way to clear out nasal passages, but if the steam is infused with a healing herb, it works even better! Fill a basin with steaming water, then add a few drops of eucalyptus oil. Grab a big towel, and use it as a tent to contain these healing vapors. Next, pop your head under the towel, and breathe deeply. Just be careful not to burn your cheeks!

allergic to. See **Allergies** for tips.

Size up your sinuses. Chronic sinusitis, an inflammation of the sinus cavities, is a major cause of postnasal drip, and you can't do anything about the drip until you fix the sinuses. When sinus blockages persist, and the lining of the sinuses swell further, the drip gets a grip. See **Sinusitis** for simple tips on coping with this pesky problem.

Use your chest. Plead with your partner to give you a soothing chest rub at night. The vapors will drift up to your nose while you sleep. Tom's of Maine makes a great one you can buy in drugstores nationwide. Or create your own—see **Colds** for the recipe.

Wallop those polyps. Sometimes polyps develop from chronic sinusitis, and these can cause an irritating, persistent postnasal drip. If you suspect a polyp may be behind your particular drip, consult an otolaryngologist, who will examine the interior of your nose. A fiberoptic scope, a computed tomography (CT) scan, or x-rays can pinpoint the offending polyp, which can then be treated with medication or surgically removed if necessary.

Pot Belly:

Suck In That Gut . . . Permanently

Look at that Britney Spears, showing off her belly button! Shame, shame, shame!

Indeed, it's a shame we all don't have nice, flat tummies like that! Age and gravity have a way of turning the sleek into the slack. But with a little work, it's possible to get rid of that pot and not only look better but feel better as well. In fact, it's none other than strong abdominal muscles that protect your back from injury, says Miriam Nelson, Ph.D., a fitness expert and author of *Strong Women, Strong Bodies*. Here's how to lose that pot—and protect the rest of your bod:

O·D·D·B·A·L·L OINTMENT

Lemon Balm Your Belly

An abdominal massage can help you release nervous tension and emotional stress, both of which are often held in the belly. Just add 4 to 6 drops of essential oil of lemon balm (*Melissa officinalis*) or chamomile (*Matricaria recutita*) to 1 tablespoon of massage oil. Using gentle pressure, smooth the oil over your abdomen in wide circles. Begin at your belly button and, making small circles with your fingertips, massage in a clockwise direction in gradually bigger circles.

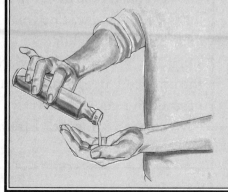

It's crunch time. The very best exercise for flattening that pot belly is the crunch, which tightens up the abs underneath and streamlines your midsection. Simply lie on the floor with your knees bent, your feet about 18 inches apart and your arms crossed over your chest. Keeping the small of your back flat on the floor, curl your upper body off the floor toward your knees. Hold for a few counts; then *slowly* let yourself down. Begin with just a few curls—5 to 10—and work up to three sets of 10, twice a day.

Lose that worry waist. If you're a woman who is eating a healthy diet and exercising regularly but gaining weight in your middle, take a look at the stress in your life. For most women, calories go right to the hips. But for stressed-out women, calories take a detour, and pile up at the waist.

It's called visceral fat, and this stubborn poundage results when you are releasing high levels of the hormone cortisol, reveals a new study out of the University of California at San Francisco. While you can't prevent stress, you can lower cortisol production by getting enough sleep and exercising regularly, the study suggests.

Calm down and relax. Although valerian (*Valeriana officinalis*) is often thought of as the sleep-aid herb, it also has a great reputation for relieving the side effects of stress and for calming the nervous system. Make valerian tea by simmering 1 heaping teaspoon of the root in 1 cup of water for 15 minutes. Sip ⅓ cup of valerian tea before each meal. The tea can be stored in the refrigerator.

Is Your Fat Not Really Fat?

Some women can develop a pot belly that has nothing to do with fat. Rather, it can be the result of osteoporosis. When the spine shrinks, the intestines are forced outward, causing what is known as kyphosis. If you are a woman over 45 years old, check with your doctor before starting abdominal crunches, which can harm some people with kyphosis.

Pregnancy Discomforts:

Making the Long Wait a Little Easier

Creating a new life and bringing a child into the world is one of the most wondrous experiences a woman can have. That said, being pregnant seldom means a non-stop glow. Those 9 months of growing anticipation also often include growing discomforts, such as nausea, backache, and hemorrhoids. Sure, you're awaiting a blessed event, but sometimes, you might wish you could escape into another blessed body!

Thankfully, there are many simple ways to ease the moans and groans and get back to marveling at the miracle of pregnancy. Here are some of them:

Less is more. Morning sickness is usually gone by the third month of pregnancy. But until it is, eat less food at a sitting but eat more often. And if you need to, nibble on dry crackers during the day to add sustenance, suggests Lila Wallis, M.D., a specialist in women's health based in New York City.

Have a minty mouth. Chew peppermint gum, suck on mint candy, or drink a cup of peppermint tea. These minty remedies may help quell some of the nausea.

Stay out of the kitchen. At least until the cooking odors are gone. Strong food odors often make you even more nauseous than you already are. So, if someone's in the kitchen boiling up cabbage soup, make like Elvis, and leave the building.

Holy heartburn! Even when those morning woes have passed, other gastrointestinal conditions can crop up as your baby starts to take up more of your abdominal space. Again, eat small, frequent meals so you never feel full. And avoid spicy and fried foods, which can be hard to digest and can trigger heartburn or acid reflux.

Speed up the sluggish plumbing. The hormonal changes of pregnancy, the pressure of the fetus, and the slowing of digestive functions can make your innards pretty sluggish. Avoid backup by drinking lots of fluids, eating lots of fiber, and getting regular exercise, says Dr. Wallis. For most of us, that means 32 ounces of water, 35 grams of fiber, and 20 to 30 minutes of moderate exercise every day.

Baby your bottom. Unless your baby's breach, her head will press on the veins surrounding your anus, causing them to swell

POWERFUL POTION

ACHY LEGS TONIC

Leg aches and muscle cramps often worsen in the last half of the pregnancy, when the baby's long bones are developing. But eating foods rich in calcium and magnesium will help stave off those aches. To get both, make your own pregnancy tea by stirring 1 teaspoon of blackstrap molasses into 1 cup of hot water. Drink 1 cup daily.

and turn into tender hemorrhoids, which can itch and bleed if you strain while moving your bowels. My advice: Raid your baby supplies—for you. For example, Desitin is used for diaper rash, and you will need it for the baby. But it contains zinc oxide, which may calm your itching. Baby wipes can also soothe those bulging veins. And ask your doctor about whether or not stool softeners or bulking agents are right for you.

Cool it. Sit on some ice to dull the pain of hemorrhoids. If ice is too cold, use a cool compress for a while. Wet a towel in ice water, wring it out, and put it against your bottom to ease those painful veins.

Try Hazel's compress. Witch hazel (*Hamamelis virginiana*) is a powerful astringent that helps shrink swollen hemorrhoids and relieve their itching and burning. Keep it in the refrigerator; then drizzle some on a sterile gauze pad, and gently hold it against your hemorrhoids.

Use a bigger lift. As your pregnancy advances, your breasts will become engorged and quite tender. The best solution is simply a larger-sized bra. Choose a comfortable style with ample support and wide straps that will not cut into your shoulders.

Don't hoard fluids. Your feet, hands, and even your face may swell during pregnancy, when you are more prone to fluid retention. Elevate your legs as

---

O·D·D·B·A·L·L OINTMENT

Hemorrhoid Healer

Break open a vitamin E capsule, and apply the oil to the freshly washed anal area to help heal and soothe inflamed hemorrhoids. This treatment is most effective (and convenient) when done before bed.

often as you can to avoid leg swelling. Do the same for your face, elevating your head on a pillow or two while you sleep. And grab every chance to exercise or simply float in water—this will minimize edema, says Dr. Wallis. Also cut down on salt, which stimulates your body to retain fluid.

Rest your legs. Veins in your legs dilate during pregnancy and sometimes, they become tender and painful. So avoid standing still for long periods of time. Keep on the move, even if you're just treading in place (walking is always better than standing). And while you're seated, wiggle your toes and heels to give your circulation a boost.

Sleep on your side. Falling asleep can be difficult when you can't get comfortable because of the changes in your contours. Sleeping on your back, for instance, can aggravate back pain and make it more difficult to breathe. So try the pregnancy-friendly position: Sleep on your side with a pillow between your knees. A full-length body pillow's especially great for this.

Keep the comfort of sex. Because you're producing more estrogen, you'll probably feel sexier, too. And according to Dr. Wallis, there's no reason to abstain from intercourse just because you're pregnant—with a few exceptions: If you've had a previous spontaneous miscarriage, it's best to avoid vaginal penetration in the early months. Other than that, however, there's no reason not to enjoy a little lovemaking. As the baby gets bigger, of course, you may need to experiment a little to find more comfortable positions for intercourse. But that can be fun, too!

Rashes:

Ditch the Itch

My friend Angie is a neat freak. One day, she decided to scrub the walls and woodwork of her immaculate kitchen. She bought a detergent specially made for tough jobs; then dumped the recommended amount (plus a little extra) into her bucket. Whistling as she worked, she scoured the place until it was operating-room clean.

Hours later, her hands started to burn, itch, and sting. The next day, the skin between her fingers cracked and split. She went to see the doctor, presenting him with hands that looked as though they were little red gloves.

"Contact dermatitis," he said. "Whatever you used in that

bucket irritated your skin. From now on, protect your hands with rubber gloves, and you'll be just fine."

That's what he thought! Several weeks later, Angie attacked her backyard deck with a scrub brush, carefully pulling on a pair of latex gloves beforehand. That night she couldn't sleep because her hands burned and itched. "Guess what?" said the doctor. "You must be allergic to latex."

Poor Angie. She got two rashes for the price of one! Some people just weren't made to live in the modern world. Now more than ever, the universe is filled with things that can make you itch, burn, or break out in blotches, including all of the following:

✔ Food
✔ Stress
✔ Metal
✔ Chemical additives
✔ Hair dye
✔ Fabric softener
✔ Perfume in soap
✔ Medication

The most common types of rashes include contact dermatitis (like Angie's), eczema, and heat rash. Most of the time, we know what causes dermatitis, or a skin rash, because it occurs soon after contact. But what we don't always know is why the substance aggravates our skin in the first place.

Most rashes respond to time and self-treatment. Sometimes,

POWERFUL POTION

SLIPPERY ELM SOOTHER

If your rash is wet and oozing, here's some help: Wash your skin; then dry up the rash and prevent secondary infections by dusting it with an herbal powder. Mix equal parts of slippery elm (*Ulmus fulva*) powder and goldenseal (*Hydrastis canadensis*) powder. Gently dust the powder mix on the rash for soothing relief and quick healing.

Flax Oil Rub

People with skin conditions such as eczema are often lacking essential fatty acids. Ideally, you should be getting these kinds of fats (found in nuts, seeds, and cold-water fish) from your diet, but you can get quick relief by applying them directly on your skin as well. Rub a small amount of flax oil into eczema before going to bed and after bathing, and sweet relief will soon be on its way.

however, a rash can be a sign of a serious infection, such as chicken pox, measles, Rocky Mountain spotted fever, or infectious mononucleosis. If your rash enlarges and spreads despite your treatment, or if the itching is driving you nuts, consult your doctor.

DON'T DO ANYTHING RASH

If your skin is prone to unexpected rashes like Angie's, here's how to keep it clear:

Lose the heavy metal. Earrings with nickel wires and posts commonly cause rashes in people with metal allergies. You'll know if you're one of them: A metal allergy will make you itch within 20 minutes, and a rash will usually appear in a day or two. To avoid both, use only stainless-steel needles for ear piercing, and buy earrings with stainless-steel posts. Although stainless steel does contain some nickel, it is bound so tightly to the steel that it is safe, says the American Academy of Dermatology. In addition to your jewelry, check buttons, fasteners, and zippers. If they touch your skin, they can cause a rash.

Avoid extremes. Very hot or very cold temperatures can aggravate a skin rash. You won't find the perfect environment anywhere, except maybe in the next biosphere. But if you can, avoid exposing your skin to extreme heat and cold. Also, avoid sudden changes in temperature or humidity, which can trigger a rash.

Use hypoallergenic cosmetics. Mascara that I had used for years suddenly made my eyelids puff up and itch. It turned out that the company had changed the makeup's chemical ingredients without telling me. Imagine! Fortunately, there are many hypoallergenic cosmetics on the market.

EXORCISING ECZEMA

Eczema is called "the itch that rashes," because the itch comes first; then when you scratch it—voilà—the rash appears!

Red, dry, itchy patches can show up on your face, behind your knees, in fact, almost anywhere on your body. There's no known cause, but it is more common in people with a family history of allergies.

Research from the National Institutes of Health indicates that 15 million people have some form of eczema. The bad news for them: It cannot be cured. The good news: It's not contagious, and it can be managed pretty well. Here's what you should do:

Know your triggers. There are no standard itch triggers for eczema. The culprits are different for everyone. But you should be able to identify—and avoid—your own triggers fairly easily. Since food allergies are strongly associated with eczema (especially dairy, soy, citrus, and wheat), be careful when handling fresh fruit juices, raw meat, soaps, and disinfectants, all of which can trigger an itch. Also, upper-respiratory infections and stress can be triggers, too.

Cream it! Hydrocortisone cream is an anti-inflammatory steroid cream that is safe for self-care, says the American Academy of Dermatology. It blocks the allergic skin reactions that trigger eczema rashes, and it can speed healing of inflamed or cracked skin, regardless of the cause. If your rash appears infected, however, ask your doctor about antibiotic remedies.

Use the nonsoap solution. Try special-formula cleansers that may help prevent itching for up to several hours. These products

O·D·D·B·A·L·L OINTMENT

Marigold Lotion

For do-it-yourself rash relief, fill a glass jar with dried marigold blossoms. Douse the flowers with olive oil, and stick the jar (sealed with a lid) on a windowsill that will get plenty of sunshine. After 2 weeks, strain out the blossoms, leaving the oil. Refill the jar with a new batch of dried blossoms. You may need to add a tad more olive oil. Reseal the lid, but this time, put it inside a brown paper bag and then back on the sunny windowsill for another 2 weeks. Strain out the blossoms and pour the oil into a dark glass bottle. Add the contents of a vitamin E gel capsule (800 International Units), cover the jar, and store it in the fridge (where it will keep for 2 to 3 months) until you're ready to use it. Apply liberally as needed.

are better than soap, because they allow more of your skin's natural oils to remain and build up, which is crucial to the prevention and treatment of dry and damaged eczematous skin. Look for the Aveeno cleansing bar or their bath treatment soothing formula.

Roll in oats. Eating oatmeal is a healthy habit, but if you itch, you may want to consider using it on the outside, too. Colloidal oatmeal baths and cleaners remoisturize your skin and help control the itching of eczema.

Lock in the moisture. Moisturizers can help prevent flare-ups of eczema. But among the different types, the American Academy of Dermatology says that ointments are best, creams are less helpful, and lotions, because they are mostly made of water, are least helpful. Whichever one you choose, use it within 3 minutes of bathing to lock in the moisture from the bath.

Be a moisture magnet. While moisturizers coat your skin to prevent evaporation of your own body moisture, humectants actually draw moisture from the air into your skin. One such product is called Eucerin. It contains mineral oil and lanolin, to provide moisture, and sorbitol and propylene glycol, which are humectants, making it particularly effective.

Help your skin cells multiply. If your skin is covered with flakes and crusts of eczema, look for products labeled "keratolytics," which break down dead, thickened skin and help remove the flakes and heavy crusts of eczema. Keratolytics, such as Eucerin Plus, speed up the natural skin-healing process and expose the healthier skin below more quickly. Use them in combination with moisturizers and humectants to keep your skin hydrated.

Leave the wool to the sheep. Coarse materials can make anybody itchy. So take care to avoid itch-inducing fabrics like mohair and other wools. Stick with cotton and silk instead.

COOL OFF HEAT RASH

Prickly heat is a common rash that pops up in extremely hot, humid weather, or when your body is overheated from exertion or fever. The rash occurs when your body's sweat ducts get blocked, causing tiny red dots to appear. Here's what to do:

Get out of the heat. Stay in a cool place, and the rash will diminish, says the American Medical Association.

Wash off the sweat. Keep the area clean and sweat free. Whenever you find yourself soaked with sweat, take a quick shower and air dry. Let it all hang out!

Slip into loose clothing. The more air that gets to your skin, the less likely you are to break out.

Rectal Itching:

Stop the Squirming

The itch that you absolutely cannot scratch can be as baffling as it is embarrassing. What's, well, *behind* this problem? There are several possiblilities: Exposure to irritants, a sexually transmitted infection, a skin disorder, dry skin, poor hygiene, even spicy food. In children, pinworms are the most common cause of a rectal itch, and for that, a doctor's prescription for medication is needed. If the problem lasts more than 1 or 2 days, see your doctor. Otherwise, here's what may relieve your discomfort:

Inventory your irritants. Ask some questions: Is the laundry deter-

---

FABULOUS FOLK REMEDY

Create a Critter-Free Zone

Ideally, the gut is an inhospitable environment for critters like pinworms. To help it become even more so, eat plenty of garlic and pumpkin seeds—both substances known to be hated by worms!

IT'S AN EMERGENCY!

If your discomfort is accompanied by bleeding from the rectum, call your doctor. There could be a systemic reason for the itch. Don't ignore it.

gent or fabric softener causing your underwear to irritate your skin? Is your toilet tissue perfumed or color dyed? Do you use scented bath oils or shower gels? Make a list of all the items that come in con-

tact with your intimate parts. Through a process of elimination (no pun intended), you may discover the cause of your curious itch and be able to toss out the offending product.

Tuck it up. While you're in the discovery process, relieve your itch with Tucks or another brand of medicated pad.

Save your skin. If that miserable itch is caused by a skin disorder or even just dry skin, see if a hydrocortisone cream or an ointment like zinc oxide can provide relief. They're usually found near the hemorrhoid medications in your drugstore.

Be a butthead. That's right, Beavis, give your nether regions some thought. Remember to wash the itchy area with mild soap when you shower. Also, remember to clean up after a bowel movement with a soft tissue and cool water.

POWERFUL POTION

A DAILY DIGESTION TEA

Rectal itching is often a sign of poor digestion. Boost your digestive power by drinking ½ cup of dandelion (*Taraxacum officinale*) tea before meals. To make your own, steep 1 teaspoon of dandelion root in ½ cup of hot water for 20 minutes. Sip warm before meals. **Caution:** Dandelion is rich in potassium and should not be taken with potassium tablets.

Take the best sitz in the house. You can buy a special sitz bathtub from your pharmacy or medical-supply store, or you can sitz in your own tub. Either way, the idea is to immerse the rectal area in warm circulating water or a mild saline solution. The commercial sitz tub is a shallow basin that can be placed over your toilet seat. It has a tube you can use to direct warm water over the area while you are seated. To use your bathtub, simply sit in shallow warm water, and paddle the water toward the itchy area.

Wave adios to jalapeños. Obviously, what goes in has to come out, so you might want to reconsider before pigging out on that five-alarm chili. Avoid spicy foods if they are the culprit, because they can make you pay later by burning their way through the membranes in your digestive system.

Moon the sun. Sun is a wonderful remedy for itching and dry skin anywhere on your body, including your anal area. Because of our social restrictions, your bottom rarely gets its place in the sun. Never mind nude bathing, just look for a private spot where you can let it all hang out, so to speak.

POWERFUL POTION

SQUIRT THE OREGANO

Too much yeast in your system can cause rectal itching and burning. To soothe the area, make a strong infusion of oregano (*Origanum vulgare*) by steeping 1 heaping tablespoon of fresh leaves in 1 cup of hot water, covered, for 15 minutes. Strain, and pour the liquid into a peribottle (available in drugstores). Keep the bottle by your toilet, and after each visit to the bathroom, squirt your bottom with the oregano solution.

Reflux Disease:

More Than Indigestion

Mmmm. That spicy, extra-cheese, extra-large pepperoni, garlic, and anchovy pizza tastes so good going down! But how about when it's coming back up—and toting a big bucketful of burning acid with it? Reflux isn't simple heartburn—it's heartburn's homicidal cousin! No need to panic, though. There's a lot you can do about reflux, once you understand it.

The digestive disorder known as gastroesophageal reflux disease (GERD) stems from a problem with your lower esophageal sphincter (LES), the muscle that connects the

Make Like an Early Bird

That's right, pretend you're a retiree, and eat your dinner while the sun is still shining—or, at the very least, 2 to 3 hours before bedtime. According to Lila Wallis, M.D., a New York City-based internist, dining early may ease a reflux problem by giving the acid in your stomach time to ebb and allowing the stomach to empty a bit.

esophagus (the tube leading to your stomach) with the stomach. When your stomach contents reflux—or back up—into your esophagus, it means the sphincter is weak or relaxes at the wrong time, according to the National Institutes of Health. But obesity and pregnancy, both of which crowd the esophagus and stomach, can also cause reflux disease.

The most common symptom is acid indigestion that feels like a burning chest pain behind the breastbone and moves upward toward the neck and throat. As if that weren't bad enough, however, if left untreated, reflux can lead to more serious conditions, including esophagitis, bleeding, ulcers, and even esophageal cancer. Here's how to make sure that doesn't happen:

Identify the problem. Since you have to identify which part of your digestive system is acting up before you can figure out what to do about it, your first step is to see your doctor, says Paul Miskovitz, M.D., a New York–based gastroenterologist. Fortunately, there are a variety of ways to test the condition of your LES and stomach acid to find out if your discomfort is heartburn, a hiatal hernia, or reflux disease. Most likely, your doctor will suggest that you have a small tube inserted into your digestive tract so that he or she can take a look at what's going on. Sometimes, x-rays are also needed.

POWERFUL POTION

GET HIP TO ROSES

Reflux can sometimes be caused by food sensitivities and allergies. If you suspect that this is the case, drink 1 cup of rose hip (*Rosa canina*) tea before meals to help reduce your reaction. Steep 1 heaping teaspoon of rose hips in 1 cup of hot water for 15 minutes. Strain, and enjoy.

Be anti-antacid. Long-term use of over-the-counter antacids can lead to side effects like diarrhea and a change in the way you metabolize calcium. They can even cause a buildup of magnesium. With this in mind, if you use antacids for more than 3 weeks without relief, ask your doctor about medications to treat chronic reflux or heartburn that won't have this effect. Some of these drugs reduce stomach acid, while others increase the strength of the sphincter muscle. Usually, heartburn can be relieved with diet and lifestyle modification, but if your LES is not functioning properly, you may need special medication or even surgery.

Check your meds. Long-term use of some medications make you more vulnerable to gastric reflux. For instance, nitroglycerin and asthma medicines, like albuterol, are suspect, and so is Valium and a class of intestinal medications called anticholinergics. Ask your doctor if any medications you take for other conditions could put you at risk for reflux disease.

Make less work for your LES. Certain foods and beverages like chocolate, peppermint, coffee, fatty foods, and alcoholic beverages can weaken the sphincter and also overtax the muscle. Go

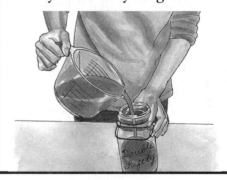

FABULOUS FOLK REMEDY

Grandma's Marshmallow Tea

Marshmallow (*Althea officinalis*) tea, a remedy that must be used by half the world's grandmothers, soothes the gastrointestinal tract all the way through. Soak 1 heaping tablespoon of marshmallow root in 1 quart of cold water overnight. Strain, and drink throughout the day to soothe your gut.

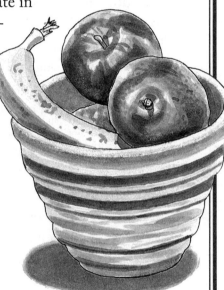

easy on such foods, and decrease portion sizes in everything that you eat. Also, if you smoke, quit now. Smoking is known to weaken the LES, says the National Institutes of Health.

Forget about fat. High-fat meals stay in the stomach longer than low-fat meals, says Lila Wallis, M.D., a New York–based internist. And as a result, they cause more acid to accumulate, slowing the digestive process. Follow a sensible diet that's low in fats, moderate in proteins, and high in complex carbohydrates (fruits, vegetables, and cereal, for example), which are easily digested.

Keep your head up. Elevate the head of your bed on 6-inch blocks, or sleep on a special wedge—foam rubber or pillows—to allow gravity to minimize the reflux of stomach contents into the esophagus. You can find the wedge at drugstores and medical-supply shops nationwide.

Repetitive Stress Syndrome:

The Mouse Is Mightier Than the Pen

I thought I was getting old and feeble when I found myself dropping things. Every so often, my left hand—the one that operates the mouse and the pen, not to mention the sword—would cramp up like a crab. Then I realized that I was having a reaction to the repetitive stress of writing all day, hitting keys, pushing the mouse around, and editing hard copy by hand.

Sure enough, I was dropping things and having cramps just as I was facing a deadline. Clearly, I was so engrossed in my work that I was forgetting to come up for air. I sure was happy to find a better reason for the dropsies than aging! Even if it was a repetitive stress injury (RSI).

Millions of people have RSI. Its cause is exactly as its name implies—performing the same action repetitively over a period of time. Everyone from auto-workers installing the same car part on an assembly line to data-entry clerks pounding on their keyboards to butchers working at meat-packing plants is susceptible to this injury. But, those of us who spend our days working at computers now make up one of the larger groups of sufferers. Usually, poor equipment design and not taking needed breaks contribute to the problem. Here's how you can avoid it:

Heed the signs. You can sidestep the serious pain and injury of RSI by taking note of any clues that crop up along the way. For instance, you may feel clumsy and crampy, as I did. You also may feel tingling, loss of strength, or less coordination in your hands. And you may feel this way hours after completing the task that caused the symptoms in the first place.

Work a 50-minute hour. Many short breaks are better than a few long ones, says Emil Pascarelli and Deborah Quilter, who experts on how to avoid computer-use injuries. Every half hour, take a minute to get up and stretch, they suggest. Loosen your neck and shoulder muscles. Then, every hour, take a full 10-minute break.

FABULOUS FOLK REMEDY

Black Willow Relief

Black willow (*Salix nigra*) contains salicylates (the active ingredient in aspirin) and has long been used as an anti-inflammatory and pain-relieving herb. Make a tea by simmering 1 heaping teaspoon of black willow bark in 1 cup of water for 10 minutes. Strain, and sip 1 to 2 cups a day.

Be ergonomically correct. If you work at a computer station, be sure your chair, desk, and computer are all ergonomically in synch. Don't make your body accommodate your workstation. It should be the other way around.

Sit up straight. Sit with your thighs level or angled slightly downward and your feet flat on the floor or a footrest. Keep your back straight but your shoulders relaxed, your upper arms at your sides, and your forearms horizontal or tilted slightly downward. Your knees and elbows should form right angles. Your keyboard should be level or have a slight negative tilt (the top row should be lower than bottom row). And the top of your screen should be at about eye level.

Don't look down. If you're stretching into awkward positions to read material as you hit the keys, you're straining your back, neck, and shoulders as well as your eyes. Give your upper body a break by using an upright copy stand if you are working from printed material, so you don't have to slump to see it.

Cushions Kill Cramps

I've never had writer's block, but I have had writer's cramp. And I've found that using a pen that has a cushion around the shaft, giving the pen a larger, more comfortable grip, can help prevent it. Either buy a ready-made pencil cushion at an office supply store, or run your regular pen through the hole in the foam cover of a plastic hair curler. Three addition tips: Write big, so you'll use the large muscles of your upper arm. Don't grip the pen too hard. And write on a slanted (slightly inclined) surface, so you're not bending your neck.

O·D·D·B·A·L·L OINTMENT

Magic Meadowsweet

Meadowsweet (*Filipendula ulmaria*) contains anti-inflammatory salicylates and, unlike aspirin, which also contains salicylates, may be taken safely long term. Make a tea by steeping 1 teaspoon of meadowsweet in 1 cup of hot water for 10 minutes. Strain, and drink 1 to 2 cups daily.

Learn to type. I've been typing since the eighth grade, and I can't imagine not typing properly. But I see people with their hands bent at awkward angles, using all the wrong fingers on the keys. Get an instruction book with a chart that shows you where all your fingers go. Don't rest your hands on the table or pad. Keep them suspended over the keyboard, and let your fingers do the walking. The rest of your body will love you for it.

Keep your hands warm. I used to wear an old pair of woollen, fingerless gloves in winter because my office was so cold. When you rest your hands, put them on a heating pad or warm towel. The National Institute for Occupational Safety and Health (NIOSH) says there are gloves called OccuMitts you can wear for warmth and flexibility as you type.

Voice your thoughts. The latest speech-recognition equipment allows you to voice your thoughts directly to the computer, no typing required. While this technology is still pretty expensive, if your arms and back are showing signs of RSI, you may want to give it try. Just be sure to enlist an expert to help you shop, since you'll be spending beaucoup bucks for this system.

Pray for no pain. Here's a neat way to stretch the muscles of your hands and wrists from time to time, and it really feels good. Put your hands together in a prayer position. Gently push both hands to one side, hold the position for 15 to 30 seconds, then gently move to the other side. Keep your fingers straight and your fingertips together. You can move your hands in this position to point upward or downward.

Get a headset. One of the worse pains in the neck—literally—is cradling the phone between your neck and your ear while you write messages or work at your keyboard. Get rid of that potential RSI by wearing a telephone headset. Get one for your cell phone, too—especially if you frequently make phone calls while driving.

> # Toss the Mouse!
>
> If your computer mouse is the cause of your pain, toss it to your cybercat; then check out this peculiar rodent—the foot mouse! Frankly, I cannot imagine controlling the cursor with my foot. But then, I can't walk and chew gum at the same time either!

Sagging Breasts:

Refitting Your Low Riders

As a budding preteen, I couldn't wait to wear a bra, because it meant I was finally a woman. Then, once it dawned on me that it was a torture similar to Chinese foot binding, I couldn't wait to get rid of the darn thing!

True liberation came in the 1960s when I was first in line to burn my bra. But I've put on a little weight since then, and my breasts are definitely pointing southward. So I've finally relented and returned to the world of foundation garments.

The Two Things Exercise Won't Lift

Get over it. There's no exercise that actually hoists your breasts back up. The only muscles in your breasts are the small muscles of the areola and lobules. So be wary of any "breast exercise" claims. Yes, you can make your breasts look a little higher with that old standby isometric—pressing your palms together at chest level. But it's your chest muscles behind the breasts that produce this minor lift. Push-ups, which exercise the chest's pectoral muscles, will also help your chest look well toned. But only plastic surgery actually lifts the breasts themselves.

There is, however, no real physical reason to wear a bra, according to Susan Love, M.D., author of *Susan Love's Breast Book*. The popular belief that wearing a bra strengthens your breasts and prevents sagging is mistaken. Sagging has nothing to do with going braless. It happens because of the changing ratio of fat to the rest of the tissue in your breasts, and no bra can undo that math, says Dr. Love.

On the other hand, while bras don't prevent natural sagging from the weight of years, they do make your breasts look as though they had certain antigravity properties. So if you crave that perky, youthful profile, your best bet is to wear a really great bra. Here's what to buy:

Use a prop for that pop. Displayed like oysters on the half shell, breasts are pushed up and out by a Wonder Bra. (I used to achieve the same effect by stuffing rolled-up socks inside my underwear.) Fortunately, we now can find a wide range of bras with wires and pads designed to create the illusion that we're well

O·D·D·B·A·L·L OINTMENT

Butter Up!

One of the signs of sagging breasts can be the appearance of stretch marks. To keep your breast tissue supple, massage your breasts daily with cocoa butter. Simply melt a small amount of cocoa butter in your hands, and massage your breasts in a circular direction, always ending at the upper outer corner by your arm pits.

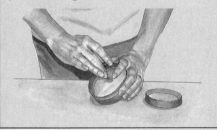

endowed. In Julia Roberts's award-winning role as Erin Brockovich, she seemed to have a different color push-up bra for each day of the week. But try 'em before you buy 'em. These push-ups have different degrees of comfort.

Go sporty to beat the bounce. Your breasts' milk ducts and lobules, which store and carry milk to the nipples, are suspended in connective tissue that is strained when you take off your bra. It's this tissue that hurts when you jog or run. For activities that involve running or bouncing, wear a sports bra that holds your breasts close to your body. A good sports bra will take out the bounce and you'll be more comfortable in motion.

Sciatica:

Help for the Hot-Wired Leg

Yow! Your sciatic nerve is not only your body's biggest nerve, but it can produce one of its biggest pains. If you've ever had sciatic pain (also called sciatica), you'll understand why it hurts where it does: The nerve travels from your back, through your buttock, down the back of your thigh and outer edge of your leg to your feet and toes—and can produce a white-hot flash of pain all the way down. Sometimes, a muscle deep inside the buttock is pressing on the nerve. But more often, the pain results from a herniated disk in your lower spine.

A disk is basically a round, flat cushion that keeps your bony vertebrae from scraping

---

FABULOUS FOLK REMEDY

Centaury-Old Relief

An old-fashioned remedy for sciatica is centaury (*Centarium erythraea*), probably because it relieves sluggish digestion and constipation, which can compound the pain of sciatica. Steep 1 teaspoon in 1 cup of hot water for 5 minutes. Drink ½ cup before meals.

against one another. When one ruptures—usually in response to an injury—the soft stuff either squishes out or simply causes a bulge in the side of the disk. The squishy stuff, or bulge, can then press against spinal nerves, including the sciatic nerve—creating some of the worst misery known to humankind.

POWERFUL POTION

MOTHER NATURE'S HERBAL HEALER

The tension that often accompanies prolonged pain only creates more pain. To help yourself relax, combine two of the following herbs in equal parts, and steep 1 teaspoon of the mixture in 1 cup of hot water for 10 minutes. Strain, and drink 2 to 4 cups daily. Here are the herbs: Black cohosh (*Cimicifuga racemosa*), passionflower (*Passiflora incarnata*), meadowsweet (*Filipendula ulmaria*), chamomile (*Matricaria recutita*), and Jamaican dogwood (*Piscidia erythrina*). **Caution:** People with ragweed allergies may be sensitive to chamomile. Also, do not use with any prescription medication.

HOW DO I KNOW IT'S SCIATICA?

The intensity of sciatica varies. You may experience only pins and needles, or a searing burning sensation. Your back may be "locked" when the sciatica is severe, or you may have only a dull ache that increases when you move. Here are the clues that typically signal disk trouble:

✔ Your leg pain gets worse when you sit and better when you stand or lie flat in bed with a pillow under your knees.

✔ The pain may be worse in the morning.

✔ Bending forward hurts, but bending backward doesn't.

If the herniated disk causes loss of bladder or bowel function, progressive muscle weakness, or the inability to lift up your foot,

Why Your Sciatica Is Worse in the Morning

You mave have noticed that the pain caused by a herniated disk is more intense in the morning. That's because your spinal disks absorb water during the night, while you are lying flat. And as a result, they press harder on the surrounding nerves. During the day, gravity pushes the water out, making the disks flatter—and less likely to pinch any nearby nerves.

surgery is needed to remove a portion of the disk and relieve compression on the nerves.

HOW TO SEND PAIN PACKING

You should be under a doctor's care with sciatica; but short of surgery, most of the treatment is really going to be up to you. In 80 percent of patients with lumbar disk injury, conservative, non-surgical therapy works while the disk has a chance to shrink, says Emile Hiesiger, M.D., a New York City–based neurologist who specializes in treating pain. In effect, the body heals itself. Here's how to keep sciatica pain at bay while it does:

Take drugs. The inflammation of the nerve is a major cause of leg pain, says David Borenstein, M.D., a Washington, D.C.–based rheumatologist. Take nonsteroidal, anti-inflammatory drugs (NSAIDs), such as aspirin or ibuprofen, to decrease inflammation surrounding the disk and nerve. This will help reduce pain and shrink swollen tissues.

Hit the sack on your back. Prop a pillow under your knees, or rest on your side with a pillow placed between your knees. Both positions take your weight off the inflamed nerve and decrease pressure on the herniated disk, says Dr. Borenstein. If you still can't sleep because of sciatic pain, lie flat on a rug on the floor with your feet and calves on a chair. Your knees should be bent in a 90-degree angle. Trust me—it works.

Take a walk on the mild side. As soon as possible, start walking on a flat surface. Take it slow and easy, and gradually increase your distance. Climb stairs with caution, however, so your weakened leg doesn't cause you to fall.

No strain, no pain. Don't lift anything, including your baby, says Dr. Hiesiger. If your sciatic pain is caused by a herniated disk, any straining will aggravate it. Take steps to treat colds and allergies, so you don't have coughing or sneezing fits—they will hurt. Even straining for a bowel movement can aggravate your pain, so if you are constipated, do something about it.

Acupuncture, anyone? Although no one has yet figured out exactly how acupuncture helps sciatic pain, studies show that the insertion of acupuncture needles just under the skin at certain key points is frequently effective against low back pain that involves the sciatic nerve. If you're interested in acupuncture, ask your doctor for a referral to a practitioner in your community. All acupuncturists should be certified and should use disposable needles.

Work with a massage therapist. A well-trained massage therapist who has formally studied the body's musculature is worth his or her weight in gold. He or she can frequently relieve muscle spasms that are pinching the sciatic nerve faster than your doctor can write a prescription. How to find said miracle worker? The certificates on the wall aren't always helpful. Instead, play 20 questions. Any experienced therapist should be able to name every single muscle in your body, tell you what it does, what damages it, and what strengthens it.

EXERCISE FOR STRENGTH

Try these simple exercises to strengthen your lower-back muscles and prevent sciatic pain:

Lower back stretch. Lie on your back, bend your knees, then move your knees toward your torso. Elevate your hips a bit. Hold this position for 30 seconds, then lower your feet to the floor. Repeat 9 more times. Next, pull your knees toward your torso, one at a time. Repeat 9 times with each knee. As your strength and flexibility improve, gradually increase the number of repetitions you do until you can do three sets of 10 twice a day.

Seated stretch. Lean forward, letting your head hang down between your legs. Your upper body should be resting on your thighs. Hold this stretch for 30 seconds, then relax. Repeat several times, gradually boosting the number of reps you do as your flexibility improves.

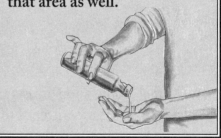

Seasonal Affective Disorder:

Lighten Up Those Winter Blues

The snowbirds sure have the right idea. In winter, these intrepid folks, often retirees, leave their dark, cold northern cities and fly south to the sunshine of Florida, just like migrating birds. As a result, they're less likely to develop seasonal affective disorder (SAD), a type of depression that is also called winter depression.

The symptoms are similar to those of other depressive disorders and include lethargy, a change in appetite or weight, and lack of interest in social situations. (See **Depression** for more symptoms.) No long-term research has yet been completed, but doctors do know that SAD is a very real disorder. It affects more women than men and, logically, more people in the north than in the south. In fact, SAD is seven times more common in Washington State than in Florida, according to the American Academy of Family Physicians.

Fortunately, wherever you live, there's a lot you can do to keep your winters from turning you too blue. Here's how to begin:

See your doctor. SAD is more than just a case of the blahs, assures Gila Lindsley, Ph.D., a psychologist in Massachusetts. The symptoms, like those of any type of depression, can affect your entire life and well-being. Some people, she says, even experience suicidal thoughts. So take your winter blues seriously, and ask your doctor to refer you to a psychiatrist or psychologist, who can evaluate the disorder and recommend medication if it's necessary.

Order a BLT to go. In this case, BLT is not a sandwich. It's a remarkably simple yet effective treatment called broad-spectrum light therapy. BLT involves simply sitting in front of a desktop light box equipped with special, high-intensity bulbs for about 30 minutes each day, generally in the morning. If BLT works for you, your doctor will likely recommend that you continue it throughout the winter. The timing and length of exposure are highly individual,

POWERFUL POTION

BLUES-BEATING TONIC

For an herbal mood lifter, combine equal parts of St. John's wort (*Hypericum perforatum*), kava (*Piper methysticum*), passionflower (*Passiflora incarnata*), betony (*Stachys betonica*), and vervain (*Verbena hastata*). Steep 1 teaspoon of the mixture in 1 cup of hot water for 15 minutes. Strain, and drink 2 cups daily. **Caution:** Kava has recently been linked to liver toxicity. So do not use this tea without consulting with a qualified health practitioner first—especially if you're taking antidepressant or anti-anxiety medications.

FABULOUS FOLK REMEDY

Flax to the Max

People who are depressed often have low levels of essential fatty acids. Take 1 tablespoon of flaxseed oil once or twice daily during the winter to head off the cold weather blues.

however, so be sure to ask your doctor for guidance.

Plan active events ahead of time. While it's easy to have fun in the summer sun, be sure to plan vacations, trips, or special events that will keep you happier in the winter months, too. Make firm commitments well in advance, so you'll have something to look forward to when the blahs set in. And if you can, take your annual vacation in the winter rather than summer, then head for the sun.

Light up your life. Use as much light indoors as your budget allows, suggests Dr. Lindsley. You might even try the full-spectrum light bulbs that include all the colors of the rainbow. Their light is much more like natural daylight, and they can lift your home's indoor mood. They're energy efficient, too, so although each bulb costs more, they last much longer than standard light bulbs.

Push back the dark. The temptation to hug the fireplace and become a couch potato in winter can overwhelm you if you prefer warmth and sun. But if you're not up to joining winter sports-lovers on the slopes or frozen ponds, head for the warmth and light of your local fitness center. Get 30 minutes of regular exercise a day to keep those endorphins circulating, and you'll more easily combat the depression of a long, cold, dark winter. Just be sure to begin your physical activity before the blahs get under way, warns Dr. Lindsley.

Stay away from tanning salons. Don't choose a tanning salon for do-it-yourself light therapy. These light sources are high in ultraviolet rays and can cause serious harm to your eyes and skin, warns the American Academy of Family Physicians.

Sexually Transmitted Infections:

Safe Sex at Any Age

Don't get shy on me, now. Because the truth is, whether you're a wild young thing or a swinging senior citizen, if you're sexually active, you're at risk for infections, period. Let me say that again: No matter what your age, you are at risk.

Women are more vulnerable than men to sexually transmitted infections (STIs) because of female anatomy. The interior of the vagina is a warm and comfy place for bacteria to stake a claim and multiply. As a result, genital infections are more easily passed from men to women than the other way around. But regardless of your sex, if you have more than one sexual partner, you are also at higher risk of infection. Microbes thrive in semen, blood, and sometimes in saliva. Genital herpes and warts can be spread simply by contact with an infected person's skin. And hepatitis B can be caught simply by sharing personal items such as razors.

Most sexually transmitted infections—the HIV infection and AIDS excluded—can be cured if they're treated early. The problem is, the symptoms often aren't noticeable until damage has been done.

Should you give up the joy of sex? Not at all! With the right precautions, you can still enjoy sex safely and greatly reduce your risk of dire complications. Here's what to do:

Be on the alert. There are a number of infections that cause different degrees of discomfort and risk. Among the more common are chlamydia, herpes, gonorrhea, trichomoniasis, and human papillomavirus. Be aware of the symptoms—including an unusual discharge, odor, genital or anal itching, a burning sensation when urinating, sores, swollen glands in the groin, pain in the groin or lower abdomen, vaginal bleeding, testicular swelling, flu-like symptoms, and painful intercourse. And if you spot them, get medical attention early.

Get tested routinely. If you are sexually active, get tested at least once a year for any sexually transmitted infection. Most women get an annual gynecological checkup and Pap smear. Let your doctor

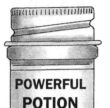

POWERFUL POTION

AN HERBAL PERIWASH

While STIs should be treated with conventional medications, you can relieve symptoms of burning and itching with a cooling periwash. Make an infusion of echinacea (*Echinacea* spp.), comfrey root (*Symphytum officinale*), and goldenseal (*Hydrastis canadensis*) by combining the herbs in equal parts, and then steeping 1 heaping teaspoon in 1 cup of hot water for 15 minutes. Cool, and strain into a peribottle. Leave by the toilet, and rinse yourself two or three times daily.

know you want to be routinely checked for any infections, too. Ask your partner if he or she has ever had an STI or has been tested.

Get shot. If you are sexually active, you're at risk for the hepatitis B virus, which can result in liver failure. Ask your doctor if you should be vaccinated against it.

Use condoms. Until the test results are in, and you are absolutely certain you and your partner are not infected with an STI of any kind, use latex condoms—for at least 6 months. Most doctors say that if you have been mutually exclusive in your sexual relationship for at least 6 months, and you both have tested negative for STIs, it is probably safe to have sex without using a condom as protection against disease. Just don't forget to use birth control if you don't want to become a parent.

Eat well. Support your healing with nature's pharmacy of immune-supporting, nutrient-dense foods. Make sure your diet includes plenty of garlic, dark leafy greens (like collards, chard, and kale), orange and yellow vegetables (such as squash and pumpkin), and seasoning herbs (like thyme, oregano, and rosemary).

POWERFUL POTION

IMMUNE SYSTEM STRENGTHENER

While you're being treated for your STI, you can help strengthen your body's immune system from the inside out. Combine equal parts of echinacea, goldenseal, and licorice root (*Glycyrrhiza glabra*). Steep 1 heaping teaspoon in 1 cup of hot water for 15 minutes. Strain, and drink 2 to 3 cups daily. **Caution:** Licorice root should not be used by people with high blood pressure or kidney disease.

Shingles:

If Only You Could Leave 'Em on the Roof

Shingles is a booby-trap disease. It's completely hidden, just waiting for something to spring the trap. Then down you go into a spiral of searing pain.

It usually shows up in folks over 50, so it's often considered a disease of the aging. But it's really a reminder of youth—specifically, the time when you were a kid with chicken pox, and the *Varicella* virus took up residence in your body.

Of course, if you have shingles, you're probably too busy hurting and itching to care much where it came from. But understanding the blister rash, called herpes zoster, which affects the nerve roots in your spinal cord, can help you treat it successfully.

Here's what you need to know:

When you first had chicken pox, your immune system may not have destroyed the entire virus, and what remained has lain dormant in nerve cells near your spinal cord and brain. Now, many years later, age, illness, medications, or stress can activate that little bug. It then travels along sensory nerve fibers to your skin and surfaces as a line of small blisters. The blisters march around your chest or back, but they can also appear on your arms or legs, your face, and even inside your mouth. You may feel a burning sensation or have a slight fever and lose your appetite.

A bout of shingles usually lasts 10 to 14 days. Sometimes, the virus will continue to hurt even after the rash is gone due to activity along the nerve fibers. This pain is known as postherpetic neuralgia, and it can cause depression, in-

FABULOUS FOLK REMEDY

Valerian Tea

Valerian (*Valeriana officinalis*) sedates the nervous system and helps put a damper on the pain of shingles. This is especially useful when you are having difficulty sleeping because of the pain. Steep 1 heaping teaspoon in 1 cup of hot water for 10 minutes. Drink 1 cup after dinner and before bed. **Caution:** Do not use with any other pain relievers, antianxiety, or antidepression medication.

Consider Yourself Typhoid Mary

Shingles is contagious to people who have not had chicken pox or been vaccinated against it. Most adults had chicken pox as children, but the chicken pox vaccine came into use only after the U.S. Food and Drug Administration approved it in 1995. So, if you have shingles, stay away from children—especially infants who have not yet been vaccinated.

POWERFUL
POTION

SHINGLES TONIC

To concoct an immune-stimulating and pain-relieving tea, combine 2 parts of echinacea (*Echinacea* spp.) with 1 part *each* of St. John's wort, skullcap (*Scutellaria lateriflora*), lemon balm (*Melissa officinalis*), and oatstraw (*Avena sativa*). Steep 1 heaping teaspoon of the mixture in 1 cup of hot water, covered, for 10 minutes, then strain. Drink 3 to 4 cups a day. **Caution:** Consult with your doctor before using this tea if you're taking antidepressant or antianxiety medication.

somnia, and weight loss. Although you can't prevent shingles, you can do a lot to recover more quickly and minimize the pain. Here's how:

Nail down shingles early. Although shingles can run its course without treatment, see your doctor early to head off any possible infection. Starting treatment with antiviral drugs within 3 days of an outbreak can shorten the duration of the rash. These medications also help prevent the pain that can follow shingles, according to the Mayo Clinic. In addition, early treatment lessens the length and severity of the outbreak. So see your doctor promptly at the onset of any symptoms.

Take two aspirin, and hold on till morning. Over-the-counter remedies can also help control the pain from shingles. Take non-steroidal anti-inflammatory drugs (NSAIDs) such as aspirin and ibuprofen according to your doctor's instructions.

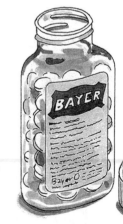

Keep 'em clean. Wash the blisters twice a day with regular soap and water. Resist the urge to cover them up with a bandage. And hang in there—the rash will usually run its course in 3 weeks or so.

Run hot and cold. Apply cold compresses to the rash to cool the itch and hot compresses to ease the pain.

Take it to the tub. A leisurely soak in a tub of lukewarm water will ease the discomfort of shingles. But if you add oatmeal or baking soda to your bath water, you'll get even more relief.

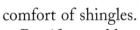
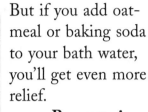

Be pretty in pink. After you dry off from your shower or bath, apply calamine lotion to your skin. The pink salve is a wonder for soothing the itch and pain of shingles. Apply it more than once a day, if it helps.

Rub them right. If the touch of your clothing against your skin drives you crazy, here's a way to defuse the sensitivity, courtesy of the docs at the Mayo Clinic: Rub the area with a clean towel for several minutes—*after* you've gotten the okay from your own doctor.

O·D·D·B·A·L·L OINTMENT

Hot Pepper Salve

Rubbing hot pepper ointment on your shingles may not sound as though it would put out the fire, but apparently, it does. The American Academy of Dermatology says that ointments made with capsaicin, the element that provides the heat in hot peppers, help some people with shingles. Substance P is the active ingredient, and it works on pain close to the surface of the skin. Apply it three to four times a day, and within 1 or 2 weeks, the pain should gradually ease. Commercial brands include Capzasin-P, Dolorac, and Zostrix. Check with your doctor about what strength to buy. And when you apply it, be *very* careful not to get the ointment near your eyes, genitals, or any broken skin.

Sinusitis:

Clogged Caverns in Your Head

Almost everyone I know who has a chronic sinus problem also has chronic frustration! Sinuses clog and hurt for so many different reasons that finding the right remedy is often difficult. Some frustrated docs have even been known to refer to sinuses as a "design flaw"—but we do need them. Without these complex, hollow spaces in our cheekbones and nasal cavities, our heads would be so heavy, we wouldn't be able to hold them up!

Sinusitis occurs when the mucous membranes lining your sinuses become inflamed, creating nasal congestion and bacterial infection. The inflammation is usually triggered by allergies, bacteria, fungus, viruses, pollu-

---

FABULOUS FOLK REMEDY

Time to Horse Around

Nothing clears your sinuses faster than a bite of horseradish root (*Armoracia rusticana*). Eat $\frac{1}{4}$ teaspoon of prepared horseradish three times daily, or make your own by grating 1 teaspoon of fresh root into 1 cup of hot water. Steep for 5 minutes; then strain. Drink 3 cups a day.

tion, stress, and genetic disorders, although smokers often have bad sinusitis because all that burning chemical junk constantly irritates their sinuses. People with frequent upper-respiratory infections or who have major postnasal drip are also more vulnerable to sinusitis. When it's bad, you may also have a fever, swelling, discomfort in the neck, and an earache, not to mention the all-too-familiar stuffy nose.

If you're unsure what's causing your sinusitis, check with your doctor. Likewise, if you have sinusitis more than three times a year, if the time between episodes is short, or if it doesn't clear up in 7 days, see your doctor for medical treatment. You may have an intense infection.

YOUR STRATEGIC DEFENSE SYSTEM

An array of weapons can wipe out sinusitis, including prescription antibiotics, antihistamines, decongestants, steroids, and sometimes—particularly if you have nasal polyps—surgery. Once it's cleared up, however,

O·D·D·B·A·L·L OINTMENT

Sinus Oil Solution

To open your nasal passages, use a sinus oil once or twice daily. First, soak a washcloth in hot water, and apply it to your face to increase circulation to the area. Keep the cloth in place for 5 minutes, resoaking it in hot water to keep it as hot as you can tolerate. Then apply a thin layer of olive oil to your frontal bone, above your eyes and your cheekbones, below your eyes, and onto the bony part of your nose. Next, place a couple drops of eucalyptus oil onto your fingers, and rub it into those same areas. Finally, place the hot washcloth over your face again, and rest for 15 minutes.

Kitchen Counter Cures

Nose clogged up so you can't sleep? There's no need to go to your local drugstore. Keep your pajamas on, and head to the kitchen instead. It's probably well stocked with such natural decongestants as garlic, onions, chilies, and horseradish.

In the mood for a midnight snack? Try a lean roast beef sandwich with a dollop of horseradish. Stuff a pocket pita with lettuce, tomato, and a heap of chopped onions and chili peppers. Or heat up a can of tomato or minestrone soup, tossing in a few diced cloves of garlic and a generous sprinkle of chopped chili. Now that's some tasty medicine!

here are some ways to prevent its return:

Employ an old salt. Use a saline nasal spray several times a day to remove mucus, which could harbor bacteria. If you can find one that contains eucalyptus, so much the better! Eucalyptus kills bacteria.

Turn up the heat. When your sinuses are acting up, place a damp hot towel over the top half of your face, and let the heat penetrate into your nasal cavities. Leave it there for 15 minutes, and repeat three or four times a day to promote drainage and increase blood flow to the area.

Create a jungle in there. Inhaled steam is one of the best ways to clear clogged sinuses. Make a tent over your head with a towel, and sit over a pot of boiled water. Breathe in the steam, being careful not to scald yourself. Add a few eucalyptus leaves to boost the penetrating power.

Keep your nose out of it. When it's cold outside, always wrap a wide scarf around your neck and lower face to cover your nose. This will protect your mucous membranes from drying out and also prevent a painful rush of cold air from reaching your tender sinuses.

Use hydropower. Drink at least eight glasses of water and other fluids a day to thin out your nasal mucus.

Lay off the cow. Stop drinking milk and eating milk products, such as cheese or yogurt, while your sinuses are inflamed. Milk creates mucus, and you already have enough of that clogging up your sinuses.

Call for an air raid. Keep your environment as dust free as possible with an air filtering system. If you can, keep your home and car air-conditioned to help filter out the pollens and allergens in the outside air. Your sinuses will thank you for it.

Pretend you're a Navy SEAL. Use nose plugs in the pool. Chlorine in swimming pools can be irritating to your nasal membranes, so don't go in the water without nose plugs.

Treat allergies. If your sinusitis is usually a by-product of allergies, dry up the drip with antihistamines before it can clog you up.

FABULOUS FOLK REMEDY

Fried Salt

Here's a remedy from my Russian neighbors: Heat some salt in a frying pan; then spread it on a towel or clean cloth. Fold up the cloth, and put it over the bridge of your nose. The heat will open your sinuses.

POWERFUL POTION

WASABI: INSTANT SINUS DRANO

Dab some wasabi on your sushi or sashimi. This powerful Japanese horseradish, which could blow the lid off a manhole, will empty your sinuses. It's available at Asian restaurants and groceries, as well as some natural-foods stores.

Sneaker Feet:

Shoe-ing Away Funky Foot Breath

Does your dog faint when you pull off your sneakers? Do the neighbors call the town hall, asking about the release of noxious gasses? Do shoe salespeople gladly sacrifice their commissions to avoid waiting on you? If the answer to any of these questions is yes, then you've got funky feet!

Some people simply have more potent body chemistry than others do. When they coop up their sweaty little tootsies, they can create a great big stink. If this sounds like you, here's what to do:

Free your feet. Peel off your pantyhose as soon as you get home from work, and bathe your feet. Walk barefoot every chance you get.

Stamp out the damp. Foot funk is often caused by bacteria that thrive in

---

FABULOUS FOLK REMEDY

Sole Tea

Move over, *Chicken Soup for the Soul*—here's a tea for the *sole:* Brew a cup of any black tea, which contains tannic acid, renowned for keeping overactive sweat glands in check. Swab it on the bottoms of your feet, let it dry, then slip into a pair of socks. Just don't walk on a white rug!

damp places. So set your hair dryer on low, and dry your feet thoroughly after bathing. Odds are, your conair will do a better job getting moisture from between your toes than your towel.

Dust well. Make your own dusting powder to help keep odors at bay and your feet feeling fresh all day. Combine 2 parts powdered calendula (*Calendula officinalis*) flowers with 1 part *each* powdered slippery elm (*Ulmus fulva*), lavender (*Lavendula officinalis*) flowers, and aluminum-free baking soda. Sprinkle on your feet before slipping them into your socks and shoes.

Right Guard your tootsies. While you're rolling your underarms, spray or rub some deodorant on the bottoms of your feet as well.

Play the sock market. What will they think of next? Reebok now makes an antimicrobial performance sock (about $10 a pair) that has received rave reviews from all my sporting friends. Soft and comfy, they also do a great deodorizing job. Look for them at your local sporting-goods store. Plain white cotton socks may be a lot cheaper, but they won't kill the smell as well as the antimicrobials.

Be a sport. The team doctor for the Nebraska Cornhuskers, Rodney Basler, M.D., recommends routinely wearing athletic socks that wick moisture away from your skin. As an added plus, these socks will also help keep your feet blister free.

POWERFUL POTION

CHLOROPHYLL CLEANSING TONIC

Chlorophyll is a potent odor eliminator. First thing each morning, drink a glass of water with the juice from 1 lemon and 1 teaspoon of chlorophyll stirred into it. This will help cleanse your system from the inside out.

Sore Throat:

Put Out the Fire

It hurts so much to swallow, you'd think your tonsils were made by Gillette. And as if that weren't enough, your morning orange juice stings like hydrochloric acid, and your voice sounds like a bullfrog singing in a swamp.

Lots of things can leave your throat sore—allergies, infections, a physical injury, too much smoking or talking. Whatever the cause, however, you can count on there being inflammation, pain, and an itchy or a scratchy feeling.

If your sore throat is accompanied by white spots in your mouth and throat or by difficulty swallowing, see your doctor immediately.

FABULOUS FOLK REMEDY

Violet Flower Tea

Violets (*Viola odorata*) are not only beautiful, they're medicinal, too, helping ease the pain of a sore throat caused by a cough. Simply steep 1 heaping teaspoon of violet flowers in 1 cup of hot water for 10 minutes. Sip slowly, 2 to 3 cups per day.

Tonsillitis Got You Down?

Used to be, tonsillitis was strictly a kid's disease. Your grade-school-age tonsils would get infected, the doctor would yank them out, and that would be that. As a result, few adults even had tonsils until recently.

But then, in the 1970s, doctors discovered that tonsils were our first line of defense against bacterial infections, so they started leaving them in. Fortunately, our immune systems tend to get stronger as we get older, so our tonsils are less likely to take the brunt of an infection. But some adults still get tonsillitis. Here's how to tell if you're one of them:

Your tonsils are located in the back of your throat. If they're infected, they're usually dark red and swollen. They may even be dotted with white specks and accompanied by an extremely sore throat, difficulty swallowing, fever, and swollen glands. If you suspect you have tonsillitis, see your doctor for some heavy-duty antibiotics right away. If the infection gets past your tonsils, it can spread to your heart and result in a life-threatening condition.

You may have a strep infection, which can lead to serious complications if not treated appropriately. If you don't have any accompanying symptoms, however, here are some things you can try at home to find relief:

Pucker up. No cough drops or candy handy? Soak half a lemon in salt water, and suck on it for a while. This treatment moistens your throat and relieves soreness.

G-g-gargle. Gargling with salty water helps dissolve mucus, cleanse your throat, and add some astringency to your body chemistry to reduce swelling and inflammation. It also helps minimize postnasal drip. Here's what you do: Put 1 teaspoon of salt in 8 ounces of hot water, and gargle four or five times a day. Don't be heavy-handed with the salt. The gargle should taste a little salty, but not overwhelmingly so. Too much salt will irritate your throat.

Minimize the pain. Pop aspirin or another nonsteroidal anti-inflammatory drug (NSAID) to dull the pain. Take as directed, until your throat feels better.

Get plenty of fluids. Drink lots of water and other fluids to keep yourself hydrated and your throat moist. Also, sip warm liquids, such as salty soups, to help fight the inflammation.

Suck lozenges. Use throat lozenges or hard candies to keep your throat moist. Look for cherry lozenges with benzocaine to numb your throat temporarily and help with swallowing. Slippery elm lozenges are popular, too.

Don't say a word. The less work your throat muscles and membranes have to do, the better

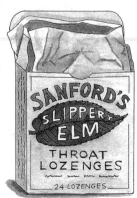

you will feel. Save the speeches until your throat has healed. Better skip the choir rehearsals, too.

Wrap up your throat. Soak a clean washcloth in warm water, wring it out, and place it around your neck. The warmth will help relieve any soreness.

Wear a carrot. Some naturopaths suggest wrapping your throat in a carrot poultice. Grate a large carrot, and spread it on a clean cloth. Wrap this around your throat, covering it with a scarf to keep it in place. You also have the choice of placing either an ice pack or a hot compress over the poultice to make it even more effective.

Steep something soothing. To relieve sore throat pain, stimulate your immune system to do what it does best. Combine equal parts of sage (*Salvia officinalis*), echinacea (*Echinacea* spp.), agrimony (*Agrimonia eupatoria*), and cleavers (*Galium aparine*). Steep 1 heaping teaspoon in 1 cup of hot water for 10 minutes. Sip the hot tea slowly, boosting your immune system with 3 to 4 cups per day.

IT'S AN EMERGENCY!

If a sore throat is accompanied by difficulty swallowing, you may be having a life-threatening allergic reaction. Call your community's emergency response team immediately.

Splinter Removal:

A Thorny Issue

Yikes! Isn't it amazing how much a teeny-weeny, hardly-nothin', sliver-of-somethin' can *hurt*? Yow. Ouch. And maybe even *$#@!! Here's how to get rid of the little trouble maker:

Tweeze it out. Sterilize a needle or metal tweezers by holding it over an open flame; then have at it. If the splinter is sticking out of the skin, tug it out gently, making sure to pull it out in the same direction that it went in.

Loosen your flesh. Yep, that's what I said. If the splinter's under the skin but not

---

FABULOUS FOLK REMEDY

Potato Poultice

Strange as it may sound, you can coax a stubborn splinter out with a potato. Use a potato poultice or, in the case of a finger or toe, simply carve or hollow out the potato for a custom fit. Leave the spud on overnight, and you'll be able to pluck the splinter out easily the next day.

deeply embedded, you can ease the splinter out by first loosening the skin around it with a sterile needle. Then use the needle to try to ease the splinter out.

Let it bleed. Squeeze the wound around the splinter so blood will wash out the germs.

Rinse with herbs. Wash a deep splinter wound with the following herbal infusion: Combine equal parts of calendula (*Calendula officinalis*), echinacea (*Echinacea* spp.), and comfrey (*Symphytum officinalis*). Steep 1 heaping tablespoon of the mixture in 1 pint of hot water for 20 minutes. Strain out the herbs; then wash the wound in the infusion.

Prevent complications. When the wound is dry, dust with goldenseal (*Hydrastis canadensis*) powder to prevent complications.

Be alert. If the splinter breaks off inside the skin or is very deeply lodged, or if the wound becomes infected, seek medical help immediately. You may need a tetanus shot.

POWERFUL POTION

SPLINTER REMOVER

The powerful salicylic acids in wart removers can also help you get rid of a splinter. The superficial layers of skin break down and become soft from contact with the acid. Use wart remover disks because they have a higher salicylic acid content than the liquid removers do.

O·D·D·B·A·L·L OINTMENT

Marshmallow Magic

Marshmallow ointment can coax a stubborn splinter to the surface of your skin. Dab some ointment on the site, bandage it, and leave it alone for a few hours. When you remove the bandage, the splinter will have inched close enough to the surface for you to easily pluck it out with a pair of sterilized tweezers.

Sports Injuries:

Work Up to Working Out

Denial. It's often the sign of a sports injury about to happen. It might start with a quick game of hoops with your kid. *"Sure, I'm in shape! One game won't kill me!"* Or one of those midnight moments when you watch one too many skinny people in Spandex promise you a perfect body in a week or so—as long as you sign up for their aerobics class. So you whip out your credit card and get ready to buy now and pay later.

Unfortunately, you're *really* likely to pay later if you're a Baby Boomer. So many of us are injuring ourselves while trying to get back in shape or after joining a weekend tennis match that *boomeritis* has

---

FABULOUS FOLK REMEDY

Ye Olde Epsom Salts

Epsom salts baths relieve the pain of almost any sports injury. Add 1 to 2 pounds to a tub of warm water, and soak those aches and pains away.

become an emergency-room byword. Trouble is, most of us weekend warriors don't bother to warm up and work our way into an athletic activity gradually. We jump in—and get injured. In fact, the number of sports injuries in our age group jumped 42 percent in the last decade.

Fortunately, most of the injuries are preventable, says Robert Stanton, M.D., an orthopedic surgeon at the Yale University School of Medicine in New Haven, Connecticut. Here's how:

Warm up. Muscle tissue becomes less flexible as we age, says Dr. Stanton. Warm up by walking for a few minutes; then slowly begin stretching your back and legs. These few minutes of mild exercise will give your muscles a chance to get ready for more intense movement.

Work up to it gradually. Try not to cram all your action into the 2 days of the weekend, chides Dr. Stanton. Increase your activity in increments of no more than 10 percent a week.

Perfect your technique. Some sports injuries happen because you're not making the right moves. Tennis elbow, for example, can develop when you're not using the racquet properly. If you're intent on playing a game you don't know,

POWERFUL POTION

A NATURAL SPORTS DRINK

Make your own sports drink by mixing equal parts of dandelion leaf (*Taraxacum officinale*), nettles (*Urtica dioica*), gingerroot (*Zingiber officinale*), peppermint (*Mentha piperita*), and oatstraw (*Avena sativa*). Steep 1 heaping teaspoon in 1 cup of hot water for 15 minutes. Strain, and pour into a 1-liter jug along with the juice of 1 lemon and 1 tablespoon of pure maple syrup. Fill to the top with water. **Caution:** If you take potassium supplements, talk to your doctor before using dandelion leaf. And remember to wear gloves when handling fresh nettles to avoid their stinging hairs.

Tingling Tootsie Tonic

Numbness, tingling, and burning on top of the foot during exercise may signal the development of a Morton's neuroma—a little tumor along the nerve extending over the ball of the foot that makes wearing lace-up footwear particularly uncomfortable. Use alternating hot and cold foot baths to reduce the inflammation, and apply St. John's wort (*Hypericum perforatum*) oil two or three times a day.

get some coaching—even if it's only from a video or a book.

Wear the right stuff. Even a quick foray into a sporting goods store to buy shoes can be an overwhelming experience. Do you need basketball shoes, running shoes, soccer shoes, or cross-trainers? They all look pretty much the same, yet each meets a different need. So when you plan to devote time to a sport, find out what shoes are best. Ask other players, the coaches, and the sporting goods stores. The proper footwear will protect you from falls and injuries to your Achilles tendon and your legs and feet in general.

Wear a helmet. Here's a scary fact: Did you know that adults are *twice* as likely as kids to die from a head injury? If you ride a bike, swing a bat, or in-line skate through town, always wear the headgear, advises Dr. Stanton.

Pad yourself. Wear shin guards, knee guards, wrist guards, or other padding to keep you safe for your sport.

Don't be a martyr. How often do we root for the hero as he or she limps back into the game to score that final winning point and then watch as that athlete collapses in a heap? If winning the game puts you on the sidelines for weeks, your body, your psyche and, yes, your team will be the losers. I can't say this enough: If you're hurt, stop playing!

Sprains and Strains:

Fast Relief with RICE

O kay. Here's a test. What's the difference between a sprain and a strain? Answer: A sprain is an injury to the ligaments that support your joints, and a strain is a pulled or overexerted muscle.

A sprain usually occurs from overextending or twisting your arm or leg beyond its normal range of movement and tearing or seriously stretching a ligament. You end up with pain when you move the limb, as well as swelling and pain in the involved joint. It feels tender to the touch, and you'll probably get black and blue. And exactly like a strain, it hurts like the dickens.

If you are uncertain if an injury is a sprain or a break, always treat it

---

FABULOUS FOLK REMEDY

A Comfy Comfrey Wrap

Comfrey (*Symphytum officinale*) wraps work wonders for speeding recovery. Blanche two to four leaves, and place over the sprain. These can be worn all day underneath an elastic bandage.

POWERFUL POTION

A WITCH'S BREW

Witch hazel can help shrink the swelling from a sprain or strain. Brew a tea (minus any spooky spells) by tossing 1 teaspoonful of dried leaves or 2 inches of root into 1 cup of boiling water. Let it steep for 10 to 15 minutes. Drink 2 to 3 cups per day.

like a break until you get medical help, advises the American Medical Association. Then, when you know it's a sprain or a strain, here's what you do:

Remember RICE. The most important thing to do when you strain or sprain yourself is easy to remember RICE. *R*est it. *I*ce it. *C*ompress it. *E*levate it. In other words, stop the activity, and rest the injured body part. Apply ice wrapped in a towel or a cold compress to decrease swelling. Wrap the injured limb in an elastic bandage or a splint or sling. And then keep the injured part elevated above the level of the heart. Don't use heat until at least 24 hours after the injury, when the swelling is gone. And by all means, seek medical attention if the pain or swelling is severe.

Use an herbal ice pack. For a cooling, heating, and healing experience all wrapped into one, add essential oils to your cold pack. First, fill a bowl with ice-cold water. Sprinkle several drops of essential oil into the water—try camphor, eucalyptus, chamomile, or rosemary. Next, soak a clean washcloth in the bowl, and wring it out well. Lay the washcloth over the sprained area, and cover with an ice pack. Limit the ice phase to 10 to 20 minutes to avoid frostbite!

Banish pain. Bromelain and turmeric are powerful partners when it comes to reducing inflammation and pain. Take 250 to 500 milligrams of *each* between meals, three times daily. **Caution:** People with sensitivities to pineapple should avoid bromelain.

Stress:

Tear It Down!

There goes my neighbor Ann, streaking down the street in her SUV. She's late for work (as usual) because her daughter couldn't find her shoes (as usual). And she'll be in trouble (as usual) with her supervisor. My neighbor really is a good person, but she's totally stressed out. And no wonder: Her to-do list would choke a giraffe.

Ann is hardly alone on the best-stressed list, according to a recent survey by the Gallup and Harris organizations. In fact, 25 percent of those participating in the survey said the stress in their lives was bad enough to put them on the verge of losing their temper—if not actually going postal!

While a little stress can

5 Minutes to Heaven!

Prayer is an invaluable tool for stressful times. Don't wait until your world falls apart before you make it a regular part of your day. Instead, begin now. Spend 20 minutes each morning and night centering yourself and reconnecting with your Maker.

improve productivity, the hormones generated by extreme or chronic stress can damage physical and emotional health. "It's difficult to think of any disorder in which stress could not play an aggravating role," muses Paul J. Rosch, president of the American Institute of Stress.

In fact, studies show that your risk of a heart attack is tripled within 2 hours of an extremely stressful incident or major meltdown. What's more, the flood of stress hormones can actually warp your brain!

Yikes! Here's how to keep stress at bay:

Have a girls' night out. If you're a woman, head to the park with your best pals or join the local women's bowling league. Women "tend and befriend," revealed a study by University of California at Los Angeles researchers. In many species of mammals, females respond to stress by seeking social contact with others, especially other females, or by nurturing their young. Both seem to be big-time stress reducers.

Ask yourself four questions. The Internal Revenue Service just told you that they want to audit your taxes for the last 5 years. Now that's stressful! Redford B. Williams, M.D., director of be-

POWERFUL POTION

TENSION-TAMER TEA

Choose one of the following herbs to make your own tension-tamer tea: lemon balm (*Melissa officinalis*), chamomile (*Matricaria recutita*), passionflower (*Passiflora incarnata*), vervain (*Verbena hastata*), betony (*Stachys betonica*), or skullcap (*Scutellaria lateriflora*). Try them each for 1 week at a time until you find your favorite. Then every time you feel stressed, steep 1 teaspoon of your favorite herb in 1 cup of hot water, covered, for 10 minutes. Strain, and drink 1 to 3 cups a day.

The 5-Second Stress Reliever

Lots of people clench their teeth when they're uptight. Here's an easy exercise to relax your jaw, face, and neck, courtesy of Elaine Petrone, a fitness and stress expert. Take a deep breath, and drop your jaw right now. Next, open your mouth and exhale with a long *haaaaaaa* sound. Finally, gently close your lips. Repeat this exercise throughout the day. You'll soon become aware of how often your jaw clenches—and how that tightness moves tension down into your neck and shoulders.

havioral research at Duke University, suggests asking yourself these questions whenever you're in a tough spot:

✔ Is this really important to me?
✔ Would a reasonable person be this upset?
✔ Is there anything I can do to fix the situation?
✔ Would fixing it be worth the cost?

If you answered yes to all questions, then take action, says Dr. Williams. But if you answered no one or more times, then just ride out the stressful situation.

Switch gears. If you are strumming your fingers on your desk as you pore over a report that is already late and not as good as you'd like it to be, get up and walk away from it. Just take a break, and shift to something mindless—even if you're on deadline. You'll come back less stressed and better able to concentrate.

Get rubbed the right way. Get a professional massage whenever you can, even once a month, if you can afford it. According to researchers at the University of Miami, massage can cut cortisol levels, ease blood presure, and boost immunity. To find a licensed therapist near you, contact the American Massage Therapy Association (www.amtamassage.org).

Move that bod! Studies have consistently found that even a single exercise session can make you feel less stressed. A simple morning walk at a brisk pace enhances the flow of brain chemicals that block the effects of stress. In a pinch, even a dash up and down some stairs will help.

Eat Chocolate!

Get out the Godiva, girlfriend! The good news is that research has shown that chocolate—yes, chocolate!—helps release endorphins, those brainy chemicals that control your mood. According to a report published in the *Journal of the American Dietetic Association*, some people may crave chocolate to compensate for a magnesium deficiency. It turns out that stress stimulates the body to excrete magnesium, which, in turn, causes a depletion of endorphins.

Symptoms of Stress Overload

✔ Rapid breathing
✔ High blood pressure
✔ Tingling in the hands and feet
✔ Headache
✔ Digestive problems
✔ Vulnerable to colds and other illness
✔ Unable to concentrate or make decisions
✔ Feeling sad or irritable with no good reason

✔ Sleep problems
✔ Prolonged anxiety
✔ Change in appetite
✔ Unable to cope with even minor setbacks
✔ Unable to enjoy things that are usually enjoyable
✔ No interest in sex
✔ Accident prone

Stroke:

Reduce Your Risk

Of course, it's scary. The prospect of a stroke—either your own or one befalling someone you love—is immensely frightening. But here's something important to keep in mind as you face down those fears: There are only *half* as many strokes today as there were 30 years ago. Why? Because scientists have finally learned how to prevent this devastating problem.

DIFFERENT STROKES FOR DIFFERENT FOLKS

There are two kinds of stroke. The most common is ischemic stroke. It occurs when blood cannot get to the brain, usually because a clot or fatty deposit is blocking a blood vessel. An ischemic stroke is frequently heralded by a mini-stroke—what doctors call a transient ischemic attack (TIA)—in which blood flow to the brain is blocked for only a few moments before it's resumed. Risk factors for this type of stroke are smoking, high blood pressure, high cholesterol levels, and a family history of stroke. The less common kind of stroke is called a "hemorrhagic stroke," and it's directly tied to high blood pressure. It occurs when a blood vessel bursts in the brain.

REWIRING THE BRAIN

Fortunately, people who suffer a stroke these days are frequently able to recover, but it's typically a long road back. That's why the best way to deal with a stroke is to prevent it in the first place. Here's how:

Calling all couch potatoes. Get up! Get moving! I'm sure you already know this, but the more you move your body, the stronger your cardiovascular system gets. This helps you prevent stroke. Being sedentary only adds to your risk. Begin by getting your doctor to give you a clean bill of health. Then take off by going for a brisk walk every day. It doesn't have to be far—just to the corner and back. Gradually increase your distance and time until you're exercising—walking, running, biking, swimming, even dancing—for 15 to 20 minutes a day.

Eat your cruciferae. Learn to love broccoli, Brussels sprouts, and other cruciferous vegetables. Researchers at Harvard analyzed the diets of more than 100,000 people for as long as 14 years and found that participants' risk of stroke was lower the more fruits and veggies

POWERFUL POTION

STROKE-PREVENTING TEA

A number of studies associate black tea—that's the regular kind you find in the supermarket—with reduced risk of heart disease and stroke. More than 800 elderly Dutch men who drank 4 or more cups of black tea a day had a 69 percent lower risk of stroke than those who consumed less than 2.6 cups of black tea a day, according to a report in the *Archives of Internal Medicine*. Scientists believe black tea works because the antioxidants in it maintain the health of the circulatory system and reduce the risk of blood clots. Perhaps it's time to have a spot of tea!

they ate. In fact, these cruciferous foods may be as effective as controlling blood pressure and engaging in physical activity for preventing stroke, says Ralph Sacco, M.D., a stroke researcher at Columbia University in New York City and a spokesperson for the American Heart Association.

Bone up on the B's. Homocysteine, an amino acid your body makes as it digests protein, has been linked to stroke and heart attacks for a long time. But new evidence is coming to light. A 2001 meeting of the American Stroke Association revealed that homocysteine is involved in actually causing a stroke, not just making you more vulnerable to one. One way to lower homocysteine is to increase your intake of foods high in the B vitamins, specifically folic acid, B_6, and B_{12}. A major study—Vitamin Intervention for Stroke Prevention (VISP)—is now under way to find out if these vitamins ward off new strokes in people who have already had them. In the meantime, however, it can't hurt to get some more of those big B's— whether you've already had a stroke or not. Eat lots of whole grains, poultry, legumes, and fresh fruits and vegetables.

Be a melon head. Add some cantaloupe to your diet. It's a

O·D·D·B·A·L·L OINTMENT

Lovely Liniment

A warming herbal liniment may help increase circulation to paralyzed muscles. Mix 2 ounces of powdered rosemary (*Rosemarinus officinalis*) leaves, 1 ounce of powdered lavender (*Lavendula officinalis*) flowers, and ½ ounce of cayenne pepper (*Capsicum minimum*) in 1 quart of rubbing alcohol. Let stand for 7 days, shaking well each day. Decant, and store in a clean bottle. Use once or twice daily.

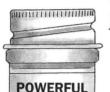

great source of potassium, and, according to the U.S. Food and Drug Administration, diets rich in potassium and low in sodium may reduce the risk of high blood pressure and stroke. Other good potassium sources are bananas, prune juice, dried peaches, plain, low-fat yogurt, Swiss chard, dried apricots, orange juice, cooked squash, spinach, and tomato juice.

Keep your spuds covered. A potato baked in its skin packs 903 milligrams of stroke-lowering potassium—tons more than any other food. But take away the skin, and you'll get only 641 milligrams. So buy organic potatoes, scrub them well, bake them in their jackets, and eat every bite.

Fish for more omega-3s. You may want to take up fishing—or at least get friendly with your local fishmonger. The results of the 14-year-long Nurses Health Study, published in the *Journal of the American Medical Association*, revealed that women who ate fish two to four times a week reduced their stroke risk by a whopping 27 percent. Fish that are rich in omega-3 fatty acids include salmon, tuna, mackerel, halibut, cod, and flounder.

POWERFUL POTION

CHINESE MUSHROOM MAGIC

Chinese tree-ear mushrooms may help prevent stroke. One study showed that a single tablespoon of the soaked mushroom, taken three to four times a week, may be as effective as a daily aspirin in preventing strokes and heart attacks. And the mushroom won't irritate your stomach like an aspirin. These dried mushrooms aren't available at every supermarket, but you can find them at gourmet and Asian markets. Rehydrate them in some boiling water, and use the water to add a taste of the exotic East to soups, stews, and casseroles.

Be wise about alcohol. A drink a day may keep stroke at bay. In fact, 1999 report published in the *New England Journal of Medicine* revealed that light to moderate alcohol consumption reduced the risk of stroke for both men and women. A second study, published in the *Journal of the American Medical Association*, found that up to two drinks a day helps prevent stroke. Too much alcohol, however, can actually *increase* your risk for stroke, so ask your doctor to help you decide how much is right for you. And if alcoholism runs in your family, don't add even a drop of alcohol to your diet.

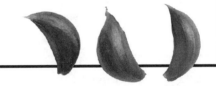

Control high blood pressure. If you're not keeping your blood pressure under control, start now. It's crucial for preventing a hemorrhagic stroke. Work with your doctor to monitor your blood pressure, take any medication regularly, and make all the lifestyle changes necessary to keep your blood pressure off the ceiling. See **High Blood Pressure** for more tips.

Don't let diabetes go too far. Diabetes is another condition that can cause a stroke if it's not controlled. Make sure you understand how to keep your blood-sugar level down. Follow your doctor's advice, and stick to your eating plan. See **Diabetes** for lots of help.

Kick the killer habit. Smoking constricts your blood vessels and only adds to your problems, especially if you already have high blood pressure. Join a support group, get medication from your doctor, use the

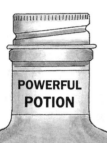

POWERFUL POTION

GINKGO TEA

Ginkgo (*Ginkgo biloba*) can reduce platelet stickiness and increase the microcirculation of the brain—both of which can help you avoid a stroke. Steep 1 teaspoon of ginkgo in 1 cup of hot water for 10 minutes. Strain, and sip. Drink 1 cup a day to help prevent stroke. **Caution:** If you're on blood-thinning medications or aspirin therapy, don't take ginkgo.

IT'S AN EMERGENCY!

If you suddenly experience weakness or numbness in your face, arm, or leg on one side of your body—all hallmarks of a stroke—head to an emergency room right away. Also, get help if you have difficulty speaking or understanding others, dimness or impaired vision in one eye, an unexplained dizzy spell, or a severe headache with no apparent cause. Even if the symptoms pass, get immediate help, because you may have had a mini-stroke, which is a sign that another such incident could occur.

patch—try everything you can to quit. Most experts say the best approach is a combination of behavioral techniques and medication.

Control your weight. The more you weigh, the more work your heart and circulatory system must perform—and the greater your risk of suffering a stroke.

Sunburn:

Preventing the Peel

When I was young and foolish, I used to play hooky from work on a perfect summer day. I'd don my purple bikini, lie on the beach, and burn. I'd sun myself systematically: 15 minutes on each side, and back again, as if I were browning a pot roast.

Today, we know how dangerous tanning is, and those burning days may yet come back to haunt me. So for some years I've been fanatical about using the proper sunscreen, wearing a wide-brimmed hat and donning wrap-around shades. (And the bikini is long gone!)

I hope you're careful, too. But just in case you do get a burn, here's what to do:

Cool it down. Fill your tub with cool to lukewarm

FABULOUS FOLK REMEDY

A Cooling Lavender Spray

Lavender is an antiseptic, cooling herb that can relieve burning and protect against secondary infections. Fill an 8-ounce spray bottle with cold water, and add 6 drops of essential oil of lavender. Shake well, and spray on the sunburned area.

O·D·D·B·A·L·L
OINTMENT

The Morning-after Sunburn Remedy

An enzyme called photolyase, which is made from ocean algae, is said to be the magic elixir for a painful sunburn, reversing some of the critical DNA damage caused by soaking up too much ultraviolet light. In fact, studies have shown that photolyase reduced redness and DNA effects by as much as 45 percent. It's scheduled to become an ingredient in some sun remedies and is headed for the market soon. Check labels to find it.

water. Add some baking soda or oatmeal, and soak long enough for your skin to feel soothed. Or place cold, damp cloths on your skin (but don't rub!). If your sunburn is severe, submerge your burned skin under cold water instead of lukewarm water, and stay under until it stops hurting, says the American Medical Association (AMA).

Chug. Drink plenty of water to help heal your overheated skin. Avoid drinking alcohol or caffeinated drinks, because they are diuretics that will steal much-needed moisture from your skin.

Try some mallow aloe. Ointments made with the fresh gel of aloe or a paste from the Indian herb country mallow are Ayurvedic remedies for sunburn. Rub one of these on your sunburned skin—but only if your skin is unbroken and there is no chance of infection. Another remedy involves the paste or oil of sandalwood. Just put some on your forehead, and—it's reported—it will cool your entire body.

Be cool as a cucumber. Soothe the burn by placing chilled

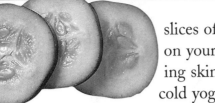

slices of cucumber on your simmering skin. A dab of cold yogurt or a splash of vinegar will do the job, too.

Munch on antioxidants. To help your skin heal itself and to protect yourself from the free-radical damage that can cause skin cancer, include five to six servings of antioxidant-rich foods in your daily diet. Berries of all types are tops, followed by citrus, mango, papaya, dark leafy greens, broccoli, Brussels sprouts, nuts and seeds, whole grains, and legumes.

Ease the itch. Scratching, which will only make your skin hurt more and encourage infection, is out of the question. So try cold compresses to ease any itching as your skin heals. Calamine lotion works, too, says the AMA.

Deal with the peel. When your skin peels or the blisters break, gently remove dried fragments, and apply an antiseptic ointment or hydrocortisone cream to the skin below, advises the AMA.

O·D·D·B·A·L·L OINTMENT

Super Sunburn Soother

For mild sunburns, mix your own soothing oil by adding the contents of six capsules *each* of vitamin A and vitamin E to ¼ cup of flaxseed oil. Apply frequently to the sunburned areas. You may also add this combination to ¼ cup of aloe vera juice, and smooth it over your skin.

IT'S AN EMERGENCY!

Call your doctor if you experience chills, fever, nausea, swelling, or blisters along with a sunburn. You could have second-degree burns or sunstroke, both of which require medical care. And never use any ointments, antiseptics, sprays, or home remedies on a severe burn.

Tick Removal:

Out Damn Spot!

My family had a big shaggy sheepdog when we kids were small. At the time, we lived in a wooded area that was full of ticks, and our nightly summer ritual included a body search of kids and dog for ticks. Unfortunately, the dog had so much hair that we often didn't find the ticks until they had sucked enough blood to become as big as black cherries. Then, of course, they dropped off and grossed us out.

Today, getting grossed out is the least of the problems ticks can cause. Lyme disease, on the rise

---

FABULOUS FOLK REMEDY

Clever Clover

Red clover (*Trifolium pratense*) is a traditional blood purifier that has an affinity for the skin and helps support the overall constitution of the body. Make a cup of red clover tea by pouring 1 quart of boiling water over ½ cup of fresh flower heads. Steep for 10 minutes, strain, and then sip throughout the day.

How to Remove a Tick

If a tick has attached itself to you, grasp it firmly with fine-point tweezers, and pull straight up—not at an angle—or the head might break off and stay imbedded, warns Joseph Piesman, D.Sc., chief of the Centers for Disease Control and Prevention's Lyme disease section. The tick will still be alive, so seal it in a vial or wrap it in tape before disposing of it. If you think you have contracted a disease from a bite, see a doctor immediately. (And take the tick with you, if you still have it.)

since the 1960s, when suburbs began expanding into deer territory, is now the leading pest-borne illness, and deer ticks can be found anywhere in the country, according to the Centers for Disease Control and Prevention (CDC). A tiny deer tick, the size of the period at the end of this sentence, causes flu-like symptoms and joint pain. Caught early, Lyme disease can be treated with antibiotics. When it's left untreated, however, it can cause severe illness.

Rocky Mountain spotted fever is carried by a half dozen varieties of ticks. It causes a measles-like rash that spreads from the arms and legs to the palms and soles of the feet. It hits children hardest and must be treated quickly with antibiotics.

TAKING TICKS TO TASK

Unless you want to spend the summer months hiding in the living room, it's wise to learn how to protect yourself from diseases caused by ticks.

Cover up in the countryside. Ticks will cling to your legs if you walk through the grass, and they'll drop from the leaves of overhead trees. If

O·D·D·B·A·L·L
OINTMENT

Pennyroyal Oil

Pennyroyal is an herb that has been used since Roman times to keep fleas away. The good news is that ticks find it obnoxious, too, because pennyroyal contains pulegone, a heavy-duty, insect repellent. To use pennyroyal, just pick a bunch of leaves, and rub them on your skin and clothing. Or, you can pick up a bottle of pennyroyal essential oil at the health-food store. Rub a few drops on the tops of your shoes and on your socks. Just don't rub the oil directly on your skin, because it can irritate it.

you're walking in the woods or grasslands, tuck your pant legs inside your socks or boots to keep the ticks off your legs. Be sure to look for tiny hitchhikers on the outsides of your socks when you get home. And wear a hat and a long-sleeved shirt when you're in tick territory.

Use the dress whites. Ticks are just tiny black spots, so you'll have a hard time finding them on dark clothing. Instead, wear white and light colors, so they'll be easier to find.

Make yourself repellent. Before you go into tick-infested areas, spray your clothes with an insect repellent that contains DEET. Read the labels to make sure the bug spray you select targets ticks.

Use the middle of the road. When you're on hiking trails in the woods, stay in the center of the trail. That way, you'll avoid brushing against trees and shrubs and be less likely to attract ticks.

Listen to that *tick tock tick*. While you are in tick country, keep track of time so that you can check yourself every hour or so to see if any ticks have begun homesteading on your body. Do a full-body search at night, and remove ticks right away.

Tooth Loss:

Save That Smile

We know you don't tear off the tops of beer cans with your teeth. But that won't save you from a broken tooth—not if you use your teeth to crack hard nuts, open the lids of pill bottles, loosen knots, or gnaw on candy bars straight from the freezer, as many people do.

The top tooth breaker? Ice cubes, says Richard Price, D.M.D., a dentist at the Boston University School of Dental Medicine and an adviser for the American Dental Association.

Aside from getting the occasional tooth snapped off in the throes of a ferocious ice hockey game, however, most of us lose

---

FABULOUS FOLK REMEDY

Homemade Licorice Toothbrush

Make your own cleansing herbal toothbrush. Peel a length of licorice root (*Glycyrrhiza glabra*), and chomp on it. Fray the ends for an instant mouth freshener. **Caution:** Licorice root should not be used by people with high blood pressure or kidney disease.

Tooth Repair Paste

To try to save a tooth that's suffering from gum disease, pack it with a mixture of powdered myrrh (*Comiphora molmol*) and goldenseal (*Hydrastis canadensis*). Add enough hydrogen peroxide to the powders to make a paste, and apply around the tooth one to three times daily. When pain is an issue, add a pinch of powdered cloves (*Eugenia caryophyllus*). Then check with your dentist.

teeth in more predictable—and preventable—ways: from decay, cavities, and the resulting extractions. It works just like your mom always said it did: When carbohydrate-rich foods like candy and soda remain on your teeth, bacteria grows and solidifies onto the teeth in a substance called plaque. Eventually, it destroys those teeth and your smile along with them—unless you brush up on these teeth-saving basics:

Brush more than once. Don't think brushing once a day will do it for you. Brush twice a day for 2 or 3 minutes each time. Although saliva is a natural cleanser, your body doesn't produce much while you're sleeping. So that's when plaque typically does its dirty work. For this reason, brush in the morning *before* you eat breakfast to remove any plaque that formed during the night. Then brush again before you go to bed. Plaque takes 16 to 24 hours to develop. If you brush twice a day, you won't accumulate enough plaque to do much damage.

Purl One, Floss Two

If you run out of dental floss, dig into your knitting basket. That's right! Use white wool yarn, recommends Richard Price, D.M.D., a dentist at the Boston University School of Medicine. It's thicker than floss, but it will do the job just as well as the commercial stuff and maybe even better!

Get an electric toothbrush with a pulse timer or beeper to help you know you're brushing long enough.

Be gentle. In other words, don't brush your teeth as though you're trying to scrub shellac off the floor. Hard scrubbing damages your teeth and won't remove any more plaque than gentle brushing. A rule of thumb; if your brush bristles are worn down after a month, you're brushing way too hard. Brush gently, but thoroughly.

Buy the right brush. Look for a brush with soft bristles with rounded ends (if the bristles are hard, they can wear away enamel and damage your gums), and replace it every 3 to 4 months, advises the American Dental Association. If the bristles fray, replace it sooner.

Floss the nooks and crannies. There are places your toothbrush cannot reach, and that's why you need to floss. Flossing removes plaque from between teeth and under the gum line. And healthy gums mean healthy teeth!

Make friends with a hygienist. Every dentist's office has a

POWERFUL POTION

GREEN TEA

Green tea contains tooth-loving tannin, which kills decay-causing bacteria and stops them from producing glucans, the sticky substance that helps acid-generating bacteria stick to your teeth. Check your local market for green tea. It's widely available now in tea bags and as loose tea. Drink a cup after every meal. **Caution:** Those who have clotting disorders or who take heart medications should check with their healthcare provider first.

wonderful person who loves teeth so much she (it always seems to be a she) spends her life getting off every little speck of plaque that you—you naughty person!—didn't get with a toothbrush or floss. This person is a hygienist. Get to know her, see her twice a year, and treat her with gratitude and respect. She just may save your teeth!

Beef up on folic acid.
Folic acid helps keep mucous membranes healthy. Be sure to include adequate amounts of this B vitamin by eating two or three servings of folic acid–rich foods everyday. Barley, brown rice, dark leafy greens, legumes, oranges, salmon, lamb, and dates are several excellent sources.

POWERFUL POTION

KISSING JUICE

It's been said that kissing helps prevent cavities because saliva cleans the mouth, and kissing produces saliva. How? Well, when you're actively smooching, your mouth is making up to a *teaspoon* of saliva a minute. (Talk about a wet kiss!) All of which is great unless the person you're puckering up to doesn't takes care of his or her teeth as well as you do. That's because cavity-causing bacteria may be transmitted through saliva, according to a study published in the *Journal of the American Dental Association*.

Vomiting:

Don't Let the Upset Get You Down

My friend Wayne hates to throw up. He forgets how much better most of us feel once we've done it, so when the urge hits, he clutches his stomach, closes his eyes, and moans like a beached whale. When he finally realizes that there's nothing he can do to resist his stomach's determination to heave, he runs to the bathroom; throws up the toilet seat; and alternately vomits, yells, moans, and vomits some more.

Poor Wayne. Since the stomach is one of the body's major nerve centers, it's vulnerable to upheaval—even in other parts of your body. An inner-ear problem that makes your head spin with vertigo, for instance, can also send your stomach a signal that it's time to vomit.

That said, the most common causes of vomiting are viral infections, motion sickness, migraines, morning sickness in pregnancy, food poisoning, food allergies, and side effects from medications such as chemotherapy drugs. Of course, an emotional shock can do it, too. Bad news can send anyone running to the bathroom.

FABULOUS FOLK REMEDY

Call an Angel!

Bitter carminative herbs help halt vomiting by relieving stomach spasms. Angelica (*Angelica archangelica*) is a slightly sweet, slightly bitter carminative herb with a long history of use in liqueurs and in nausea medicines. Make a decoction by simmering 1 tablespoon of stems and root in 2 cups of water for 20 minutes. Add 1 teaspoon of aniseeds for taste or when the nausea is persistent. Strain and take 1 tablespoonful every 30 minutes until your stomach settles, up to 2 cups a day.

But, unless there's a related serious illness or trauma, the most serious side effect of vomiting is dehydration, since you lose lots of fluid when you lose the contents of your stomach. And don't take that lightly: Dehydration can lead to life-threatening complications—and it can happen to children in the wink of an eye.

Persistent vomiting should always be followed up with a doctor visit, as should vomiting without an obvious cause, vomiting that lasts for more than a day and is accompanied by diarrhea or fever, and vomiting that is accompanied by signs of dehydration such as very dry lips and mouth.

Fortunately, most vomiting responds quickly to one of these do-it-yourself tips:

Make it salty, Sweetie! When you've been vomiting, avoid water or fluids without salt or sugar, because they'll usually come back up. Instead, sip clear, sweetened liquids, such as ginger ale. Clear liquids and broth will stay down better than juices and cola-based sodas.

Go for the Gatorade. Keep a few bottles of sports drinks on hand in case you need to restore electrolytes—the sodium, potassium, and other chemicals that keep body fluids in balance—lost via vomiting. If you don't like sports drinks, get an over-the-counter, oral rehydrating solution or mix, such as Kaolectrolyte. These powders are available without prescription. They come in several flavors and quickly dissolve in water. Be sure to follow package directions.

Sit! Stay! Moving about only makes you feel worse. Try to rest quietly in one place until the need to vomit passes. Just sitting in a calm spot, with a small plastic trash can in your lap and some baby wipes at your elbow can absolutely soothe your psyche—and maybe even your belly.

Snuggle up. Holding a toasty water bottle next to your stomach can help ease those heaving queasies. Although the warmth may soothe you, sometimes just holding anything next to your belly—like a teddy bear—can make you feel better.

Postpone prescription meds. Don't waste your pricey prescriptions by taking your usual medications while you are vomiting. You won't be able to keep them down. But if your stomach upset is causing you to miss rather than just temporarily delay doses, ask your doctor for guidance on what to do.

Excuse yourself. From the dinner table, that is. Let your stomach rest from its usual work of digestion. Don't eat anything or even force yourself to be around the smells of food until the vomiting has passed completely. Your belly will let you know when it's safe to eat again.

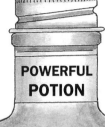

POWERFUL POTION

MINT MAGIC

The volatile oil contained in minty herbs such as peppermint (*Mentha piperita*), lemon balm (*Melissa officinalis*), spearmint (*Mentha spicata*), catnip (*Nepeta cataria*), and calamint (*Calaminta officinalis*) helps relieve spasms and may help allay bouts of vomiting. Make a tea by steeping 1 teaspoon of the dried leaves of any one of these plants in 1 cup of hot water. Strain; then take small sips while it's still warm.

Warts:

Make 'em Disappear

It's just a little bump, right? Hah! Try a pyramid, a skyscraper, Mount Everest! When I was 13 years old, I had a wart on the end of my nose. Such a horror would be unwelcome anytime, of course, but to the poor adolescent psyche . . . well, you can imagine. Daily, I considered cutting off my nose to spite my face. Instead, I'd scratch off the wart. (Now, why I thought a scab was an improvement over a wart, I can't recall.) Unfortunately, it always grew back—until I learned a few of the tricks in this chapter.

There are more than 50 types of warts that can appear anywhere on your body, but warts on the hands and feet are the most common. And, as if one weren't bad enough, they sometimes

---

FABULOUS FOLK REMEDY

Michigan Birch Bark

Folklore from Michigan suggests that you find yourself a nice birch tree, and then cut off a strip of bark. Soak the bark in water until it softens. Next, tape the bark directly to your wart. Nobody knows why it works, but folks point out that birch bark contains salicylates, the basis for some U.S. Food and Drug Administration–approved wart treatments.

Keep Your Hands to Yourself

If you have a wart on a finger of one hand, don't use the same nail clipper or nail file on your unaffected hand, because you can easily spread the warts this way. If you have a wart on your nose, don't powder it with the same puff you use for the rest of your face. In fact, segregate all your personal care tools to keep warts from spreading.

appear in groups! Touching toads or practicing witchcraft doesn't cause them, but making contact with a little virus called the human papilloma virus does. This virus stimulates the rapid growth of cells on the outer layer of your skin.

Fortunately, warts appear less frequently as we age—possibly because we develop immunity to the virus that sprouts them. Everyone's immune system responds differently to this virus, so some people's warts go away faster than other's. If a wart changes color or size, or if it morphs into a new shape or begins to bleed, however, see your doctor. You want to be sure it's not skin cancer. Luckily, most warts usually disappear without any treatment.

HOW TO PART WITH YOUR WART

In the *Adventures of Huckleberry Finn*, Tom and Huck debated about

O·D·D·B·A·L·L OINTMENT

Yellow Cedar Oil

Yellow cedar (*Thuja occidentalis*), also known as thuja, contains a potent oil in its leaves that makes an excellent wart remedy. Fill a small jar with thuja leaves, and cover with oil. Add the contents of a capsule of vitamin E oil. Let sit in a sunny window for 10 days, shaking well each day. Strain, and keep the oil in a cool, dark place. Stored in the refrigerator, the oil will last 4 to 6 months. Apply two to three times daily to the surface of the wart.

The Sole of a Wart

When a wart is on the sole of your foot, it's known as a plantar wart. The pressure of walking on it makes it grow inward. It then presses on nerves in your foot, so it hurts to walk. This type of wart needs to be removed by your doctor.

several ways to get rid of warts—most involving prowling about town at midnight. But the most effective, they agreed, was to take a dead cat to the grave of a recently deceased, "wicked" person. At midnight, they said, a devil will come to take the wicked person's body away. "You heave your cat after 'em and say, 'Devil follow corpse, cat follow devil, warts follow cat, I'm done with ye!'"

If dragging dead felines through a cemetery seems just a bit much, consider the following ways to get rid of warts:

Kill 'em with acid. Warts will disappear on their own, but if you're impatient, head for the drugstore. An over-the-counter acid solution can help, say doctors at the Mayo Clinic. You'll have to apply these remedies *twice* a day for a few weeks or they won't be effective. Look for a product that contains salicylic acid, which will peel off the infected skin. But be aware that the acid can irritate your skin. Try a 17 percent acid solution on your hands (or the end of your nose) and a 40 percent solution on your

POWERFUL
POTION

ANTIVIRAL ASTRAGALUS ANTIDOTE

The development of warts can signal a weakened immune system. Give yourself an antiviral boost with astragalus (*Astragalus membranacus*) tea. Simmer 1 heaping teaspoon of root in 1 cup of water for 20 minutes. Strain, and drink 2 cups daily.

Miracle Wart Weeds

If you have dandelions growing in your lawn, go pick yourself a wart cure. Herbalists say you should apply the sap from the flower stem to your wart three times a day for as long as it takes for the wart to disappear.

feet. If you are pregnant, ask your doctor if these remedies are okay to use.

Avoid other warts. Warts are everywhere, and you can get them easily by following in someone's footsteps in a shower, locker room, or public pool. These little growths are also acquired through direct contact with an infected person. Don't shower in the same stall or tub of someone who has warts. It takes about 3 months for a wart to appear once you've been infected, but it can also lie dormant for years, so you probably won't remember where the heck you got it.

Go with a pro. If your warts don't go away, if they are tender, or if they are a cosmetic nuisance, ask your doctor about having them removed. There are many treatments available—from freezing them with liquid nitrogen to zapping them with lasers and injecting them with virus-killing drugs. The resulting wound can be cauterized with chemicals or an electric needle.

Don't scratch. Picking at a wart just spreads the virus that causes it. And, as I learned, it will grow back—bigger and better than ever.

Herbal Wart Wizards

Basil, say folk healers, can banish a wart. Basil contains several antiviral compounds that make warts disappear faster than you can say, "Watch me pull a rabbit out of a hat!" Just crush up a few basil leaves, place them right on the wart, and cover the area with a bandage. Change this dressing every day, and the wart should disappear within a week.

Yellowed Teeth:

Polish Those Pearly Whites

Today, getting a bleach job doesn't mean a trip to the hair salon, it means a trip to your cosmetic dentist (the same peroxide is the basic bleaching agent for both processes). If fact, in the last 5 years, there's been a three-fold increase in the number of people getting their teeth bleached. Here's how you can join their ranks:

See the pro in the white coat for your new white coat. Your dentist can bleach your teeth in the office or fit you for a mouth tray and give you

---

FABULOUS FOLK REMEDY

Juice 'Em Up

Fresh strawberry juice is said to whiten teeth over time. Paint the juice on the teeth, and leave it there for 5 minutes. Follow with a rinse of warm water with a pinch of baking soda added to it.

the bleach so you can do the job at home. The in-office treatment takes two visits, but the at-home treatment takes a bit longer because it includes a milder bleach solution. The in-office treatments cost between $600 and $1,200 for one or two visits. If you choose the at-home method, be ready to fork over $200 to $600. Your pearly whites should stay that way for up to 3 years. To find a dentist near you who whitens teeth, check with the American Academy of Cosmetic Dentists at www.aacd.com.

OTC kits are the pits. You can buy a tooth-whitening kit at the drugstore for about $80, but the results won't be as good as if you visited your dentist. The teeth trays don't always fit properly, and because of poor fit, the trays often leak. So my advice to you is, save your money, and see a professional.

Give whitening paste the brush off. The commercial brands of whitening toothpastes don't work very well. There's not enough bleach in them, and a quick brushing won't leave the bleach on your teeth long enough to do much good. And boy, are they ever expensive!

O·D·D·B·A·L·L OINTMENT

Paint Some Primer

Some bleaches are okay for sensitive teeth, but if yours are extremely squeamish, you may need to prime them first. Ask your dentist about teeth primers, such as Gluma, that can be painted on your teeth to desensitize them. Or you can opt for the less expensive route, and simply brush your teeth with a toothpaste that contains potassium nitrate, such as Sensodyne, for 6 weeks before your treatment.

Zits:

Glands Working Overtime

Don't tell a teenager with a face full of zits that it's only a temporary hormonal overload. At that sensitive time of life, it's a disaster! Actually, it's a disaster anytime it occurs—as some unfortunate adults have discovered.

When the sebaceous glands under your skin work overtime, they produce more oil than your skin needs and your oil ducts can handle. The excess collects under the skin's surface, and it's there that the problem begins. Add some dead skin cells to the mix, and a hard plug forms. If it stays under the skin's surface, it's a whitehead. If it enlarges and pushes out to the surface, it's a blackhead. If it ruptures the wall of a pore, invading bacteria jump in, and

Shun the Sun

Sunlight, often thought to be a remedy for acne, may not help clear up skin. Dermatologists warn that sun and heat can increase the amount of oil your skin produces. So avoid the blazing sun at midday, and always shade your face with a brimmed hat.

When a Blemish Is Not a Zit

If you have a blemish that won't go away and appears somehow different than other blemishes, get it checked out right away. It could be something more serious, like melanoma or another form of skin cancer.

there's your zit. And if more than one zit erupts—and let's face it, zits travel in groups—there's an acne breakout.

CHAOTIC HORMONES

Acne usually results from the increased hormonal activity of adolescence—specifically, the surge of androgens that stimulate the growth of body hair. Unfortunately, this process sometimes ends up clogging pores and blocking the flow of sebum. In grownups, the sudden appearance of acne may be a sign of a hormonal imbalance or the side effect of certain drugs such as steroids, lithium, anticonvulsants, and medications with iodine. If you take any of these, ask your doctor if you can change prescriptions.

Thankfully, most acne is more of an embarrassment than a serious medical problem. But if it persists past adolescence or is particularly severe, you may need medical treatment to prevent scarring. The most effective drugs—both for topical and oral use—are derivatives of vitamin A. These drugs are safe when used under the supervision of a dermatologist, but shouldn't be taken casually because they

POWERFUL POTION

CALENDULA WASH

Calendula's bright orange flowers can be made into a refreshing facial wash. Just steep 1 teaspoon of calendula flowers in 1 cup of hot water for 10 minutes. Cool, and strain. After cleansing your face as normal, rinse it with the calendula wash.

can be irritating and toxic. Likewise, infection isn't the primary cause of acne, and long-term treatment with tetracycline and other antibiotics should be avoided.

KEEPING PIMPLES AT BAY

The best way to handle zits is to prevent them in the first place. Here's what to do:

Use lavender steam. Steam your pores open, and prevent acne with an herbal anti-septic. Just place 1 tablespoon of lavender (*Lavendula officinalis*) flowers in a pot of hot, steaming water. Bend over the pot, and tent your head, being careful not to burn your face. Let the lavender vapors steam your face for 15 minutes. Rinse your face with cool water, and pat dry.

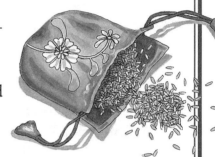

Is It a Guy Thing?

Most girls start noticing pimples around age 11, and most boys by age 13, when the adolescent body begins producing large amounts of androgen, which seems to cause an overproduction of the oils that trigger acne. Boys produce about 10 times as much androgen as girls, which is why we see many more pimply faced boys than girls in high school.

Be a soft touch. All the scrubbing in the world won't make those zits disappear—in fact, it might just cause them to spread. So wash your skin gently.

Visit your drugstore. Over-the-counter, antiacne creams contain ingredients, such as benzoyl peroxide and salicylic acid, that can be helpful in reducing acne flare-ups in some people. Use them at night, and, after a week or so, add a morning application. You should notice an improvement in about 3 weeks.

Don't dine on iodine. Most dermatologists insist that chocolate and pizza don't cause zits. However, doctors do warn that the iodine in a hot fudge sundae or a slice of anchovy extra-cheese pizza just might. Known to trigger angry red pimples, iodine is abundant in dairy products, because iodine cleansers are used on milking machines. Fast foods, salty foods, and shellfish can aggravate acne for the same reason.

POWERFUL POTION

WITCH HAZEL

Clean from the inside out. Increase circulation to your skin, and you'll help cleanse it from the inside out. All you have to do is drink 1 or 2 cups of tea each day made from burdock root (*Arctium lappa*) or red clover (*Trifolium pratense*). For burdock, simmer 1 heaping teaspoon of root in 1 cup of water for 20 minutes. Then strain, and sip. For red clover, pour 1 cup of boiling water over 1 heaping teaspoon of flowers. Steep 10 minutes; then strain, and sip.

Witch hazel, an excellent oil remover, has long been a popular item in medicine cabinets. In fact, I know of a young woman who played high-school basketball and was nicknamed Witch for this reason. She played hard and got pretty sweaty—and the oils in her skin poured out, too. So she kept bottles of witch hazel in her sports bag, her locker, and at home. Do as Witch did, and use a clean cotton ball to dab some witch hazel on your skin to help keep it oil free.

Witch Hazel

Be the leader of the laundromat. While you're in dreamland, your body is busy pushing oil and tiny flakes of dead skin off your face—and into your pillowcase. So unless you make a point always to sleep on a clean pillowcase, you spend each night rubbing your face into the accumulated dead skin cells and other debris. (Gross!)

Come clean. As at least two presidents learned so many years ago, coverups don't work! So, don't try to hide your acne under gobs of makeup—it will only make it worse. Too much foundation clogs the pores and oil glands, which leads to more pimples.

Hang loose. Try to arrange your life so that you're under as little stress as possible. (Easier said, than done, I know!) Stress alters hormone levels, which can trigger zit outbreaks.

Got egg on your face? Egg white draws out the oils from your skin. So when a zit hits, use a cotton swab to apply a little egg white to the area. A dermatologist once told me that egg white is a mild astringent and may contain some anti-inflammatory proteins, as well.

FABULOUS FOLK REMEDY

Honey–Onion Mask

Sulfur is renowned for its healing effects on the skin. Add 1 teaspoon of onion juice to 2 tablespoons of honey. Mix well, and apply to your face. Leave in place 10 to 15 minutes; then rinse with warm water followed by cool water.

Index